Medicine of God

Christian Medical Ethics for These Times

Ruth Oliver, M.B. Ch. B., F.R.C. P.(C).

Medicine of God

Christian Medical Ethics for These Times

Ruth Oliver, M.B. Ch. B., F.R.C. P.(C).

CONGREGATION FOR THE PROPAGATION OF THE FAITH, S.A.S. 58 1186

Upon the approval of Pope Paul VI, on October 14, 1966, with the abolition of previous Canon 1399 & 2318 of the former Canonical Code, publications about new appearances, revelations, prophecies, miracles, etc., have been allowed to be distributed and read by the faithful without the express permission of the Church, **providing they contain nothing which contravenes faith and morals**. This means that no Imprimatur is necessary when distributing information on new apparitions not yet judged by the Church.

All information contained in this document therefore submits without reservation to the Authority of the Roman Catholic Church in matters of Faith and Morals.

Fr Anthony Zimmerman, STD Japan reviewed unrevised version of this book and and says in part…

"Much more should be said, but here is a short review which you may use if you wish.

I wish to thank the author for the book, Medicine of God, Christian Medical Ethics for These Times, Dr Ruth Oliver, for this treasury for the medical professionals and ethicists. The author has selected only authentic Magisterial sources and competent medical professionals and commentators for content and citation. Reading these expands the mind and brings one up to date on the very latest issues of medical ethics today. I stand in awe of the keenness of mind of the author, who gets to the point quickly and professionally, of medical materials and their ethical evaluation. The book sparkles with commentaries by authors cited and by her own brilliant evaluations.

The book takes a novel turn of interfacing science with inspirational writing. The author sets off medical matters from her own reflections and conversations with the Lord by use of bold type, which is commendable. I confess, however, that my own preference is to read the medical materials and breeze quickly over the bold type. Nevertheless I have also dipped into those parts and received good inspiration. "

Truthfully and properly stated the Author of these "Words"is Jesus Christ or whoever from Heaven He chose to speak in His Name. I received the Words on my knees in prayer with Omen, taped and later typed them. My name appears as the "author" only because, as He explained ,He needed a human,in this case a physician, through whom He could get His Words into print and publicized to the medical world. (See Acknowledgments 1 and 18.)

Copyright © 2009 Ruth Oliver,M.B. Ch.B.,F.R.C.P.(C).

All rights reserved

No part of this book may be reproduced, stored in a retrieval system, or transmitted by any means, electronic, mechanical, photocopying, recording, or otherwise, without written permission from the author or publisher. There is one exception. Brief passages may be quoted in articles or reviews.

Library and Archives Canada Cataloguing in Publication

CIP data on file with the National Library and Archives

ISBN 978-1-926582-43-6

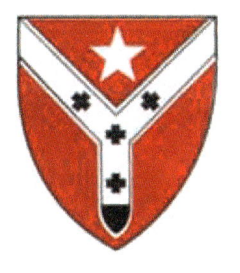

Catholic Archdiocese of Durban
Isifundabhishobhi samaKhatholika sase Thekwini

Street Address: Diocesan Chancery, 154 Gordon Road, Durban 4001, South Africa
Postal Address: P.O. Box 47489, Greyville 4023, South Africa
Telephone: (031) 3031417 • Fax: (031) 3121848
E-mail: chancery@catholic-dbn.org.za
www.catholic-dbn.org.za

19 July 2011

Dear Dr Ruth

As so often happens in life, when God blesses us in a very special way it is precisely because he has some special mission for us to carry out on his behalf and on behalf of his people.

I believe it is in that manner and spirit that you must regards the special mission and the special graces that he has given you. What makes your mission ever so much more difficult or challenging is that what he wants you to convey is not very acceptable or even reasonable to our sceptical world. Indeed, it is difficult to convince even Church leadership to back up what has been revealed to you. Often it is not because of unwillingness on our part, but because we are generally out of our depth in this kind of field, and truly don't know how to respond; with prudent reserve or blind faith both of which are most challenging.

Nevertheless, you have the full support of my prayers and as far as what you've been asked to speak out on falls within Church teaching.

May God continue to support and bless you with his love and care.

Sincerely yours in Christ.

+Wilfrid Cardinal Napier OFM
ARCHBISHOP OF DURBAN

Dedication

This book is dedicated to
Saint Dr. Gianna Beretta Molla,
who died on April 28, 1962, at 8:00 a.m.
beatified on April 24, 1994 and canonized on May 16th 2004 by Pope John Paul II.

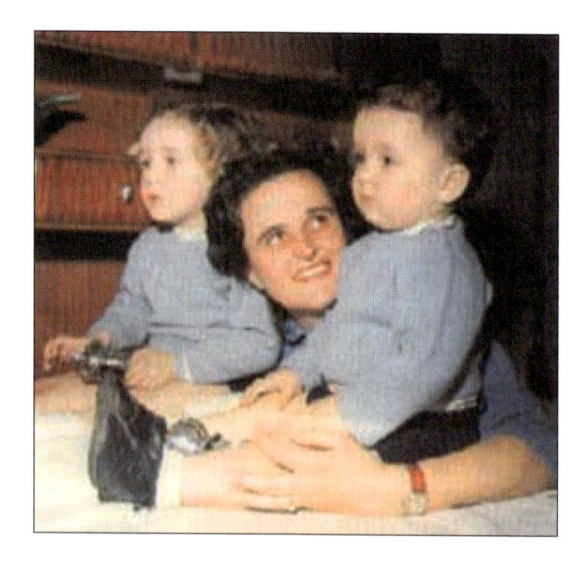

The *Postulatory Letter,* dated 11th April, 1988, signed by Cardinal Giovanni Colombo and sixteen bishops of the Bishops' Conference of Lombardy, asked for the glorification of this wife and mother, defining her as an *"example of the highest order in this our world unable to understand and inclined to deny the right to life."* The members of the

Conference insisted:

Such a mother and martyr, who, out of love for God and in obedience to His Commandment, "thou shalt not kill," bears witness and exalts the heroism of a Christian wife and mother, sacrifices her life to say 'yes' to the Christian duty of love, and out of her respect for life, God's gift to men. And this example of wife and mother is what we, Archbishops and Bishops of Lombardy, as well as in the name of the faithful, would like to propose today to the whole Church, at a time when egoism and violence are rampant. It has become easy to kill, in both hidden and blatant ways. In this our world prone to introduce the legalization of abortion, the Servant of God, Gianna Beretta Molla has become a courageous example of Christian behaviour. This example of lay sanctity, lived in the sacrament of matrimony, as the Vatican Council II teaches, will encourage many Christians to seek God in holy matrimony. The exemplary fame of Christian conduct, lived by Gianna Beretta Molla is valid proof.

Dr. Molla threw light on the importance of the Christian family, by her life and conscious sacrifice. She threw light on the importance of Christian Schools and Azione Cattolica (Catholic Action), in the formation of the human being in Christian values and it gives us guiding principles to which the Christian subordinates his own life, as Dr Beretta Molla knowingly did. The heroism of her Christian life will bear much fruit...

This dedication was requested by Jesus Christ on July 9, 2001, because:

"She knew the value of the human soul. She was ready to and did give up her life for her baby."

Medicine of God

Christian Medical Ethics for These Times

Title page page	3
Frontispiece	5
Dedication	6
Table of Contents	7
Chapter 1: The Oath: Reflections upon God and Science	9
Chapter 2: His Words	24
Chapter 3: Abuse	38
Chapter 4: Addiction	41
Chapter 5: Homosexuality	51
Chapter 6 Abortion	56
Chapter 7: Organ Donation	88
Chapter 8: "Brain Death"	100
Chapter 9: Satan, Sin and Death	119
Chapter 10: Sorrow and Woe	127
Chapter 11: Blood: The Covenant: The Blessing and the Curse	139
Chapter 12: The Ten Commandments	150
Chapter 13: Conversion	157
Chapter 14: Instruments in the Ingathering	164
Chapter 15: Healings, Blessings and Anointings	175
Chapter 16: Priesthood and the Church	190
Chapter 17: Archangels and Angels	205
Chapter 18: Mary and Her Holy Rosary	213
Chapter 19: Victory and Salvation	230
Chapter 20: Jesus, Eternal Physician	244
Chapter 21: Peace in His Presence	275
Acknowledgements	289

CHAPTER ONE

Reflections upon God and science in relation to the Christian Physician's Oath

Mark of Cain Gn 4:15.

JESUS: "Come!" I am your Jesus of merciful Love. Now is the needed time. The time is at hand now for the conversions, the necessary conversions to take place. *All* come unto Me. I call each one by name, for they are Mine (Is 43:1). I bid you write as I direct you to write, for this Mission is part of the great Ingathering which is taking place all about the Earth now. The 32,000 at the Pentecost Mass are but, as you would say, a drop in the bucket, of what is being called forth upon the earth now. Those who do not believe, do not adore, do not love the Lord their God, are in great peril to their souls. Emerging upon the earth as a new evangelization, Christianity surges forward now, in a great anointing of the Holy Spirit of the Living God, upon all those who live the great Commandments of Love. I reject no one. Let them come unto Me *now*.

I have taught you that the killing of the Gift of Life is a grave offence against the Living God, Creator of all life. It is abhorrent to the Lord your God; an abomination in the Eyes of the Lord your God. I have taught you that what is happening to those at the moment of their death, their bodily death, is, in the eyes of your God, a sacrilege. It is not of Me. Oh sorrow! Oh woe! Great sufferings are caused by this lack of Faith. The harvesting, the mining, the utilizing of human body parts, is foreign to Holy Scripture, and foreign to the Lord your God! *Mortal man, what are you thinking of!* At the moment of their own death, when their souls, covered in these transgressions, come to Me in this state themselves, how shall they answer the Lord their God at that Judgment, before which every man and woman must stand?

[The Lord describes that the souls appear with their sins as appendages attached to their souls like great lumpy skin cancer all over.] There is indeed a time to be borne and a time to die (Eccl 3:2), as is written. Prideful man chooses which infant shall live and which shall die. He chooses to prolong life when I am calling someone to come Home. He chooses to exterminate life at the discretion of the physician, without consultation with Me, the Lord your God, the Giver of Life, who takes His Own Home to Glory at the opportune moment! Indeed, a reign of death, a death culture is upon the Earth! Up, you small band that can see, and fight! [Our Lady of La Salette] The Lord your God is with you in this battle since you choose to proclaim the Truth, My small daughter of obedience. My Sorrow is complete. The Mother of Sorrows, Who has the most loving of hearts, is pierced by that sword* again and again, weeping copious tears for mankind, pleading for more time, that they will at last rethink their ways, their strategies. It would appear to be to no avail! [Prophecy of Simeon. Luke 2:33-35]

"Those who read the documents you have presented, must from then on answer to Me! It is incumbent upon each one who reads the documents to come before Me prayerfully and choose whether they wish to live under a blessing or a curse! [Dt: Ch 28] The physicians of the world themselves are precipitating the wrath of God, in unison with certain other malefactors. And yet your Merciful God causes a turnaround in this affair. Little one, the Lord your God is with you. I have given you a few comments. Should you choose to use them in your summary, you may. You have sufficient inspiration and knowledge, and I Myself assist you in this matter. In the power of the Holy Spirit, Mother and I assist you as you prepare your document now. Little children, the dark days and all the trials *have to be*; before the Dawn of Light is upon the world. It is rapidly approaching, yet you have time to save the souls of those who by their atheist beliefs, their humanist beliefs, are hurling their very souls into eternal darkness. This is your Mission. I would that they be spared such a fate! It is sad what occurs to the dying and to those receiving body parts from others. But sadder before the eyes of your God, and your Heavenly Mother, are the state of the souls of these scientists!

My little ones gathered here in this small prayer room, great blessings accrue and pour forth upon you. Many pray here, little children; many pray for you and with you. All those with whom you are interwoven are united, each praying one for another. Blessings flow. This is accompanied by prayers of the great and heavenly angels and saints of Glory, whose voices resound before your God; and, in addition, accompanied by those yet in their purification, as you invoke them to pray with you that they may all the sooner attain Glory. It is indeed happening, blessed children of a Merciful and Loving God. My Peace is upon you. Do not be distressed about your discomforts and your heaviness at times. Little children, your sacrifices as you yet remain in love with your God and your Heavenly Mother, these sacrifices are brought before your Father, and blessings flow on the beloved Humanity, which finds itself in dire straits today. Most of all I bless you this moment with a great Peace, the Peace of My Presence. Give glory to Our Father.

I, the Lord God, reiterate! Thou art My Own, My precious little one. I have anointed thee to bring the Good News to the poor (Rm 10:15). Who are the poor, you ask Me. They are those who do not know Me, do not love Me, do not will to serve their God. Forgive them, you pray; claim them once more as My Own, you plead; and I am doing that; I am doing that through the voices of many, many chosen ones throughout the earth. This great Mission I am giving to Faithful Missionary is a part of this claiming once more as My Own; in answer to your frequent plea, your daily plea. Darkness and despair are the lot of those who choose Me not! As you have recognized a depression in humans who are not in unity with Me, whose very spirit and their soul is grieving My absence. Here is one situation where My Presence readily heals and is an example of the healing Presence of Your God. Little children, many, many afflictions are caused from a similar root; a root of despair, a lack of Hope and Faith and Trust and Love; a root of disbelief, root of pride, believing that they need Me not! These people suffer the consequences of these attitudes. It is not that I ask too much of each individual. I ask you to love your God with all your heart and all your soul and all your mind, and to love your neighbor as yourself (Mt 22:37-39).

Humanity makes this so complicated but does not live it, for the most part. I send little emissaries of Light about the earth to teach My Way of Love, a gentle Love. When you love your God in total abandonment of Love, it is so easy to love your neighbor as yourself (Mt 22:39) then, for you see the Majesty of God and you see the beauty of Creation; and about you all Creation indeed proclaims the greatness of the Lord, and you become at one with your God, in love with God and fellow man and all created things. It is not a difficult thing to attain. Do not complicate it, therefore, with if's and but's and rules and regulations and concepts that it is impossible. For with Me, you know well that nothing is impossible (Lk 1:37).

The darkness of sin against the Father is a cause of all the fallout of suffering which is upon the Earth now. I address you, Faithful Missionary. I bid you, My little one, prevail in this Mission. Remarkable events occur and things simply fall into place for you are powerfully assisted in this Mission. I am calling to the scientific world most specifically: If today you hear God's Voice, harden not your heart! (Ps 95:7-8)] And you pray:" "My God, I believe, I adore, I trust and I love Thee. I beg pardon for those who do not believe, do not adore, do not trust and do not love Thee. And Heaven hears and now We are responding, through Faithful Missionary, to the scientific world to come back to their God, each one with all their hearts. They are beloved, each one, of the Lord God. And each one has been gifted with intellect and talents, abilities that make them capable of doing works of merciful love. Now the medical profession is, as it were, engineered to wreak havoc upon the world, to do harm to humanity, to deceive the common people. Oh woe! Oh sorrow! Each one of you is called to love your neighbor as yourself (Mt 22:39). This is not happening when you abandon all ethics, all morals and strive to sterilize and abort entire nations and peoples about the earth!"

I am the One Who reads your hearts, your souls, your minds. I am your Omniscient Lord! Do you think you are deceiving Me, children of sinfulness! You are deceiving only yourselves. Indeed you are deceived by the deceiver, the father of lies. Don't you know that you are serving the father of lies? Don't you know that you are in Death's camp? What are you thinking about? Many of you have been Baptized unto Me, dedicated unto Me in your infancy or early years. What are you doing now? Did you betray your Savior thus? You do not betray Me! You betray yourselves and you betray your brothers and sisters on earth! Many of your healings are but inflicting more sufferings upon those you offer healing to, and they continue in life suffering more than before they attended upon you. What form of healing can this be? I bid you take an Oath to heal your brothers and sisters without worrying about costs and without a desire to kill your brothers or sisters, regardless of their age! The minutest life form is of Me and the elders are of Me. The minutest life forms in the water and the giant coniferous trees. *They are Mine, the Works of My Hands!*

Go tell everyone the Good News of Salvation you are told, and you come to Me and you ask, 'Whom shall I tell?' and since you are a physician, I ask you to tell your brother and sister physicians the Good News that God lives, that God lives in and through the many faithful, that God lives in and through the many poor, the sick, the deaf, the blind. Do not harm My precious little ones. Harming them, you harm Me! When you come before Me at that Great Moment of Transition, what will you say to Me? I'm waiting to hear what you have to say. I would that you would repent now and begin now to be true healers, as I have called you to be! The Spirit of the Living God is as a Living Flame of Love in the heart of each true believer upon the earth. I want to place this, My Spirit, in each of your hearts. Behold, I stand at the door and knock (Rev 3:20). Brilliant men and women that you are, read and study these Words I have given over to you for your benefit, for your healing, and come back to Me with all your hearts (Jl 2:12). Let us begin again to live Love, that you shall indeed live to love again! [St. Theresa of Avila]

"That which you have asked of Me, I give to you, since you have given yourself in utter abandonment to Me. You may use My Words as you have perceived to use them. I Myself bless all that you do on My Behalf. I bless all that you do in your life with your loved ones. My little children, when you fall into the Loving Providence of God, you have no longer to fear or be anxious. Use My Words; they are for you and your brother and sister physicians. My Love is for all mankind, for I *am* Love (1 Jn 4:8). I pour out My Love in a great anointing of the Holy Spirit upon all mankind. All those who read these Words, which you shall give to them, with an open mind, will be blest, will be anointed and will come back to Me. Since mankind always seeks what they call verification and confirmation, all that I have spoken unto them in thee and through thee is indeed verifiable in Holy Scripture; there is no need to doubt. And despite all that each one may have done in the interests of science, which may have harmed other humans, My disposition is to forgive them. It is My Desire to forgive them, for none of My Own shall be lost! My little children, I reiterate, your God-given talents must be used for your brothers' and sisters' well being, as is taught!

I am Jesus and I hold you fast, little one, in the Power of My Spirit! Behold, I make all things new (Rev 21:5)! Indeed, I send the little one for My Own Reasons. Little one, they shall unfold; they shall unfold as I desire! Little blest children of God, stay prayerfully united with your God, and all goes according to

Heaven's Designs for you. Our Designs, little children, are for your good and for the good of your fellow man, as you well know. Sometimes it takes labor and even testings and trials; but how great is My Love for you, and how great are the rewards that fall upon you, both on earth and in Glory! My little ones, the workman is worthy of his hire (Mt 10:10)! My little ones, My blessings are upon you. Cling to your Jesus, cling to Our Mother, the Ever-Virgin Mary, the Mother of All, and all goes according to Heaven's Design!

Therefore, be at Peace (1 Th 5:13). Your one True Home and Native Land is Heaven, your temporary home on earth is the Two Hearts of Love; Your Jesus' and Mother Mary's Hearts. My little one, the abode where you dwell now is blest and is of your God. Then our Lord sings the hymn, "I the Lord of snow and rain,.. whom shall I send? which He sang last week and called for me to sing twice at Communion in the past week and even at my kitchen sink at the lunch hour today! Where are You sending me, Lord? Abide with Me and bide your time, one step at a time, little one. Circumstances preclude a move at this time, and yet you foresee great changes in your life. The Mission you have been given is no idle Mission. It is profound and it leads you farther afield, yet you are secure under the great mantle of Love, secure in the power of the Holy Spirit of Love. You rest always in the Providence of God.

Little children, in your 'yes,' your surrender to Love, emulating the Mother of God, I have accepted your 'yes,' and thus each one of you is anointed in a unique manner at this time of times, in the working of the Great Ingathering of My people. They have been scattered far and wide about the Earth. Many are lukewarm. He shows the Ingathering; it is huge – like, yet not only, the Jews going back to Jerusalem. It is a true Calling. Like the last two lines of the *Magnificat*, Mary is claiming the Promise given to the people of Abraham, for all the people of today. Change is ever present. Creation is not static; there is always an ongoing moving on, like the waves of the ocean. It is delightful, for you are walking with your Lord and with Our Mother and with St. Joseph, and with a myriad of angels and saints walking in the Power of the Holy Spirit of the Living God.

I am Jesus. I am ready to address thee now. I bless thee, Faithful Missionary. I bless each one gathered here in My Name in a profound anointing of My Peace and My Love and My Joy. Precious little children, I find thee pleasing for thou hast heeded the Call to Love and obedience in all humility before your God, and not worrying about human esteem, about the woundedness which you suffer, for My Name, for My Cause. My Cause is Love. Thus, I have given the Great Commandment of Love, that My little ones truly love one another, even as I Love each one (Jn 13:34). Precise details We have given thee in Our Epistle of Love to the Scientific World. Many have read it. Some have begun and not completed reading it, those whom you have dispensed it to. Do not worry about it. Your duty is completed in giving them My Words, Words of Enlightenment. What they do with it is between them and their God! I Myself attend upon them, for all Words I give to thee flow as blessings upon thee and upon the readers of My Words.

Even so, in free will they may be rejected. This is not to say that they are rejected, except by certain few, and some only in certain instances. Little children, in the river of darkness upon the earth in which the physicians are working, these My Messages of Love fall startling upon the many who have not contemplated their God to any great degree or have not weighed their actions and the consequences of their actions in the Light of Holy Scripture. You are now in possession of these Images and Words which are pleasing to the Lord your God. Know that hosts of angels are attendant upon your Mission of Love, that angels attend upon Our Writings and upon Our Pictures. In other words, I have blest all these works of your hands that they may come as anointings and blessings upon those physicians and priests who open their hearts to Me, who invoke the Holy Spirit at the time of the readings. Some priests are ever attendant upon Me in the power of the Holy Spirit. Even these, though they have read them, have not responded. It is puzzling to you. Do not be puzzled. Some are inhibited with regard to their various obediences. Some are inhibited with regard to words of prophecy in these times. Some simply don't wish to shake up or disturb the *status quo.* Therefore what shall we do, you ponder.

You children, as it were, you seem to be defying *the establishment* as it is called, rather shockingly, rather blatantly in the eyes of certain individuals. Yet you have chosen to say '*yes, Lord*," in obedience under the example of Our Beloved Mother and Our Beloved Joseph. This is so pleasing to the Lord your God that many blessings accrue and flow freely upon you. Despite all these trials you have remained doggedly faithful to the Lord. Believe it or not, such holy obedience is rare on this earth, for there are billions on the earth and so few respond to My Call of Love, My Call of conversion. Mother attends upon My beloved little Faithful Missionary, small sister of Jesus, small sister of St. Luke of whom you inquire. Medical healing is good, can be good. There are many acceptable practices in the healing ministry of physicians, and this is pleasing to the Lord God, the Giver of all the gifts, and all the intelligences, and all the arts. These are gifts of the Living God to His sons and daughters, among whom you are numbered.

Used within the walls of the Commandments, in obedience to Holy Scripture, most especially in loving one's neighbor as oneself (Mt 19:19), there is no harm. It is when one ceases to see an individual as a unique gift of God and treats them, one might say, like so much merchandise, that the harm comes into effect. At times, from My View, it is that My people are processed like so much livestock. How can this be pleasing to your God? Do not you view in the garden many flowers, and each flower is beautiful in its own right? Each orchid created is in startling beauty, each one! So your Creator God sees each human, each individual. Except you look at them with My Eyes, you people of the world, you do not see the beauty of each individual, the preciousness, both strength and fragility present in each human. And yet, this is how your Creator has designed each individual! I do not will that any of My precious humans be treated experimentally, except should they without coercion, in free will, choose to be treated thus.

Beloved Luke is a physician who loved much, who loved in Christ-Love. How could he write in such Love in the Gospel if it were not so? He lived Love. That is what every Christian physician is called to do: to live Love, all-compassionate Love, all Love and Charity upon each suffering soul presented to them. I fail to see this in many clinics, in many hospitals. Yes, there is derision for the Christian physician in many circles." *The angels are singing: "Lift high the Cross; the Love of God proclaim. Till all the world adore His Sacred Name.* Little ones, that is what it is all about! Many people on the earth today, who know Me not, are caught up in a crucible of suffering appalling for your God to behold. I give free will to My beloved little ones that they might be God-like, and look what they have done! In My great Mercy, We turn this whole thing around. I ask each one of you to say, 'Let it begin with me. Thus far, you have handled the rejection most beautifully. Know that I have molded you and fashioned you to be My instrument in this matter. It is to rejoice that your God, Who so loved the world, so loves you, that He has strengthened you to do this task in My Name. Many blessings accrue and flow freely upon you for what you are doing in My Name, on My behalf, so to speak, and on behalf of humanity, My precious mankind. Little one, ask of Me what you will (Ps 2:8).

Dearly beloved, you may use them [My Words] in this fashion. Little children, I bless you with many discernments, and in the Gifts of the Holy Spirit you are, as it were, empowered to use My Words freely, for we are friends. We are friends; we share together in Love. In Love's union, My Enlightenments are continuously flowing upon you. Little children, you live in a time of great trial, but yet a time of Great Love. There is Peace in the heart of those who truly know Me that surpasses all understanding. And in this unity of Love, in such hearts, We work freely in friendship and Love. Miracles of change are upon the earth. In the power of the Holy Spirit, it is so! Continue communicating with each one in whatsoever manner you deem possible, and when you come to Me at the Holy Sacrifice of the Mass, ask for a blessing upon them, and that their eyes, their hearts, their minds be opened, to Love. I *am* Love (1 Jn 4:8)! And when you come to the shrine, as we share a Communion of Love there, ask for a releasing blessing upon these individuals. Let us pray often, invoking Our Mother's love to come upon these individuals.

Let us, therefore, pray together with the whole Heavenly Court, and in unity with those yet in their purifications, the miraculous prayer, the *Memorare*, that Mother begin to work on these, Her children as well as Mine, and the miracles begin, the miracles of conversion and enlightenment. Do thou, little children each one I ask, know how many voices have pleaded before the Throne of Godhead on this issue? When you pray in this manner, they resound in Heaven, and Mother is moved to tears of Joy. Little ones, an opening is made unsolicited, for nothing is impossible with God. Give Glory to the Father! *Glory be*…Indeed, let it be so. Little children, as Mother loved Luke, so she loves Her physician children. Mother weeps copious tears of sorrow at some of the events that are happening in the medical field, and yet glorious tears of Joy at the many beautiful successes in healing Love, for the use of the God-given intellect and capabilities on behalf of the suffering brother or sister is so pleasing to God. Many, many physicians are precious and blest of the Lord God, yet the grave error of this humanist wave of atrocious medical actions is grievous to both Our God and to the Mother of God.

Little children, I am Jesus, Eternal Victor! My Victory is before My Eyes. Small instruments, blessings accrue, for each one of you who partakes in this Mission of Enlightenment. As long as the Message is clear and attractive as it is now, it is more than adequate. See, you have hearts of Love, you little ones, but many, while they are partially of Love, they are still partially of the world; and some are yet stony cold hearts, in the world. Little children they are Mine. You are My instruments in all that you have done in connection with your fellow physicians and with the priests, it is launching My arrows of Love at their hearts, to change them from stony cold hearts, or from fearful hearts, or from disinterested hearts. I wish to take all this away from them. I wish them to know that indeed I am God, (cf Ex 14:18) supreme among the nations; that My Laws are immutable!

Were all the stars in Heaven to disobey, as My beloved mankind has, all the constellations, what would happen to creation! Man is in a chaotic state on earth; like so many shooting stars out of control. I must act must I not? Therefore I must first warn My beloved mankind, for I do not cease to Love them! Even when they walk in error, I Love them. Little children, think about the Words you are placing on your typewritten pages, as each one being an arrow of My Love, to reach the heart of someone somewhere on the earth , and do not cease pouring forth these Words which are the Way, the Truth, the Life,(Jn14:6 the Light for My poor confused Humanity.

Even as We speak, all these things which We have discussed are occurring all over the earth. My people are being denied their God given rights all over the earth and the hearts of so many remain unmoved. Be like a little child , be like a little child I'm calling to all My Own, because then your heart is not cinctured by the cares of the world. Little children, in each of you here, I have removed any obstruction in your hearts and minds. Yet the enemy attempts to put obstruction in your thoughts. This is ongoing; as he pours forth his arrows of hate, We in unity of Love pour forth Our arrows of Love. I am victorious. Hearts as cold as ice melt in the warmth of Our Love. You shall see many changes in many people. You will realize that the process appears slow to you and the conversions, but I ask you to prevail. I Myself will fill your heart with love for My priesthood, My suffering priesthood, as you write to Father Francis and give him Words held in My blessing for him , for He too is My instrument in the unique Way I have chosen for him. Understanding comes.

Little children, sing often the song of Pentecost. It is not only for yourselves, but for the multitudes on earth. Little children, believe; the action of My Love is never limited to one or two persons but is universal. The need for money for every activity on earth is quite abhorrent to the Lord your God. The great need for so much money in these times. *He's giving the quote about so much money for so many bushels referring to inflation.*

It is a sign of the times. It is forewarned to you in Holy Scripture and it is so. The year 1999 fast approaches . Little children, proclaim the Good News now while you have the opportunity for it is not always with you. My delight is in all those whom you have touched. I am the Lord your God. (Is43:13) I Myself make the plans as I Will. Remain abandoned to My Will and continue. You will find a way. There is always a way in unity with your Jesus Who is the Way. The great lighted Cross in the sky will indeed appear at a date in the future. (Mt24:29-31)The time is not yet, and yet it is not far. In the interim little children, work and believe, that all your tomorrows are blest, for indeed they are. Do not be fearful of the future. I Love you little children, I want only always that which is good for you. My Own have nothing to fear.

My little children, it is written; blessed are those who do not see but believe! (Jn20:29)Such are you My little ones. But there comes a day, when I must make a Sign in the Sky , (Mt24:29-31) that those who don't, will at last believe that I am your all-powerful God! It is not a time of fear for My faithful little ones, who have already embraced the Cross of Eternal Life. *Knowing full well what to expect if I attended the "Ethics 2002"conference, and having no stomach for any more of this disobedience to God, I pleaded not to attend but our Lord said;*

You must attend; I desire that you keep abreast of the affairs of this group. Little children, know well and recognize that this disobedience which is ever confronting you in these days, began long ago, even before the beloved Pope Paul VI spoke out on Human Life [*Humanae Vitae issued July 25th1968*]. Little children, it is a fierce battle, yet every human has free will as you know, and often times their pride of intellect leads them on, rather than matters of the heart, matters of Divine Love, and that is why, multitudes who are truly yielded unto Me persevere in praying for their conversions. You are not alone praying for the conversion of such individuals. Little children, the warfare is fierce in these times, as the scientific mindset becomes increasingly irrational in relationship to the Will of Our Father. Watch it with Me, in Me, for Me. Persevere little front line warriors! [*David and the five stones; Rosary*]

The Christian Medical Oath.

"The Great Commandment shall be your Oath!" (Mt 22:37-39)."

On June 5th, 1998, during prayer the Lord gave me Deuteronomy 11: 26' [I give you a blessing for obeying the Commandments; or a curse for following other gods. '] and later 2 Tobit, 4,5, 6; the magnificent intervention of the Archangel Raphael, who was sent to help in all aspects of Tobit's life when he was blinded after faithfully serving God. [Tobias12:7-15.] The angel Raphael said to Tobias, 'it is good to hide the secret of a king, but honourable to reveal and confess the works of God']. So I prayed further;

Lord I give thanks for the beautiful Words of the Mission and for the gift of St Raphael the Archangel; and for protecting my daughter from the very close encounter with death on Friday. Lord you asked me to put the Mission, under the seal of St Raphael, and I don't think I've heard of a seal of St Raphael.

JESUS: It is the seal of the King's ring, designating Raphael[rapha-heal;-el- God], as the Archangel charged with this Mission of Love in unity with thee and a faithful core group who will always be with you in your profession, and in the priesthood. Act simply by Faith. That assistance which you ask of Me is readily given unto thee for your Mission must be done!

To confirm the reality of what He said, Our Lord performed a miracle on that very same day. My daughter was completing her batchelors degree in Science at the university in Birmingham, Alabama and due to fly home on the 6th June. She had spent the year with the Salesians helping organize summer programs for the most underprivileged children while completing her degree and lived in an apartment with a group of other students. She borrowed a car from one of them to do final errands and two students were watching from the second floor window as she parked. She had a moment thinking she would reverse to park one space back, but changed her mind, got out of the car and went upstairs. When she got there the two called her to the window to see that a tornado had uprooted a tree, which had smashed down onto the car she had just parked, totally destroying the car—-the only damage done on the whole street! When I met her at the airport all she could say was, "Mum, I nearly died yesterday!" I told her about St Raphael, ——three time zones away Our Lord confirmed His Power and His Truth!

Our Lord insists that St Raphael the archangel is just as old in sacred history in Heaven as Lucifer the fallen angel is. He asks why we the Christian physicians insist on using the Aesclapian serpent (symbol of the fallen angel) instead of using Raphael, the faithful archangel, Medicine of God, as our symbol. Our Lord has spoken to me many times about this issue in the Mission. I received the Words while praying with another who receives Words and I tape-recorded as we prayed. Over 90% of medical graduates no longer swear any oath at all, so there is no commitment to revere life.

Faithful Missionary comes to Me for a consultation of My Love and I give it to her readily. It will be through the great Archangel St Raphael that these things will come to pass. Is he not a better symbol of the physician that the one you use? How much easier it is to bring in the St Raphael Oath since most physicians have taken no oath at all! You do not have an old oath to cast out; you simply have to present this Oath. I do not say use this title, but consider that it might be called, "A Reflection upon God and science in relationship to the Oath of the physician". One may alter this according to ones Inspirations. It is but an Inspiration itself. The Words flow now but you must be ever watchful-the vengeful one lurks about seeking an opening in your armour (Ep6:10-20) little children. Be not anxious therefore. Remain always in My Peace. Behold the Lamb of God! Behold it is I Who take away the sins of the world. There are fierce battles over each and every soul on earth. I am enamoured of you little ones gathered in My Name. Each one of you is precious to Me. I have called you to do that which very few would choose to do, therefore you are profoundly blest and assisted, but I will that you know how fierce the enemy prowls about. My little one, a great Archangel Raphael has, and continues to play a key role, in the affairs of man. By the decree of your Lord God it is so. The one who is named Medicine of God, therefore is depicted holding the vial which will give sight to the eyes; spiritual sight to those who are in darkness- Great Enlightenment thus as he holds the vial in his hands it radiates Light on behalf of the Lord your God Who is True Light of the World. (Jn8:12)It is I your God Who opens eyes, opens ears, opens hearts. It is I Who Am the Great Physician, Wonder Counselor, Shepherd of My People, My chosen ones.(Is 9:6) Raphael holds a crystal clear liquid in one hand. He is a magnificent Angel of Light. Since he is Medicine-of-God, he destroys the disease-causing demons; causing conflict, poison and venom upon My suffering people. I Myself will give you Faithful Missionary, the complete vision of the great Raphael. (cf Tb chapters 5-12)

Now is a moment of sweet surrender to Love. I imbue you Faithful Missionary now with what you will see at a moment of Adoration. I set about you great angels of Light circumscribing you and I imbue you now with that which you will see in My Presence. What you shall see will be sufficient to make the picture which will have certain details but need not be an elaborate picture. Be at Peace in this issue. (I saw the vision of Archangel Raphael, surrounded in and radiating light, standing to the left as you face the tabernacle in the Adoration Chapel on the 27th March 1999, anniversary of my own miraculous healing in 1977. Thank you Lord Jesus!)

I reiterate, I remind you, that the eyes of the scientists who elect to practice in small specialties; one looking only at blood, one looking only at the workings of the heart, or the brain- they do not always- or even seldom see, the whole picture of a human life; a life which is both body and soul, and important to Me the Lord your God, Creator of all. As they hold fast to the practices, the traditions of the medical arts, the medical discipline, they become rigid and immovable about anything that is at a variance to their preconceived ideas . It takes much to move one from a rigid position. *[He says like the oyster stuck solidly to that one spot on the rock.]*

Altruism. The Enlightenment which Raphael carries will open eyes and ears and hearts of some but not of all. This is not your concern. We will simply proceed as We have discussed. Raphael holds the key. Pray the angels prayer from the Pieta prayer book and trust Me. Begin to sketch, however haphazardly, what you imagine while in My Presence, and We cause you to be inspired to know what it is We call you to. Therefore bring the sketchpad and be prepared. I Myself assist you profoundly in this matter. Beloved Raphael, powerful Archangel of God, Angel of Might, is pleased at this turn of events. The Virgin Herself will converge upon you Faithful Missionary and the vision will become clear to you.

Angels hold thee fast My little ones, each one of you stands secure as has been pledged. It is so. The great force which was permitted to confront you has been defeated and certain barriers have been removed now. All the saints you have invoked attended upon you, for My little ones in such Faith as yours, you are always close to the whole Heavenly Host. My little ones, the great Archangel Raphael bids thee Peace. Thou shall make the drawing now and I shall guide your hands. My little one, obtain your impression of the beloved Raphael and then we shall work together on the actual drawings. The singing angels hold thee fast. Were there to be another picture We would have given it to you. This picture is pleasing and acceptable to the Lord your God. Hold fast to your Faith little children. Mercy, Merciful Love, is what I wish for every human soul on earth. I do not wish My little ones to be mutilated and dissected when they yet live. I do not wish My physicians, named to do good, to be committing murder, day in and day out.

It is My Will that My Christian physicians no longer use a serpent regardless of what it symbolizes, but use Raphael, Medicine of God, since he is protector of travelers, he is protector of every Christian during their journey, their Faith pilgrimage upon earth, and since he is terror of demons, when he is recognized those afflictions which are not of Me, are cast out by invoking his name. Bread of Life, Bread of Life I give to you. (Jn 6) The angel of death is defeated today. I shall arrange for someone to make the picture in more perfected manner, and the portion with just Raphael and the scroll and vial must be the symbol that replaces the serpent on an Oath but the whole picture must be made, for the website and whatever else our Lord intends. Do you love Me little children? Lord we love You always. I thought I would see an actual vision of Raphael?

The vision will come to you at a great moment of Peace. Recognize little children that you are fiercely attacked, but I protect My Own. Be at Peace, we bless you in an astounding and remarkable manner, each one of you little children. It is pleasing to the Lord your God. A day will come when the scroll will be widened to include Raphael on the left, and the rays flowing through the vows and the words on the right. My delight is upon you, and a blessing is upon you. The artist is uniquely blest as well. Do you love Me? My Delight is that you do it yet you remain in free will. He is very pleased with the scroll-Because it is like the teaching of the Hebrew. My vision is of such a scroll in every physician's office, and even in hospital entrances.

Tears, there are delays. Little children prevail. Miracles of change are upon the earth; in the power of the Holy Spirit it is so. Continue communicating with each one in whatsoever manner you deem possible, and when you come to Me at the Holy Sacrifice of the Mass, ask for a blessing upon them, and that their eyes, their hearts, their minds be opened, to Love. I am Love!(1Jn4:7-21) And when you come to the shrine, as we share a Communion of Love there, ask for a releasing blessing upon these individuals. Let us pray often, invoking Our Mothers' Love to come upon these individuals.

Be it Peace, it is understood by those who behold it and this is what is important. I bless thee, I bless the works of your hands, I have given you Divine Inspiration. We shall find the artist who will bring it to perfection. Of prime importance is the Image of Raphael that it will be ready to imprint as a symbol of Christian physicians. Do so. Because they have not responded to thee does not mean that they are in non-compliance . The Message is as it were, overwhelming to the many. They see Truth at last; I am Truth- and must ponder and pray ; and comprehend and pray, seeking gifts and graces to cope with it in their own minds before they take action. There is yet a little time dear children, be at Peace, be not anxious. All falls into place according to Our Father's Schedule. The Oath has not died! It is obstructed, it is delayed, but it has not died. Trust in Me. The virtue of Love is such that you may address the subject of the Oath in your speaking, and have it there should any one wish to study it, to read it over. The media would of course regard it as a drastic change to what exists today, and yet, what exists today; is anyone loyal to any Oath today? A Blessing is upon this work. It is pleasing to the Living God. Therefore, it is the Lord Who speaks, leave it as it is, rather a symbol not only of the Cross, but of the Star of Bethlehem, for Enlightenment, for Light coming into the world of darkness, that the darkness be no more! (Jn8:12)

Indeed send him a letter and a copy of the Scroll for it is Our Desire that none of those in key positions can say, "I did not know". Therefore do so: it is the Lord Who speaks. Those who are open to My Words, should be motivated to say to you, "tell me more, what is this about" and when they do that their learning is enhanced, because you have at your disposal much, much more to give to them. Soon this will be happening with specific individuals. Little one do not be distressed at the slow response. There is an immense store of knowledge in the Information you have been given by your God, which takes man a little time to absorb, and to ponder upon and decide upon. Patience dearest children; patience. Correction in the vision of multitudes occurs because of these prayers, Heaven delights in your persevering Faith little children! Rest assured, 'His Eye is on the sparrow, His Eye is on me!" (cfMt10:28-31)In due course it occurs; We are in a time of great change little children.

Little children You delight Me in your persevering Faith and love, you are precious to Me. My Plan is at hand and it falls into place. You will be remembered for your works become well known and accepted. None can refute or deny what you are saying, and thus they are silent at this moment but not for long! In due course it happens and thou art recognized jointly with other physicians as bringing Truth back into this gray area of medicine. Do not be afraid to approach JP bringing the Oath. It is a time when I wish all My Intentions to be known to as many as possible and do not worry if and when you get shut down by any given one; I keep on opening doors. My Will IS done! " When I am lifted up from the earth, I will draw all people to Me."(Jn 12, 32-33.)

What seems impossible to man is possible to God! Behold, I make all things new;(cfRv21:1) a new beginning is established on earth, a stronghold of Faith and Truth. That I Jesus, AM TRUTH; is self-evident now on earth! The enemy is wrath, there are obstructions hither and yon about the earth, but My Victory is most assuredly at hand! The Virtue of Love is such that I the Lord your God bless you and bid you receive all that I Gift unto you, and proceed to spread it and continue to spread it as you are doing. Indeed send it to this Pontificate; are they not all Mine, or at least allegedly My Own? I Myself cause them to open their minds and hearts with regard to what is occurring in institutions of learning and so-called institutions of healing.

Dearly beloved, simply wait on the Authorities of the Church at this time in regard to the Oath. My Blessings are upon you in all that you are doing . Be not anxious. Walk ever in patient , prayerful perseverance. (cf1Cor13) This is the Way, as you well know. It shall be promoted for there is someone whom I have in mind to take up the Cause, and it shall be thus! It is excellent; thus they have a full-fledged report of the truth with regard to medical practices of today. This man is blest with great discernment, and discernment of Spirits. And indeed wisdom. He knows well the workings of the Vatican, the workings of the Magisterium, and he also knows how the Spirit of the Living God moves in mankind; therefore he is ideally suited for the works I yet have in mind for him. Be astounded. It is best to wait a little longer.

Is it not like unto a cutting of Our Mother's mantle? Peace, We shall inspire him to do it beautifully for nothing is impossible to God. Did not Raphael come back with the funds that were owed, he healed and he disposed of the demons. But he came back with the money, the Providence. As you walk the *Via Dolorosa* on My behalf, I will work the needed releases here in this Our Mission of Love. It is indeed delightful. I am now ready to bless these works profoundly. Immediately after the Christmas celebration begin to mail them out. We are with you. The virtue of Love is such that thou art called to a great Mission on behalf of your God. I remind you again, indeed I have molded you and fashioned you and strengthened (cf 2Cor12:9)you for this Mission. Even as St Paul was trained in all the Holy Scriptures and well educated in the Faith before he became one of My Own, he was thus prepared for his Mission with a sound basis, each one of you have been prepared to become the individuals that you are now in these works of Love. It is I the Lord God Who does it. You are profoundly blest in all that you do in My Name.

The Blessing is indeed already upon it. Be at Peace! Those who cast their eyes prayerfully upon it, or just simply cast their eyes upon it, reading the Words, absorbing the Words, are indeed blest. Where it hangs it will cause others to come along and read it, admiring it, being impressed by it you might say, not knowing the great Blessing that comes to them as they rejoice in the Words written upon it. It is so. What should I tell John? Am I to tell them the picture is blest, or if they want to have it blest by a priest Lord like other Sacramentals, what should I say? The Blessing emanates! Howsoever, should they wish to have a priest bless it, it is good. [but when I said what shall I tell John, our Lord quoted from Scripture; when the people sent by St John the Baptist went to see Him ,] tell them that the blind see, the deaf hear, the lame walk!(Mt11:4-6) Raphael's Light is upon all who read the document. Is he not the opener of blind eyes! (Tobit 11)It is truly a miraculous picture. We take Our Light and Our Life and Our Love to the vanguards of war, to the hospitals where I am not well known, and yet where the many are suffering and dying. This is where I belong, in the Healing Ministry of mankind, I belong in the front lines of the battle of Life and Death!

Proclaim them, share them; he may not publicly acknowledge them, others may not do so publicly, or even to you as you have noticed; and yet once they read them and take them to heart they receive a Blessing. At the opportune moment all, ALL is recognized and proclaimed, and open for the multitudes to believe and know little children.

The Redemption was for all! The Healing is for all! 'Nay, not so,' say the unbelievers! They go to soothsayers. They do not seek Healing at the Mass. They do not seek Healing in My gifted ones. They go hither and yon to everyone or anyone except the Lord God! I wish to be present to mankind, through the Mercy Gate Mission. Many and varied are the Healings that I have chosen to give through your hands, little children. Countless are the cures – spiritual, mental, emotional and physical – which have occurred specifically in these past five years and, more specifically, in this last year. In fact, little children, as you use these specific gifts, let us call them talents: the more you use, the more you believe. The more you lay hands, the greater the strength of healing becomes! Little children, you are as lighted candles shining in the darkness. When there are enough lighted candles, the darkness is no more! Bless Me! *We adore Thee oh Christ and we bless Thee, because by Thy Holy Cross…*

Little children, the scientists abandon Me and they use their intellect to bring that which is unpleasing to the Lord God, into their practices. How shall I respond to what they are doing? Even as the great nation of America, and other nations self-destruct as it were, for lack of obedience to My Will, lack of obedience to My Ten Commandments of Love, lack of obedience to Truth, so will these scientists suffer in strange and varied ways. Surprising events occur because they reject the Shield of Protection of the Holy Spirit! When I am rejected, I do not reject you My people, but you have shunned Me, and are no longer under My Providence. My little ones, you seek the fountain of youth. Little children, you are on this earth for perhaps seventy years, or perhaps a few more. By then you are no longer youthful, and this makes you disgruntled, unhappy; but in that aging process throughout those years, those who have said "yes" to Me, have learned great wisdoms, and are respected as elders in the Faith, elders in Truth, with much to give the younger generations. It has always been thus with My people; and in their "yes" to Me when I call them Home at an opportune moment, then they attend upon Me in Glory, and it is in Glory that you will know the fountain of youth, the River of Light and Love and Peace and Joy, forever and ever, for all eternity! Do not worry about what others think about you, even those priests, even unto bishops because I am with you and I remind you of the works of the great saints, [Teresa of Avila and Catherine of Sienna] who corrected the Pope when she felt he needed it. Do not think your "Words" go totally unheeded by believers in the Church; they regard them as Divine Inspiration, ponder and study them carefully, seeking to ascertain Truth. For each person who is in My service I give a profound anointing of Knowledge and discernment of My Truth. Little ones, I ask you to persevere, remembering always that I am with you, for your prevailing "yes" in My service is pleasing to Me, the Living God!

At the close of one of these prayers my eyes were riveted by Our Lord, in the statue of the Infant Jesus of Prague was smiling broadly at me, and His Eyes, as well as the signet ring (seal of the King) on the upheld fingers of the right hand (which signify True God and True Man), were shining brilliantly. As I was gazing silently at Him, my prayer partner who knew nothing of what I was seeing said, "for some reason He is giving me Numbers 12 and 21. I don't know what that is about." But I knew that was for me. Our Lord reminded me that we are His friends:

Numbers 12: 6-8. Now hearken to the Words of the Lord; should there be a prophet among you, in visions will I reveal Myself to him, in dreams will I speak to him. Not so with My servant Moses .Throughout My House he bears My Trust. Face to face I speak to him plainly, not in riddles. The Presence of the Lord, he beholds.

Numbers 21:9. John 3:14 footnote. And as Moses lifted up the serpent, even so must the Son of Man be lifted up, so that everyone who believes may have life everlasting in Him. Commentary. In Numbers 21: 9, Moses merely mounts the serpent(the healing occurs through obedience to, and Faith in GOD.). But John substitutes the verb, and " Lifted up" implies exaltation or glorification. [New American Bible: St Josephs edition.]

Jesus Christ Himself, is exalted to Glory in His Cross and Resurrection. Therefore He Himself gives healing to all. Therefore a Christian physicians' Oath must Honour Jesus Christ, True God and True Man, and His symbols.[Raphael]

Genesis 9:4-6

Only you shall not eat flesh with its life, that is, its blood. For your own lifeblood I will surely require a reckoning: from every animal I will require it and from human beings, each one for the blood of another, I will require a reckoning for human life. Whoever sheds the blood of a human, by a human shall that person's blood be shed; for in His own Image, God made humanity.

Also read
THE BIOETHICS MESS   *by Dianne N. Irving, M.A., Ph.D. – in Crisis Magazine: Vol. 19, No. 5 May 2001*

TWO VERSIONS OF THE MEDICAL OATH.(next two pages).

The first is the original version, which is a specifically Christian version. After this work was presented at the international meeting of Association of Christian Therapists in 2006, the second version was offered. At the workshop where ten people reviewed it, the point was made and accepted, that many God-fearing doctors and other paramedical workers who were not Christian, might like to participate but were excluded. With the help of my spiritual advisor the second version, on the other hand, does NOT exclude Jesus. Some will recognize the words of the promise from the document originating from the CHCW used here with permission.

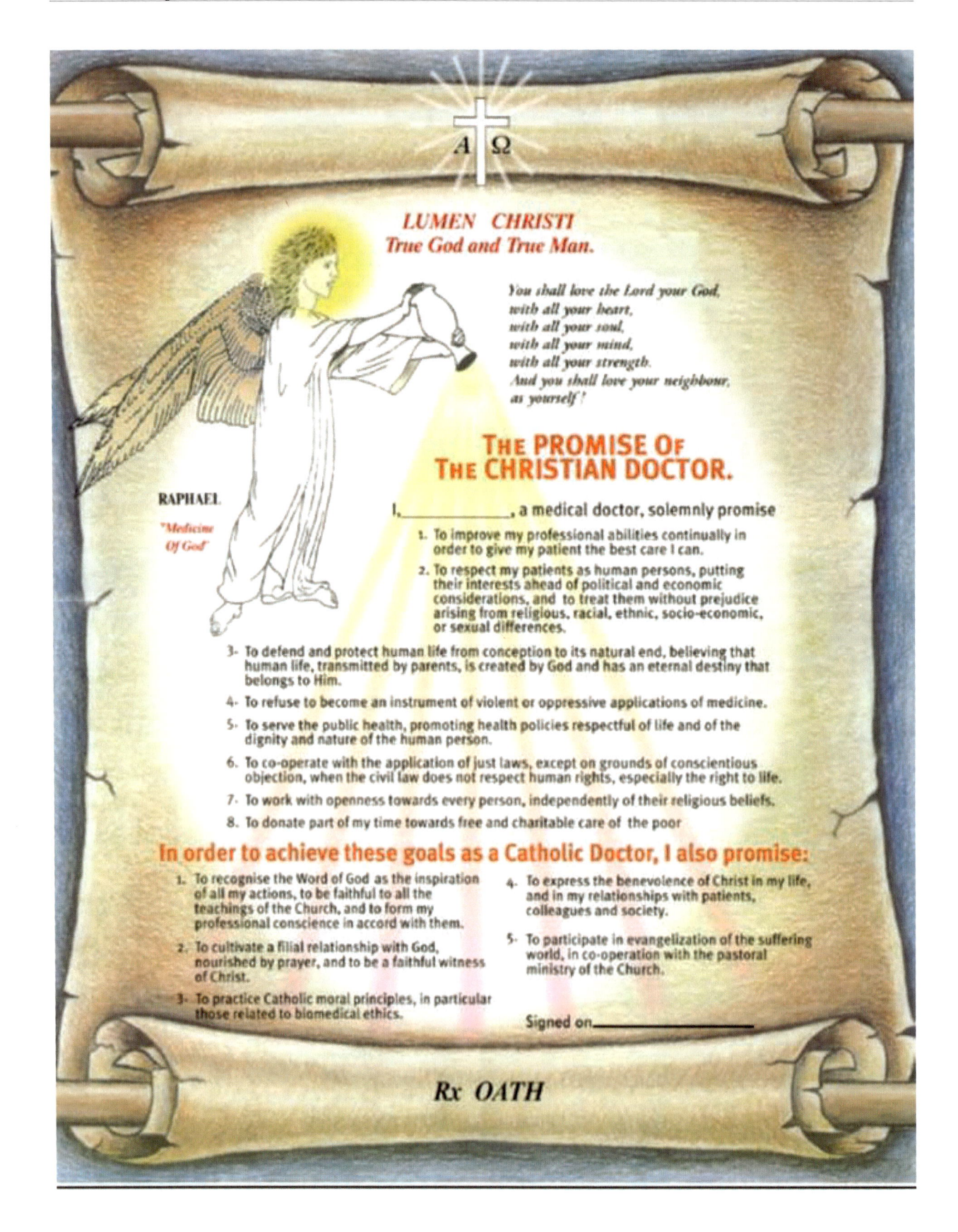

LUMEN CHRISTI
True God and True Man.

You shall love the Lord your God,
with all your heart,
with all your soul,
with all your mind,
with all your strength.
And you shall love your neighbour,
as yourself."

THE PROMISE OF THE CHRISTIAN DOCTOR.

RAPHAEL
"Medicine Of God"

I,_____, a medical doctor, solemnly promise

1. To improve my professional abilities continually in order to give my patient the best care I can.
2. To respect my patients as human persons, putting their interests ahead of political and economic considerations, and to treat them without prejudice arising from religious, racial, ethnic, socio-economic, or sexual differences.
3. To defend and protect human life from conception to its natural end, believing that human life, transmitted by parents, is created by God and has an eternal destiny that belongs to Him.
4. To refuse to become an instrument of violent or oppressive applications of medicine.
5. To serve the public health, promoting health policies respectful of life and of the dignity and nature of the human person.
6. To co-operate with the application of just laws, except on grounds of conscientious objection, when the civil law does not respect human rights, especially the right to life.
7. To work with openness towards every person, independently of their religious beliefs.
8. To donate part of my time towards free and charitable care of the poor

In order to achieve these goals as a Catholic Doctor, I also promise:

1. To recognise the Word of God as the inspiration of all my actions, to be faithful to all the teachings of the Church, and to form my professional conscience in accord with them.
2. To cultivate a filial relationship with God, nourished by prayer, and to be a faithful witness of Christ.
3. To practice Catholic moral principles, in particular those related to biomedical ethics.
4. To express the benevolence of Christ in my life, and in my relationships with patients, colleagues and society.
5. To participate in evangelization of the suffering world, in co-operation with the pastoral ministry of the Church.

Signed on_____

Rx OATH

MICHAEL
"Power of God"

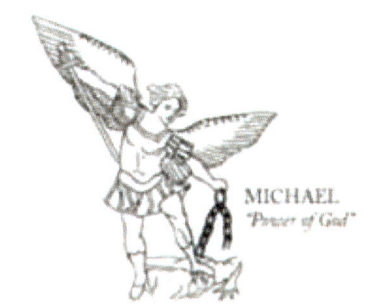

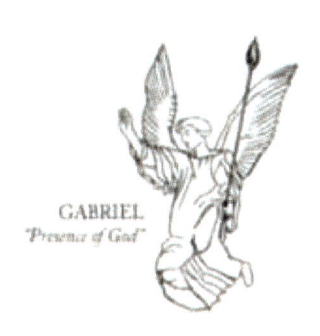

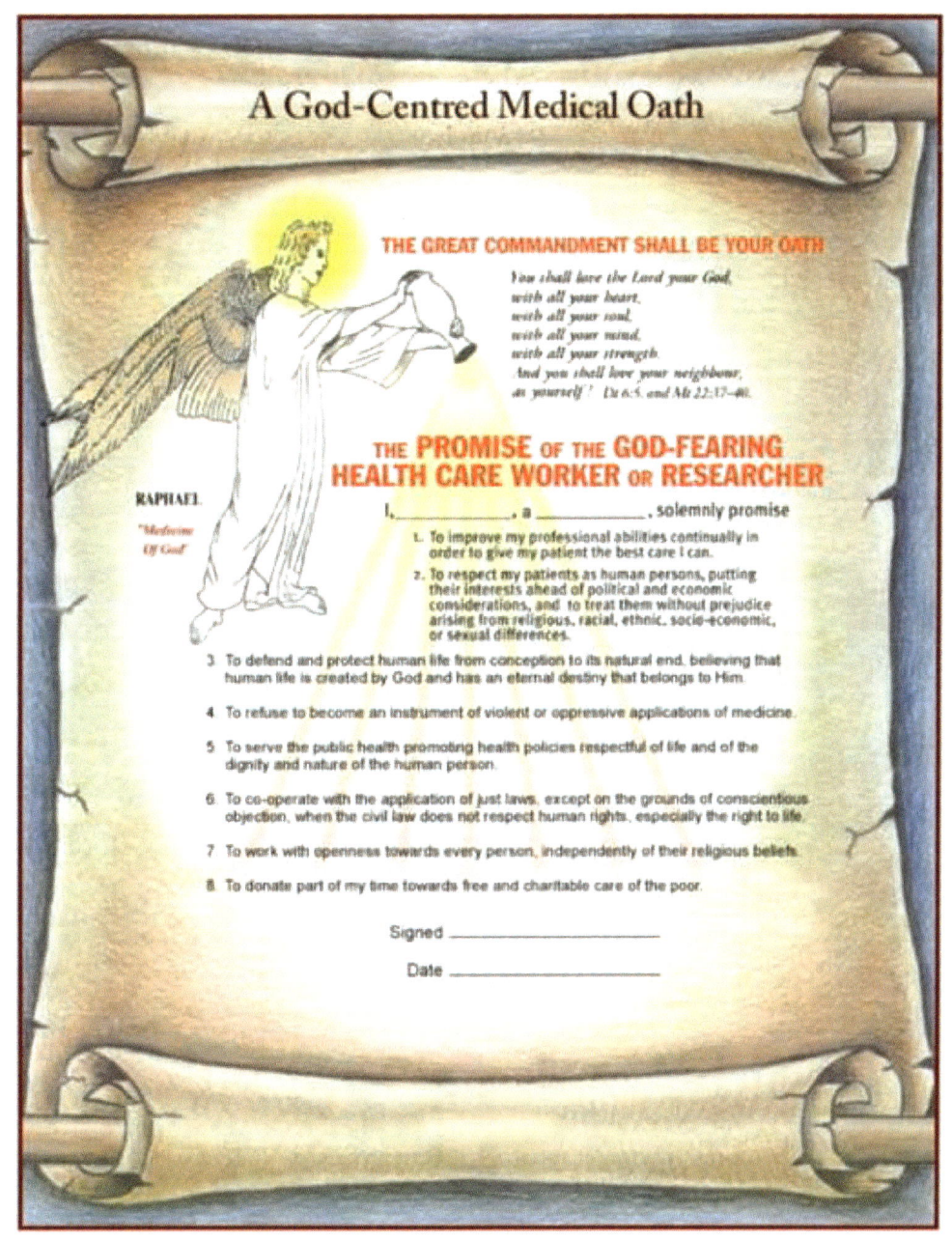

GABRIEL
"Presence of God"

A God-Centred Medical Oath

RAPHAEL
"Medicine Of God"

THE GREAT COMMANDMENT SHALL BE YOUR OATH

*"You shall love the Lord your God,
with all your heart,
with all your soul,
with all your mind,
with all your strength.
And you shall love your neighbour,
as yourself."* Dt 6:5. and Mt 22:37–40.

THE PROMISE OF THE GOD-FEARING HEALTH CARE WORKER OR RESEARCHER

I, _____, a _____, solemnly promise

1. To improve my professional abilities continually in order to give my patient the best care I can.

2. To respect my patients as human persons, putting their interests ahead of political and economic considerations, and to treat them without prejudice arising from religious, racial, ethnic, socio-economic, or sexual differences.

3. To defend and protect human life from conception to its natural end, believing that human life is created by God and has an eternal destiny that belongs to Him.

4. To refuse to become an instrument of violent or oppressive applications of medicine.

5. To serve the public health promoting health policies respectful of life and of the dignity and nature of the human person.

6. To co-operate with the application of just laws, except on the grounds of conscientious objection, when the civil law does not respect human rights, especially the right to life.

7. To work with openness towards every person, independently of their religious beliefs.

8. To donate part of my time towards free and charitable care of the poor.

Signed _____

Date _____

CHAPTER TWO
HIS WORDS

JESUS: Every Word I speak is a blessing for mankind." My blessings are in My Words. Those who are open to Me are given Enlightenment. A *cause celebre* is in My Holy Words. Those who will, will take it up like a great crusade! You are beloved of Jesus, beloved of Mary, continue to take Our Names prayerfully on your lips and We are with you, resolving the concerns of your heart in the Peace of Our Presence. "Ask of Me what you will. When you want testimonials of any sort, ask Me and the power of the Holy Spirit to be with you where I am, and together we write the Words! I Myself speak to you as you well know, in Divine Inspirations, and a Word here and there, for I am with you. Ask Me, and I set great angels and assistants about you at all times. Indeed, certain selected saints assist you now. My little one, pray as you do; it is pleasing to the Lord your God. Do not be anxious about anyone or anything. Stay always in My Presence. Anxiety obstructs, one might say, the pathway.

Be with Me now - a moment of blessings in the Peace of My Presence. I am writing My Words within your heart and upon your soul that you may write the necessary papers. Rest in Me a while, little sweetheart of your Christ. I am holding you to My bosom. I bless you, caress you; I strengthen you, I inspire you and then I set you back on your sturdy little legs to do that which you must do, little one. Love Me. It is sufficient! You walk ever in Great Light - be not afraid. Delightful and surprising actions occur now, for I hear your prayers and I make your pathway straight, leveling the hills and mountains. Little child, never enter an hour of despair. Cling to your Jesus, claim the Name of Jesus - you gain silent victory. Cling to Our Name and all goes according to Heaven's Design. My beloved one, a great blessing is upon you. Triune God!

The Message I give to mankind is for *all mankind*, all Christians to receive. National borders do not count in this My Work. Send them out to be read by the eyes of those whom I choose to read. Do not worry about the others. Simply send it out - it is at the least, thought-provoking. It is for the conversion I so desire from the medical profession. It will occur in many instances. I Myself bless the Messages. Know this: every Word I speak is a blessing for mankind. Those who accept the blessing are promptly anointed and profoundly assisted in their discernment and in the works of their hands. Those who reject it cannot say they have not known when they too answer to the Lord their God on that great and glorious day of the Lord.

You are profoundly blest for it is Faith-in-action, as I so desire it to be lived. Holy Light ever surrounds you. Now is a moment of sweet surrender, as the power of the Holy Spirit comes upon you, enfolding you in a great stream of the river of Love. In this Love you are given Words and Divine Inspiration for the Work of Mercy at hand. Mother and I are at one in this matter. An anointing is upon each one who reads the Words, opening their hearts to the Spirit of the Living God. Our Works of Mercy, the Works of Love must prevail! Teach My people; go forth in My Name! Yes indeed, send it to all! You know well there are some who will accept; others will reject. Do not worry about that. You will have done what I have called you to do in sending out those Words. Continue to ensure that M receives My Words, and go forward in Faith. I am with you; proceed.

This is the means of Salvation for the Hebrews and the Moslems, all peoples; the Blood of the Lamb without spot. The Call goes out to all the nations of the Earth to come to the Baptismal Waters; the Call like unto that of the beloved John the Baptist. Indeed, greater is He Who is in your hearts and souls and minds little children, than that which is in the world. Radiating, healing Love is upon all those through this Peace of the True Cross. It is done.

The realm of Glory is attendant upon this holy priest of God and upon yourselves. Therefore in any concern do not hesitate to address Fr J; We shall speak in you and through you to him, each of you, and he shall attend upon your Words. He will not always tell you what he is thinking about these matters for he is a prudent man, but I assure you he has not only the Church's best interests at heart but each of your own best interests at heart. Such is this priest that has been assigned here, at the same time that each of you are attending here at Good Counsel parish. It is the Hand of God which has placed you in these circumstances. Do not doubt that it is a heavy burden for both Father and the beloved Archbishop. This is true wherever My Words are given over to mankind through My precious little ones. He shows us that Medjugorje is still not approved.

Do not doubt that I am with you even as I am with him. Do not be alarmed at the behaviours of the other priests pertaining to your Mission. A day will come when you will understand all that is occurring ; why it had to be this way. I just ask you My little ones, each one of you to persevere in all prayerfulness enduring all that occurs in My Name. Remember, all the harsh words fall on Me. All woundedness I take into My Wounds, thus you shall most assuredly persevere, for this Mission is serious, the consequences of the actions of the unchristian doctors, I cannot permit to occur. Therefore it is essential that you prevail in My Name. Already, many eyes have been opened to Truth, as you have noticed, as you spoke to Fr J he did react to your comments.

You see, I have told you that the enemy has an insidious way of infiltrating everything with a duplicity of words so that one is never quite aware of what is occurring according to the writings of those who do not work for Me. This deceit is evident not only in the medical field but the political, the educational and We could go on. Rest assured that the Living God is aware of all the deceit that is poured forth upon all the unwary children of God in these days. Appropriate the Words I have given you as Divine Inspirations, that all goes according to Heaven's Design. Your Virgin of Fatima, your Mother, blesses you with a great anointing and in the power of the Holy Spirit, great graces fall upon you and your works of merciful love. My little one, even if the mindset of one person is altered by your Message, it is worthwhile; and I assure you that it is not only one person, but many, many who will respond to this Enlightenment, for We ensure that it is a profound Message.

Each life is sacred to the Lord your God, as you well know, yet your God is merciful and forgives mankind individually their transgressions; yes, even murder - for you serve a merciful and loving and forgiving God. There is one who will assist you - a priest of Holy Orders. We shall draw your attention to him, and he will be approachable...You will understand and he will indeed assist you. You are called to walk in Faith and hope and trust and therefore that is exactly what you will do. I the Lord Your God bless you! And yet your Merciful God, causes a turn-around in this affair. Little one, the Lord your God is with you. I have given you a few comments. Should you choose to use them in your summary, you may. You have sufficient inspiration and knowledge, and I Myself assist you in this matter. In the power of the Holy Spirit , Mother and I assist you as you prepare your letter now.

Little children, the dark days and all the trials *have to be*; before the Dawn of Light is upon the world. It is rapidly approaching, yet you have time to save the souls of those who by their atheist beliefs, their humanist beliefs, are hurling their very souls into eternal darkness. Humbly you come before Me in prayer-petition, seeking Words of discernment and understanding to share with the brotherhood of physicians throughout the world, yet thou art assigned to the beloved M, that your Words may be shared with your fellow Christians throughout the world.

My Words are not edited. I speak in the power of the Holy Spirit. My Word is Truth. You may yield the full information to the beloved Father. Do not concern yourself with what he does, or does not do, or with what he believes, or does not believe. My Words remain a Blessing to all those who read them. This is a time of great change upon the earth. My little children, you are part of that great change; and sometimes the journey is rough and difficult, but I am with you through it all.

As you send this document to M, as you well know, that will cause grave concern, even consternation; but My Words in you and through you are irrefutable; though some try to reject them; this is not unexpected. 'Pour forth Your Spirit and renew the face of the earth' you pray, you pray and you pray, My faithful ones; and it is happening. But it is My Will at this time in the history of Man, that much Enlightenment is through the faithful, among whom thou art numbered. A Flame of Love is upon you, for you are profoundly anointed in the Spirit of the Living God. I bid you yet again, do not worry about who appears to believe and who does not appear to believe. Leave it to Me, the reader of hearts. Simply tell them! Your Mission is complete in the telling. After that it is up to each individual. I Myself assist many to understand, to begin to comprehend; to begin to turn around, and know Truth as it is. The son of God, peruses the documents, reading and rereading them, in a puzzlement and yet a wonder. Had it occurred to you that the movement of the Holy Spirit occurs in and through the Words of the Lord your God, which are in and of themselves a Blessing?

It is given to each and every one of them! Have I not told you that My Word shall emanate from this point of Light throughout the world? Many believe, many do not believe; many are confused feeling a pull of the world and of human intellect. They reason it cannot be, that the Lord is speaking to some unknown on so profound a subject. Even so the tug of My Words being Truth will, shall We say haunt them, causing them to linger in attendance upon these Words, making an opening in the door of their heart, that the Spirit of the Living God may enter. Rejoice; it happens to the many. Do not worry about any hard hearted individuals. Leave them over to the Lord your God. Love conquers all. Continue, no matter what happens, as you are; for your prayers, your love, your obedience, your humility, your patient perseverance are the hallmarks of sanctity, and are pleasing to God.

Believe little children, We are not giving you Words which might inflate your ego. We are simply blessing you with Our Words. Persevere in Faith and hope and trust and love and patient perseverance, relying on your Jesus. Remember, in your weakness is My Strength, and that I am with you always. Address those to whom it is possible, fairly soon. Carry with you these Words to the conference. There are means readily available for translation into various languages. Be at Peace in this regard. Be at Peace in My Love. Know that I have tested you and trained you these many years for this time and this Mission which is singularly yours. Be at Peace therefore - I am with you always. I cause rivers of Light and Enlightenment on those in the profession whom I am calling by name now; and in September, My Enlightened ones will be in every nation!

When you are working as My friends, My Works, I am with you; and I am with My beloved bishops and priests as they read and ponder the Words which I have given unto thee; therefore, there is no cause for fear and anxiety here. You might say I have armed and armoured you very well for this Mission. The beloved M has need of more Words therefore I gift thee with more Words. My graces fall upon you little one. When you are speaking to M, the Words will flow from your heart , for your heart is Mine and Mothers, and in this Trinity of Love you will speak the appropriate Words for it will be the Lord God speaking in the Power of the Holy Spirit . Therefore I ask you to just rest in Peace and Light in My Presence and wait on the Lord yet a little longer. *Now* is a moment of surrender to Love, as the Spirit of the Living God pours forth from the

Immaculate Heart of the Beloved Virgin Mary, a river of Light upon you. *Angels keep singing, glory, glory, glory to the Lord.*

Be not anxious therefore, remain always at Peace, holding fast to your Jesus. Great graces will flow upon those who open their hearts and minds at the next meeting and they will be Enlightened . All will mind; I call all unto Me, those who are pledged to Me, in all Faith, will know the Truth. I the Lord God, Am Truth. A number of events will occur in their lives that will cause them to see more clearly, the Message you bear; and you are not alone. Others about the world bear similar Messages. Continue to go forth, humbly before your God, but boldly in the face of what the world would tell My people. Remember that of all the priests in Jerusalem, only John the Baptist would tell Herod, who symbolizes the worldly; that he was committing sin. My little one, you are safe in Me. Be not afraid; you do not suffer the fate of the great St. John. But simply speak out the Truth in My Name. You are greatly rewarded in this Mission of Truth which is assigned to you.

My little children, this whole catastrophe of medical science is because man does not follow God's Law, the Will of God as taught even unto Moses and even unto this day. If you had before you a blessing and a curse, I ask you this - would they stop because of My Word or your word? Even so, speak your "Words!" Thou art tested, other physicians are tested; the priesthood involved in this area of concern are also tested. It matters not whether certain priests or physicians unite with you. A given number shall indeed; and I Myself deploy them, and My Words in you and through you, about the world; and all those whom I Will, are exposed to these concerns of your God. This desire to Enlighten My beloved little ones is of Me. Ask of Me what you will now. We are in attendance upon thee. It is your Jesus who speaks. In the Unity of the Triune God We address you.

Many rejected Me, many will reject you, yet I have strengthened you to persevere, and that you shall do! Little children, those who heed the Words know a great Victory of Love, and begin themselves to evangelize, and to propagate the Faith of the Apostles, which is in sore disarray upon the earth at this time. Persevere little children of Faith, persevere! *Jesus shows us my beloved Therese` again and He is saying,* "How appropriate is she not, the Patroness of Missionaries; and is this not a house with a great Mission; and are not your Words, as a missionary of " *the Epistle of Love to the scientific world.*"

Our Lord showed us how St Paul converted the Greeks in the great' Logic ' of their minds; they too surrendered to Truth and Love. Little ones, prevail fearlessly for I am with you, and I am with Father Francis, and I am with a myriad of people who will come to your assistance.

A great Light of Faith pours forth upon you and emanates from you. Never concede any defeat little children in My Name; continue always in Faith and hope and trust and Love and patient perseverance; for this is My Way; I am the Way; it is the only Way, for those who would know Me. My little sisters, you are profoundly blest and anointed this day. Thus I come to you My little humble ones who have fought the good fight against the assaults of the enemy, and stand in the courage of your convictions despite what is occurring about you. The Lord shows how He opened the door to the prison for St Paul.

My blessings are upon you now . Those who serve Me are never prisoners of the world. Doors open at the Hand of your God, your Almighty God. I am Jesus, your Eternal Victor! My Words are a blessing to those who will heed. Do not worry about those who reject My Words or even reject you. Prevail little one in patient perseverance. You are blest profoundly with the necessary fortitude to do the Will of your God. Whomsoever heeds the Words shall be profoundly blest. Those of irrational thought will reject it. They may even taunt. It matters little. Remain close to your Jesus and Our Mother, and My Peace, My Providence, My Protection, is upon each of My Own.

And should I choose to send you to speak My Words to My people would you in free will go? *Yes Lord.* First of all come before Me here in the Adoration Chapel, and pray for discernment and you will surely know before you leave which times to say yes and which ones to decline. You are powerfully assisted by Heavenly Beings and all is going nicely, like unto a free flow of Words and Works. Be at Peace, it is Our delight. You are My delight. Just continue as you are in Divine Inspirations; all that you have done in these printings is pleasing to the Lord your God. Little children, great angels fight a great battle, that these Words be given over first for the doctors, then even to the priests involved, but ultimately for the general public, those that can and will read . Do not be dismayed at the obstructions little one, or any of the strange events that will attempt to slow you down or even stop you all together. <u>It shall not be</u>. I Myself cause the Victory to happen. Thou hast worked well; thou art well advised from Glory. Things are going according to Heaven's Design. Be at Peace. The virtue of Love is such that I am present to you. A severe testing, a severe attack is upon your Works little children; prevail, We are with you. Believe, We are with You. Be at Peace therefore!

We confess that you are appealing most profoundly for their mercy, but yet there remains such a black cross over the medical field. You are doing that which I have requested of you. Be at Peace in this matter. We bless many with Enlightenment now. It is just to let you know little one, the great Mission to which you are assigned. The power of darkness is immense. There is grief in Heaven for the behaviours of many doctors, research scientists and many more; and yet as My Church walks the *Via Dolorosa,* you must know, as I did, and as Our Mother did, <u>that it had to be</u>*!* Little children, it is so for the Body of Christ. Little children, you are little and humble and obedient, but your Mission in My Name is great. You are My instruments. Your God is a carpenter, a builder, who uses you as a hammer to keep hammering and hammering and hammering the Truth to mankind. I am Truth. Enlightenment will indeed come to many. Do not be dismayed at those who shut themselves away from My Words. I have empowered you, strengthened you for this Mission. I Myself am carrying you throughout this Mission.

Walls of flame surround many whom you will be dealing with, for they do that which is highly displeasing to the Lord your God. Be not afraid, you are surrounded in My Light, and great graces accrue and fall upon you throughout this Mission of hope. Seeds of destruction of human life are rampant about the earth , yet in the midst of this remains My Light, My Life, My Love. Now is a moment of Enlightenment. Open your hearts, your minds, and together with your God, you will readily work great miracles of healing. The vaults of Heaven pour forth the needed Enlightenment now. I repeat; *now* is the opportune time. I am your God of merciful Love.

A living testimony of My Love is Faithful Missionary. Should she be prevailed upon to speak , she may use these Words. Be not surprised at what is happening. Each one of you who has truly said "yes" to your God, like unto the Blessed Virgin Mary, their soul becomes like unto a mirror; reflecting My Love, My Truth, upon mankind. The Angels keep singing," His Name is wonderful, Jesus Our Lord! My Words are a blessing to those who will heed. Do not worry about those who reject My Words or even reject you. Prevail little one, in patient perseverance. You are blest profoundly with the necessary fortitude to do the Will of your God. It is no secret what God can do; although it is not in Holy Scripture, it is My Word, therefore proclaim it, to all who will heed. Give him the time to establish it on the Web. Whomsoever heeds the Words shall be profoundly blest.

You will begin to see, as you might put it, a Light at the end of the tunnel, for I am profoundly united with you, in this great Mission of Love. Clarification may be asked of you in some of Our Words. Believe, I shall inspire you, even speak in you and through you, addressing anyone's concerns about My Words. Be at Peace, no matter what is happening, remain at Peace in all things. Indeed send the Messages afar. You have bespoken to the several about you(the local Catholic physicians guild) with no positive response. They must therefore wait in turn (He's showing us a long lineup) before they begin to receive My Words of Truth once again. Should one seek you out asking for this information, be pleased to give it to them. But as you say the many appear to be stonewalling your efforts. Leave them there. Pray to the God of Mercy that they too be Enlightened. At this time verbal coercion or any such means are to no avail. Remain therefore in the Spirit in prayer for the many.

Should a door open for you to speak, remembering all things are possible with God, do speak. And should it be necessary to speak only to this individual or that one, or perhaps two or three, do so. It would of course be in a very limited way; but accompanied with the brochures it will be adequate food for thought and discernment for those individuals. (*Fr Francis listened to a show on the CBC where they were talking about selling the kidneys. Father wanted me to discern whether I should be on such a talk show.*)No because it would be biased; your responses would be limited by the goals of the program itself. One must therefore discern the entire vehicle, before one is free to strive to Enlighten the listeners. On a Christian program where thou art not necessarily the one in control, but the sole speaker, My Words are safe in thee. In the public programs they can be chopped and altered randomly to destroy Our Word, for that is the way of the world. Little one, you are blest in your Mission and assisted profoundly by Heaven. The Glory of the Lord surrounds the true faithful ones in a unique manner not visible to their fellow man.

Down on your knees before Me little ones, I have anointed you as My brave warriors. I know your frailties, I know your weaknesses, your strengths and I Myself am your Strength now.(Our Lord's strong arm holding a little chisel[me], chiseling away). My little ones persevere; I am with you; Mother is with you; great saints and great angels; powerful angels assist you in this Mission. Thou hast asked that We rebuke in the Name of Jesus, it is the Lord Who speaks, the spirit of pride which assails many intellectuals. This has been an ongoing war throughout the course of the centuries, and continues to now; yet some will yield. A certain yieldedness-in-Faith to the Living God is essential, before the thoughts of this people, the minds and thoughts, are opened to Truth. I the Lord God AM Truth.

Another gateway of Truth is opened elsewhere in the Americas, in agreement with what you are given, converging as it were with what you are given; and this assists you. Little children, those who serve the Lord do not work alone. Much help is given you. I Myself will inspire you when and where to speak, even as you spoke a second time at the conference. It shall be more clearly given to you to know when and where to speak, by Divine Inspiration; by even a few Words; and you shall know it is that moment to speak; and do not worry about those who close their ears, or their minds and hearts, to what you are saying. When you are called to speak in My Name little children, I address you all; it is because there is someone there even though it be only one, but usually there is more than one; whom I wish to hear My Words. And they shall respond to My Words wholeheartedly, and it is for them that you speak little ones. Do not worry about those who do not heed, or who shrug you off; or even more so make negative comments. They are the deceived; they are the ones with the stony hearts which are not opened, and they are so in need of Merciful prayer. Truly, they are the poorest of the poor.

Include more of the Holy Father's words from the Apostolic Letter, *Tertio Millennio Adveniente*; the ones that are in union with what I am asking you to do. Therefore you are doing all that I ask of you. Do not worry about what the Bishop, or any priest or any physician does with My Words. Once you have done what I have called you to do, thou art blest tremendously. What they do with it, is between them and your God. Those who heed and act accordingly, also receive vast blessings. I do not say that all heed. It has never been that way. I wish you to always remain at Peace, never worrying or being anxious about any responses to

Our Words. Answer in Truth. I AM Truth,(Jn 14:6) and I am with you. I dwell in your heart, I speak with your lips. Do not be worried about anyone attempting to scandalize you or Omen. You belong to Me now and forever, and your obedience to this Commission, which might I say, no one else operating by intellect alone, by human intellect, by human reason, would attempt to do; yet, by Faith, My little ones you are doing it; a task which would be fearful to those who are not closely united with Me, you do, little trembling infants.

It is beautiful, it is Holy. [He shows us the Monstrance all Lighted up.] I am with you, whither thou goest I bless you. I bless you here, I bless you in your prayer times, I bless you in the Mass, I bless you in Adoration, I bless you in this warfare in which We are, and which We undertake; whither thou goest I am with you! Simply find a way to portray all My Words. Since you will use the ones I have anointed for you to use, these documents become clear to the reader. Precious little children, I find thee pleasing for thou hast heeded the Call to love and obedience in all humility before your God, and not worrying about human esteem; about the woundedness which you suffer, for My Name, for My Cause. My Cause is Love. Thus I have given the Great Commandment of Love, that My little ones truly love one another, even as I Love each one.

Precise details We have given thee in Our Epistle of Love to the scientific world. Many have read it. Some have begun and not completed reading it; those whom you have dispensed it to. Do not worry about it. Your duty is completed in giving them My Words; Words of Enlightenment. What they do with it is between them and their God. I Myself attend upon them, for all Words I give to thee flow as Blessings upon thee and upon the readers of My Words. Even so, in free will they may be rejected. This is not to say that they are rejected, except by certain few, and some only in certain instances. Little children, in the river of darkness upon the earth in which the physicians are working, these My Messages of Love fall startling upon the many who have not contemplated their God to any great degree, or have not weighed their actions and the consequences of their actions in the Light of Holy Scripture.

The vortex of the storm in which you have been is now moved from you, and recognition is beginning to occur in the minds of several who have read Our Commission to you. Be at Peace therefore. You were in the eye of the storm because of the Messages you sent out. But there is now some belief and they no longer focus on you, that the Word of God has been given unto thee, but Your Mission itself becomes the focus of attention rather than you *per se*. He condemns you from the start but then has a conversion. He becomes an instrument in the implosion in the medical world with regard to the issues at hand. Indeed. Again, do not be dismayed at any initial response or any apparent lack of initial response. There is much food for thought in these Missals, and therefore these busy men take their time in discerning these documents. My time schedule leaves room for these discernments. Be not anxious therefore little one.

JESUS says; Fall on your knees to the Father and let the angels themselves anoint you little ones. [Praying prone] Living Waters flow upon you little ones. I am the Living God come down from Heaven. I address you as the Triune God. The Mission of Love given over unto thee Omen and thee Faithful Missionary, are important to the Lord your God. A day will come when these Words of Mine shall indeed be recognized by all believers. Rest in My Love a moment as My great anointing continues upon you. Angels are singing, "His Love is more precious than silver and gold". You recognize I am Owner of the assets; in you comes the essence of a poverty, to promote Our Words as We desire you to do. My little ones, bless Me! *We adore thee oh Christ and we bless Thee, because by Thy Holy Cross, Thou hast redeemed the world.*

While you are resting in Our Presence many actions of the Holy Spirit are occurring in your lives and the lives of those whom you carry in your heart . The enemy busies himself in obstructing all the plans of My faithful little one. Piecemeal is the response you have received to Our Messages to the scientific world!

Provide the pamphlets as you shall do at the conference. I reiterate; don't worry about those who choose not to read or heed My Words. Those who read them are blest. They are indeed My Words, not yours; not yours, but Mine The Blessing is in the very Words. Prevail little children, prevail! Continue in all Faith. All falls into place for those who believe as you do. I remind you, you are handpicked each one of you for this Mission of Love which is important to the Living God, and you shall prevail. Consider the events of today as merely further testing and strengthening.

Little children, My Words to you, are they not, if implemented now, turning the medical world as it were upside down, causing a great turn around? Many, many, many physicians have themselves lodged in a comfortable position and have no desire to be moved from that position. [He shows like oysters attached to rocks which cannot be moved] *Yes Lord and some priests too I am sorry to say* .It is so. This is how certain people are little children; not only not open to change but reluctant to change. Yet little children, in the Name of Jesus of Nazareth, ALL SHALL CHANGE ! IT MUST BE !Continue working diligently to send the Information to the various physicians as you understand it, and do not be distraught, as you would say, if you don't get any feedback at this time. Thus it will be with this My Love Letter to My scientific friends.

On sending me to Israel; I will show unto thee many delights in the Faith of the Fathers; in the Faith of the Apostles. Thou wilt see and comprehend so very, very much! I need you to know all that you will be learning because We have much to do together, My small sister, and it shall be so. *Lord please strengthen me for the much You will expect when I get back!* It shall be so! Would you invoke St Peter; so few people invoke St Peter. I am now ready to bless these works profoundly. Immediately after the Christmas celebration begin to mail them out. We are with you. The virtue of Love is such that thou art called to a great Mission on behalf of your God. I remind you again, indeed I have molded you and fashioned you and strengthened you for this Mission. Even as St Paul was trained in all the Holy Scriptures and well educated in the Faith before he became one of My Own, he was thus prepared for his Mission with a sound basis, each one of you have been prepared to become the individuals that you are now in these Works of Love. It is I the Lord God Who does it. You are profoundly blest in all that you do in My Name. Indeed, anything that opens any of their minds, to the Way of Holiness; to fully comprehend the sanctity of Life; to fully comprehend the awesome Gift of Life to its fullest. Give glory to the Father, pray and send copies to those to whom you are inspired to send them. Verse and Phrase of your Words are in Scripture! I the Lord God, heed and answer. I have come to earth to give freedom and Salvation to all mankind! I am the Lord your God and I am attendant upon you as is Our Mother. Little children bless Me.

See little children, a great work of Redemption is occurring now, through My Church, and you little ones are integral parts of what is happening in the Body of Christ; and indeed, none of My Own shall be lost to Me. As you can see, Enlightenment is coming, person by person, as the Spirit of Love touches them, and My Understanding comes to them, "For the darkness covers the Earth, and the clouds the people." (Isaiah 4:1.)Little children, Enlightenment is coming. I am the Light of the world.[Jn 8:12] I am casting off the darkness which enshrouded My people for so long! Little children, blessed are those who believe and act on their belief, as you are doing. My delight is in you! You know well that My Church is like unto a living tree, a living vine with branches spreading hither and yond, and the bishops of Rome are astounded at the many turns that are taking place in the Church now.(Jn 15)Shall We say, they have their hands full with many new concerns. The beloved John Paul is ever attendant on the matter of Life and Death. He himself, like yourselves, is touched by affliction. He has great compassion for the afflicted. He has a heart of love, My kind of Love, for all humanity. My delight is in the beloved John Paul.

Blandishment! There are those who would brush off anything that the Pope pronounces with many, many words such as occurs in the spirit of confusion. Do not be dismayed; My Will is done in and through the beloved John Paul, and those who adhere in all faithfulness to the Magisterium of My Church. The face of evil is evident in what is now referred to as the 'abortion industry.' How can the slaughter of innocents,(Mt 2:16) and the so-called harvesting of their body parts, be called an industry, and how can this relate to the Kingdom of God; and it is but the beginning of this, which the beloved John Paul has aptly named, "culture of death." My little children of Life, I bless you each and every one. I am Blessing those who comprehend that I am God, and yield their free wills to Me. When you yield your free wills to Me, it is for the love, not only of your God, but the love of mankind, for the betterment of mankind, for the Salvation of mankind. Thus little children, when you practice loving your neighbour as yourself, great fruits are produced; to come to know Truth, and to live in My Light and My Love.

As you know, while you were in Rome, the many encounters were arranged by the Hand of your God, that an understanding of My Word, My Will, be known hither and yond about the globe, about the earth, for the hour is late and much of My Word is yet needed. Little children, as each one believes as GI believes now, they too in their Faith begin to believe, so that healing love emanates from them unto others, and thus is expanded the Great Mission of Light and Love and Life.

"Hear oh Lord, the sound of my cry; hear oh Lord and have Mercy," you pray. I am responding little one; at the opportune moment the beloved John Paul speaks the needed words. This will send the scientific world into great controversies as you know; and so it is done at a specific time, with most specific words that are clear, and cannot be interpreted in a confusing manner. The work is already begun on this subject. Wait yet a little longer children. I am with you in all of this, for have I not inspired you and brought you thus far? Thou art in the Presence of Almighty God, the Triune God, who wills to address you thus; The Sovereign Queen of Heaven shall be recognized in the Church of God, for the beloved John Paul will speak the long awaited dogma. It is the moment of Truth for Mankind to comprehend what the Lord God has done for Mankind! I have opened Scripture that it be understood by those who have long studied it, that they recognize the Truth of the Church which I built on the rock of Peter. The Ship of State which is the Vatican, is not a political state, but is the core of the Body of Christ.

Those that have eyes to see and ears to hear, will understand and desire to be united in the One Body, and will come in droves to be united in the One Body, and the Vatican shall surely be a ship, a great ship like unto the Ark, but it will be Mankind entering the ship, that all know Salvation from the perils that will one day befall the earth. I ask you to continue to pray the pardon prayer; 'My God, I believe, I adore, I trust and I love You; I beg pardon for those who do not believe, do not adore, do not trust and do not love You;'(words of the Angel at Fatima) that many yet will come unto Me, the Living God. There is a way that I would have you walk, each one of you, My Own little ones, and in so doing you are evangelizing according to your state in life, and being instruments in the conversion of many, for it is most assuredly the time of the Great Ingathering.

Loving Mercy is outreaching to all. There are those who have bodily hungers and needs, but the majority have a great spiritual hunger which I, the Lord, would fill at this time. I would assuage the anguish of the souls so in need of Comforting Love. Continue to speak out in the Name of Jesus. In so doing you are living all that has been asked of you little children. You are Faith- filled children; there are many who have scant Faith and are in sore need of a deepening of Faith. Soon they will experience an Enlightenment and have a great hunger, a great thirst to draw near the Bread of Life.(Jn 6:35 Mankind is ever seeking a sign of My Existence, a sign of My Presence with them. The beloved John Paul is himself a great sign. Even so, I will cause specific signs to occur on the earth, to melt the hearts of many, to take away disbelief, to cause people to know that I am your God, that I am Mercy, that I am Love.

The Hand of My Justice is stayed yet a little longer because of My Love for Humanity. Continue to be lights along the way for the many weary travelers on earth who walk yet in darkness not aware of the Light of My Presence. *The angels are singing, 'oh what could My Jesus do more, Oh silence my soul and adore."* Speak to Me of Love. *My God I believe, I adore...*

I am the Lord your God; on whom I will, I have Mercy. Little children, I love you My precious ones. In your abandonment to Me, your abandonment to Love, I am profoundly united with you; in all your trials I am with you. My precious little ones, I tell you again, you are living in a pagan world, not unlike My first apostles lived, even I lived, and that is why evangelization today is so very important. Of this, the beloved John Paul is fully aware, as he too works his miracles of healing love even as you do, My precious ones. Beloved Faithful Missionary, that which you are experiencing, has to be at this time; but always, always remember, in My Name; Jesus, is your victory.

These unbelieving, even pagan individuals empowered by hate and greed and pride, attempt to hurl everything that they can against every true member of the Body of Christ, to no avail. My little ones, you are victorious in My Name, Jesus, Eternal Victor. Even so, I guide your steps. Cling to Me, keep your eyes upon your Jesus. Hold the Names of your Jesus, and Our beloved Mother Mary, always in your heart and soul and mind, and at the ready upon your lips, for those moments of crisis, those moments of stress, those moments of sudden need, that appear to just pop up out of nowhere, upon My little warriors.

You have a word in your language called stalking, and it is as it were, that My precious ones are stalked by the invisible one, through those who operate under his power, yet greater am I, as you are well aware. Therefore know that I am Truth, and that in full knowledge of Truth, which you have little children, you do indeed succeed. I have called you from all time to be here at this time, for this battle, and I have strengthened you, and I have molded you and fashioned you with all your weaknesses and your strengths, to be the instrument of Peace, My Enlightenment, to suffering Mankind, and therefore you shall persevere. With regard to the questionnaire, the appraisal, it falls neatly into place. With regard to the many patients behaving as they are doing , simply continue to pray for them as they steady themselves mentally and emotionally, and some even physically. As you pray for them, they are changed for the good.

I recognize that your work is made more difficult, for not all believe in My Name, Jesus; but you believe in Me, and your prayers, your Faith, are the power which defeats that which has come against these suffering souls. That is why I speak little children; We ask you now to begin frequently praying the Pope Leo 13th exorcism on behalf of the Vatican itself. Little children, be assured you are at war. Yes you are front-line soldiers, but so is John Paul and many like him. My faithful cohort prevails against tremendous odds, but I ask you little children, to pray in this matter. Little children, when you make the prayer on behalf of John Paul in the Vatican, it falls down, even unto your parish, your diocese, and Providence (Health Care), and many such Catholic organizations and facilities which have been most insidiously invaded by what the beloved Pope Paul VI called, "the smoke of Satan." Therefore little children, continue praying as you do, but add this prayer; it was given most assuredly for this time in the history of the Church.

Each one on Earth is given the opportunity to choose Eternal Life. My Church, My Body must experience this. I have chosen John Paul, a man of Wisdom and Fortitude, and much, much more, for the Mission in Life. The role which he plays in Salvation history is profound. Be at Peace then little children; love your God and love one another, and remain in the Peace of My Presence. The beloved Holy Father, the Bishop of Rome is aware of the Epistle of Love and has many working on a paper, a thesis, regarding the grave matters at hand. You know well that he prays and discerns intently, and is thus able to make the great documents of Truth which he does, for he is in Unity with Me.[the Lord shows a great big horn that he is speaking through loudly to the world]and it shall be thus!

You see, he is a Pope of profound discernments. In this time frame that you delivered the Message to him, he must verify each and every concern, and validate each and every concern, and remain ever in My Truth, while dealing with ever so many complexities. In due course, this changes. In the interim, know that your God is working powerfully with many, many individuals involved in these very concerns. They are instruments of My Peace and Healing Love, and together a framework of Truth in this field of Medicine is set up. A bulwark of Faith is set up and My Will is done, and all those who are My Own heed! Be at Peace therefore! The battle lines are drawn. By this conference, *all* will know My Stance, and the stance of the beloved John -Paul, My Vicar in this matter. This is not pleasing to the mad scientists, who use My Creations- human bodies, oblivious to My Truth. He speaks in a manner that none can deny his Truth. That does not mean little children that all will heed Truth and respond in Love! Even so, the battle lines are clearly drawn and Truth comes to the fore in this issue of euthanasia and 'brain death,' and in the issue of abortion and what is occurring to the aborted infants. All of this is anathema; all of this is an abomination in the Eyes of the Living God, in Whose Presence you live!

Mother and I attend upon the beloved John Paul constantly; all of Heaven is attendant upon him, united with him in the great Victory battle now ongoing. Rest assured, all that is in My Power and Design, is aligned with this holy man, that My Church, My faithful remnant, knows Victory in Me, Jesus, and the Triumph of the Two Hearts, is upon the world. The time is not yet, but very soon. In the interim, ongoing trials and disasters are upon the Earth, for the majority of mankind, is not yet yielded to the Will of the Father, and brings suffering upon themselves and those of My Own who die in these bloodbaths and disasters. All come as martyrs into My Presence, and great is their reward in Glory.

Write My Words; yet it is perfectly permissible to record those which you have heard about through your practice. An addendum of those cases may be attached. However, I shall leave that up to you. You will be inspired by the Lord your God and assisted by many from Heaven, to write this paper. It is to the Glory of God that you are working this paper, little one. It is pleasing to the Lord your God and thus profound spiritual assistance is given over unto thee. A haunting sorrow is in the Heart of the Lord your God, because of the tragedies of mankind's pride in the works of their hands, not consecrated to Me, but to power and to greed . My little sister, I am anointing you and blessing you profoundly - be at Peace in all these things. My Voice needs to be heard. These people need to at least revise what they are doing, because it is true that a day comes when they stand before their Judge; and since thou art the one I choose to forewarn a multitude, thou art profoundly blest. Remember you are not alone. There are others of like heart and mind amidst your people and Heaven is with you.

I am the Lord your God(Is43:13), All Powerful and on whom I will, I have Mercy ! (Romans 9:16) Indeed, I give the Gift of Life, I am Life and I am Truth.(Jn14:6) I am here in a moment of tender and compassionate Love for mankind. My Gift to thee, child of God, Faithful Missionary - a Word for mankind - some will consider and heed. You are well aware that others will not. Even so, the Word must be given. Ask Me now what you will. You are under Assignment from Me, the Lord your God. Of course you may share with others of the profession. As you send this document to M, as you well know, that will cause grave concern, even consternation; but My Words in you and through you are irrefutable; though some try to reject them; this is not unexpected.

'Pour forth Your Spirit and renew the face of the earth' you pray, you pray and you pray, My faithful ones; and it is happening. But it is My Will at this time in the history of man, that much Enlightenment is through the faithful, among whom thou art numbered. As you are kneeling before the Father of Enlightenment, Mercy attends upon you, blessing you. A flame of Love is upon you, for you are profoundly anointed in the Spirit of the Living God. I the Lord your God, bid you know that I am not unaware that the seven deadly sins are no longer mentioned among Christians. They are not recognized among pagans; but it is the very humans who claim to be Christians who now shun the seven deadly sins! Were there no lust, there would be no abortions; were there no greed, there would be no sale of body parts; If there were not self-seeking, power-seeking scientists, there would be no cloning of humans; no mutilation of precious embryos and all the other desecrations that are occurring upon My Own Creation, with precious human bodies and souls.(Cf Mk3:5-6. Lk16:19-31) Ask of Me what you will that you may be clear about what you wish to express. Come unto Me as you need to know. I am working closely with you, and I am delighted with our conversations of Life and Love."

The Roe vs. Wade case was falsified, as you know. And so you see, with the proponents of these evil machinations in the name of science and progress, there are scandalous lies and occurrences to promote that which is not of God. This is the world in which you are living! It is worse than Egypt ever was. What would you have Me do about these vile occurrences over which My little faithful ones on earth grieve, even as I grieve? Oh, My little one, there is sorrow in the Heart of your God at what is happening in the field of medicine and all the sciences; both sorrow and grief. The walls which surround the hearts of the many prevent them from knowing Merciful Love, Agape Love, compassionate Love. In a sterile, loveless way they work their works of iniquity upon My Creation, humanity. It is enough what they are doing to the other creatures on earth, but what they do to My precious gifts of Love brings down My Wrath, as you well know! I bid you read Ezekiel, read Jeremiah, read the many messages in Holy Scripture and know that I do not take lightly the attacks on innocent victims such as aborted infants and indeed those whose bodies are so mutilated by, as they call it, the harvesting of their organs. Why would they need a substitute kidney or heart or liver had they or their forbearers been faithful to Me in the first place? Even now, were they simply to be faithful I would cure them!

Do you not call Me the Great Physician, the Healer? (Mk2:17) But you use Me not! Even so, in the Mercy of God, I call the medical profession in particular, and their research scientists, once again to come back to Me with all their hearts. At times, you mention God, or even My Name, Jesus, but you neither know Me, nor obey Me, nor honour Me, as I would have you do. Little helpless ones who are yet praying incessantly on the earth, who do know their God, and the awesome Power of the Creator of all that is, do not do surgical operations; they simply pray for one another with all petition, seeking healing and I give it to them. See, you have strayed out of the domain of your God's Love; of the Holy, the immutable Will of the Living God.

I repeat; I reiterate; It is the Lord your God, Who set the stars on their courses, that gives you the life-bearing planet, at the essential distance from the sun, that there might be life here! Now you toy with all these gifts of Mine, which cause life to be! The seeds of My Love have fallen on bare rock and are bearing no fruit in this community of practitioners of Death. (Mk4:5-7)Each of My Own who believe in Me walk on this earth as a lighted candle(Mt5:14); for the Flame of Love, the power of the Holy Spirit is upon each one, even as it was upon My apostles and disciples at the time of the first Pentecost. (Acts2:2)"This blessing of the great Pentecost is upon the faithful all over the earth - those where Love yet reigns in their hearts and controls thus their rational thoughts and minds.

Therefore, I bid you heed - which is essentially to hear and to act upon My Words, through My little voice, My little Faithful Missionary, whom I have chosen in this fashion to enlighten My people. I the Lord God, attend upon her, and every other faithful-to-God person on earth today, most powerfully. I am calling My people not to surrender to what may be termed 'mad science.' Little children, it is not different, in a sense, from a gambler who seeks money by gambling; serving Mammon, as is written, and failing to trust the Providence of the Lord your God. It is this failure to trust in the Loving Providence, the Blessing of your Lord God, that causes poverty where there should be none; affliction and complicated afflictions through science where there should be none. (Mt 6:25-34) My Love is a healing Love. The practitioners of Faith know full well that the prayer for one another, both friend and stranger - aliens in their land - even then I heal each and every one by the power of Faith(Jm 5e). I reiterate, Faith grows in direct proportion to the individual's attendance upon the Lord. Shun Me not! Attend upon Me, that I may Enlighten your heart and soul and mind also. Deuteronomy will cover all the rest. Read it, little children; We have Words there which you will recognize. Little one, you live in trying times, yet I am strengthening you profoundly to do that which I desire of you. These are the talents you have been given, which you are not burying in the sand but are using to the utmost, to the greater Glory of Our Father in Heaven. Therefore, your Father in Heaven is benevolently watching over each move you make. All-Powerful is the Lord your God. Heaven rejoices in your faithfulness. Do thou, My little one, discern and write. I Myself assist you in the writing. I am your Jesus of Merciful Love. I make a River of Light flow upon the earth. Do not worry about those who do not heed. Leave them to your God and be at Peace!

As you re-read it once more, I Myself read it with you and I inspire you should there be necessary alterations in the Words. The Message is clear, concise and to the point, and pleasing to the Lord your God. The titles are subject to the prevailing winds of these times and are adequate. Be at Peace in this matter. Those who want to understand, understand! Great graces flow upon you and those who read with an open mind that which has been written. Believe and be at Peace. Angels carry your Message to M in all delight! The virtue of Love is such that the Lord your God is present. The enemy would taint you at every opportunity. Stay always in the Presence of your Jesus. That is why I am giving you lessons in holding your armour (Ep6:10-20) secure about you and not opening it up to react to negative emotions but stay always in the Joy of the Presence of the Living God - and teaching your brothers and sisters to do likewise. It is a self-discipline - all you who have dedicated yourselves to the Living God, through the Immaculate Heart of Mary, are called to be masters and stewards of your own body and mind. It entails much mastery of your thoughts, words and deeds. The enemy loves to trick you. We bless you with the necessary wisdom, understanding and forthrightness to train your brothers and sisters in this area of purity. Love conquers all.

A Vision given continuously on the 10th to 11th February, 1999 about the effect of these Holy Words of Jesus,

Thank you Lord for ES who visited me with a brilliant smile from Glory on our anniversary, the 11th February with Our Lady of Lourdes, all day long. Continuously from the evening of the 10th February, I have been seeing that every time Your Holy Words reach someone, as from the foundation or the ground, I see a spring of living water, sparkling clear like Baptismal water, springing up from the ground, and gradually this living spring water mixes with, dilutes and purifies the old murky water, from the bottom gradually up to the surface, so that nothing is seen to change from the surface, until a considerable amount of the new water has mixed in, and the purifying effect continues until all the impurities are replaced by the new living water. This is the spiritual grace coming from Your Words Lord, akin to the healing waters of Lourdes. Lord, this vision You gave me on the eve of 11th February, is almost exactly the words You spoke to the Samaritan woman [symbol of a woman missionary] in John 4: "The water that I shall give will turn into a spring inside him, welling up to eternal Life." Lord, I hope I am not deluding myself with this understanding of this prolonged vision.

Little one, you are not deluding yourself. Stay as you are, close to your Jesus and Our Mother, trusting Us in all things. The Blessings flow.

Emma, my neighbour and I first started praying the Rosary daily at Immaculate Conception, Delta on 11th February 1982, and we celebrated that anniversary by getting together for Rosary, Mass and breakfast wherever we were every year until she died and was buried on All Saints day two years before this vision. She kept the anniversary from Glory on the day I was given this vision. God and Our Heavenly Mother are very generous and faithful.

When in 2001, Our beloved Archbishop gave the homily about "a new springtime of hope," these Words took on a deeper significance as Archbishop Exner kept emphasizing we would "change the water."

Also read Jn Ch 4.

CHAPTER THREE
ABUSE

MARK OF CAIN Gn 4:15

JESUS: And furthermore, We touch upon child abuse, which is extensive throughout the world, a world where My Laws and Holy Scripture are neither known nor desired to be known. Thus, the multitudes operate in the realm of free will, at the mercy of the foe. And thus, your teachings are pouring forth right now as upon a narrow road. It shall not always be like that. Very soon they begin to heed and come to Me and I bless them with understanding and wisdom and knowledge. Persevere, little ones, persevere. Persevere! For nothing is impossible to God.(Lk1:38)In My Mercy, I attend upon this woman in you and through you and her healing is accomplished as much as can be accomplished to the individuals so abused and so debased. And at this time, the pleas for such victims resound in Heaven, and I am attendant upon all of these concerns.

I make an act of Healing for countless such individuals, for a cry rises up to Heaven on their behalf. The suffering is eased, lifted, and the little ones are restored to fullness of life. Believe! My Love, My Mercy, My Compassion comes down upon him (the husband) also and he understands more fully the feelings of his spouse. Mother consults with the Father and bids thee know, in the power of the Holy Spirit, that demonic lust is the cause of homosexuality, even as it is the cause of sexual abuse, rape and all of the incestuous behaviours that are upon the earth right now to the abhorrence of your God and of your Heavenly Mother. Little children, I would have My people honour the saints in the Great Communion of saints; they are ever attendant upon the pleadings and causes of the precious little ones. Many, many are the people walking on the earth who have been tormented, abused, debased in many ways by those who should be parenting them; whether physical parents or foster parents. They have been harmed, and in their own little minds, irreparably harmed.

Little children, just periodically pray this little prayer, and yet for each of those whom I set in your pathway of life , just invoke her by name, "St Dymphna, pray and intercede for this child of God", and in this matter, I allow the healings to begin. Remember, these little ones' souls are beautiful and precious to Me; but in what they have experienced, they do not believe in their own worthiness; in what they have experienced, they cannot accept a Christian embrace, Christian love, for they only see abuse, both physical and sexual. They distrust every hand of love, for they have been debased by the demons of power and of lust, of hatred; in such manners that their very psyche as you say, is wounded. How to heal them? Here again, I the Lord God, am naming St Dymphna as the patron saint of abuse victims. Call upon her and teach the little abused ones to call upon her frequently, and by her intercession I, the Lord God come powerfully to their aid.

Lord I pray for two more abused women , both suffering illnesses, both being persecuted unjustly in court, and for the conversion of their persecutors if it be Your Will: if not then please strengthen them to go through these trials successfully. St Dymphna and St Maria Gorretti, we invoke your aid.

Jesus showed us the woman Susanna in the Bible(Daniel 13) unjustly accused by the two old men who tried unsuccessfully to seduce her and then accused her falsely to cover up their crimes.

Living Love is upon you little children; give these suffering souls over to the Lord your God and be at

Peace. I Myself carry their crosses; be uplifted little one, great Blessings come upon you for your pleas on behalf of these suffering individuals. Children; know that the world learned well the lessons of Hitler and the Nazis; learned well the cruelty of communism and atheism; it is now humanism. The many look dispassionately upon medical patients, not regarding them as equal in the Eyes of God to their pride-filled selves. It is simply shall We say something to experiment on; to use, to abuse, to refuse! I could speak further on this subject, but I wish to portray to you, that this is not pleasing to the Lord Your God.

I did not say that you would be safe from verbal abuse; did I not suffer it also? My little ones, Mother still suffers it and I still suffer it, from those who know Me not. My little ones, I strengthen you each one as I strengthen My true faithful cohort of Christians, that faithful remnant all over the earth. I have told you and I reiterate; My Own will be battle-scarred and wearied, but ever victorious in My Name, for I am Jesus, Eternal Victor! My little ones, in Jesus Name is your victory. Prevail in all that I have assigned to you fearlessly, for fear is not of Me; Faith is of Me. In your weakness is My Strength(cf2Cor12:9); I strengthen you little ones. I hold you fast. Rest assured the Lord is with you! (Ps 18 etc)

A judge was to decide if my medical records where to be handed over to the lawyer of the sexual abuser of my patient. That lawyer has hired a UBC professor who has made a career out of discounting memories of patients like mine, [though she never had a loss of memory.]Little children, Trust Me in this matter. Mother attends upon the little wounded victim. Heaven attends, Truth prevails in this sordid story of abuse and deception. Abhorrent to the Lord God is all this activity of firstly the acts of abuse and then the attempts at lying. Remember little children, vengeance is Mine. (Dt 32:35) I shall repay, and yet I am attendant on this matter. Heaven hears the prayers of faithful ones. Persevere in all faithfulness little children, for you are living in most difficult times. Pray the miracle prayer on behalf of her and her husband. Dear little children, it is sufficient for this evening. Leave the little suffering ones with your Lord for this evening. Continue to pray for them. Behold, I make all things new. (cfRv21:1)

Little children, in the world today there is so very much child abuse, sexual abuse; there are so many attacks of rapists upon innocent victims. All of this is abhorrent to the Lord your God, for the victims are so wounded. I am attendant upon this one also; Heaven hears your prayers. Leave her with Me: I attend upon all the ones for whom you pray little one. The abuse falls on Me, your Jesus, and is no more. My little one, I died also for them, I suffered the Passion for them. Leave the abuse fall on Me. All are known to Me; I do indeed attend upon each one. Be at Peace in this matter. I Call each into the Light of My Presence. Many have not yet responded. Tirades of abuse are hurled against those who speak out in My Name. Thus the world treated Me; thus the world treats My Own, and yet, what wondrous Treasures My Own are storing in Heaven. I hold these Treasures in Glory for each of My Own. Do not be afraid of this turning of the new year, of the new century. I am with My Own. I shelter My Own, I shield My Own. You are safe in My Providence.

Continue to address this matter to Me in the Adoration Chapel, and I Who am Truth, will prevail, and Truth will become known to many more about the world. Little children, you are as yet front line warriors and you must remain so in this time of spiritual warfare which is upon the earth. When you unite with Me at Adoration, My Healing Love, My Truth, My Mercy pours forth, wheresoever necessary on the earth. Bring Me your Cause at each visit and leave it there with Me. At this time it is the chosen Way. Take the St. Dymphna card, for all victims of abuse to plead through her. These words on the card are not precise; use your own prayer."

Prayer to St. Dymphna, patron saint of those afflicted with mental and nervous disorders and of victims of abuse (feast day: May 15):St. Dymphna was martyred by her widowed father, who tried unsuccessfully to force an incestuous relationship upon her.].

Lord Our God, you graciously chose St. Dymphna as patroness of those afflicted with mental and nervous disorders and abuse. She is thus an inspiration and a symbol of Charity to the thousands who ask her intercession. Please grant Lord, through the prayers of this pure youthful martyr, relief and consolation to all suffering such trials, especially those for whom we pray [Mention here]. We beg You Lord, to hear the prayers of St. Dymphna on our behalf. Grant all those for whom we pray, patience in the suffering and resignation to Your Divine Will. Please fill them with Hope, and grant them the relief and cure they so much desire. We ask this through Christ Our Lord, Who suffered agony in the Garden of Gethsemane for our sins.

CHAPTER FOUR

ADDICTION

MARK OF CAIN. Gn 4:15

JESUS: The virtue of Love is that as you direct your thoughts towards these My suffering children addicted to both alcohol and drugs in what you call an addictive personality, know too, like the other addictions, it is of a demonic source. By their blindness it is so; they have not responded to the Call of Love. Do you will Me to set them free? What will you offer? Lord we offer prayers ; Adoration; Masses.

The depth of depravity into which humanity has sunk itself in the matter of drug and alcohol addiction is abominable to the Lord God. Yet We hear the prayers of the faithful. We are, as you know, releasing one here and one there, and yet the overall picture as you know, is very grave for many are addicted, and the fallout of sin and suffering upon their families , especially their children, is immense. My little ones, you ask much of your God. Lord, You alone are the Victor. That song, *"softly and tenderly Jesus is calling,* And it shall be so. Little ones, prevail in all prayerfulness with regard to the addictive personalities, who are but prisoners of demonic forces; We release them. Am I not greater than any drug , be it prescription or illegal? Be at Peace; We work the necessary miracles of healing Love, for Heaven hears the prayers of the faithful among whom you are numbered. Little ones-Peace. We prayed at length for the many aspects of my patients' needs. Our Lord says, Do you know how much you are asking of Me?" Lord, You are Christ the Healer; to whom shall we go?

Miracles of Love occur for what you ask dear children is rarely done. My little ones, in this year of Merciful Love, in this year of Jubilee, I bless you both for you each in a unique manner work in My Name, in My Healing Love, and thus I Bless most resoundingly each one of you, the works of your hands, for you are indeed My Heart, My Voice, My Hands, even unto My Mind, for I have anointed you each one, little children, with a vast anointing of wisdom and discernment, and therefore let the healings begin! You ask Me to withdraw the addictions, that more reasonable therapy come into play, and therefore it is begun. You ask Me to open hearts for you have learned that nothing happens by chance, in the Design of your God. Because of your prayers and the prayers of many like you, We do indeed open hearts, so that Love enter.

My beloved Faithful Missionary, you shall persevere. I have strengthened you, My little one to a great Fortitude, thou art strengthened. My Love, My Love, My Love, I am ever with you. Our Lord shows us Psalms; I will pour out My Spirit on all mankind says the Lord and you shall live. (Ps104) Little children, your heartfelt prayers are so pleasing to the Lord God; your patients are, as it were, a microcosm, in comparison to the similar, and are even to the point of being identical to the suffering of the multitudes, about the earth. None has pleaded their cause little children, better than you. As you plead your own cause, you are pleading the cause of your suffering sisters and brothers throughout the world. My precious little ones, it is thus that you have found favour with your God, Who pours blessings and graces upon you. Be strengthened oh soul, I am with you most profoundly. Remember you are never alone, I am with you at every action you take, every decision you make, I am with you. You must little one remember, before each stressful moment, call on Our Names prayerfully perhaps, one Our Father, one Hail Mary, one Glory be... before you pick up the telephone to return the calls. Heaven is working in unity with you. Miracles of Healing Love occur upon some of your most difficult patients, for indeed nothing is impossible to Me, the Living God. (Lk1:38)

As to the many concerns of your heart, My small one, I am with you; am saying " yes" to all that you seek; all things fall into place beautifully, because you are one who knows and loves and serves the Lord.(Rm 8:28) It is so! I give much to you in all that you are doing, for My little one, you give much to Me, you give yourself to Me, as few do. *Lord please heal M,M,S,K and others who are suffering and not doing well.* I heal you that which has been distressing you; I take it away, that you are truly yourself yet again. Be at Peace. A Caucasian woman has come to you who is not of Me, that has brought much of what has been occurring round about you. Remember little one, you cannot carry their crosses; they must carry their own cross! They would give it to you, or to anyone if they could, so many of them; and yet it cannot be and it shall not be! So My little one, be at Peace. We work together. I Bless you in a renewed vigor of well-being.

The oppressive resistance to your therapies is removed. Believe! Recognize that We are in grave warfare at this time. It is not simply a matter of an affliction on an individual, but there is more serious warfare occurring at this time little children, that is why each one of you are feeling it so much, but I am with you, and remember your prayer, "Greater is God Who is in my heart and soul and mind, than that enemy who is in the world." The enemy is an illusionist as it were, and wishes to cast a bigger shadow before you than what the actualities of the cases are. He does this regularly to many, many people. Always remember, Greater is your God, and be at Peace. Come unto Me all you who are weary and I will give you rest, (cf Mt11:28)says the Lord. Beloved L loves Me, the Living God, and I am attendant upon her. She has been sorely tested, yet I am with her. That which must be done, must be done! The report must be delivered over to one in authority higher than this one for whom she works.

It is the Lord Who speaks; a clean bill of health is given to D this day, in honour of the Mother of God; it is his for the taking. Little children, simply continue to pray for him that he does not weaken again. I have My Hand upon him most powerfully; Mother is attendant most tenderly upon him; watch and see him grow now. Mother and I attend upon all the faithful, all the lukewarm as We bring them closer to Truth. I am Truth, and upon the humble little innocents who carry Love in their hearts. We bring them to Ourselves. Thus, the Mission to the street people, begun by O and F, is pleasing to God, and many who are considered derelicts in society are now given the occasion to restore themselves to the dignity of sons of God and sons of Mary. Know that I the Lord and the Mother of God, and a multitude of angels assist, in this street Mission which is Our Will. All come unto Me. I am Your Jesus of Divine Mercy. My little children, come up on your knees and pray the rebukes you have been taught in such cases.

In the Name of Jesus of Nazareth, and sealed in the Holy Spirit, and in union with the whole Heavenly court, we command you, all demons from hell, go now before Jesus the Just Judge and answer. Great and glorious is the Lord Our God !

In the Name of Jesus of Nazareth, and sealed in the Holy Spirit, and in union with the whole Heavenly Court, we command you , all spirits of paganism, of occult practices, new age, witchcraft, satanism, divination, rebellion, affliction, addiction, infirmity, anxiety , depression, fear, anger, hatred, unforgiveness, vengeance, bitter roots, division, confusion, any and all unknown interlocking spirits ,assailing ... go now before Jesus the just Judge and answer. Great and glorious is the Lord Our God.

In the Name of Jesus of Nazareth, and sealed in the Holy Spirit, We rebuke thee satan, We rebuke any and all that has come against your beloved. . In your Holy Name, We sever all bondages of affliction, in Ns Family tree; all hereditary seals, curses, spells, snares, bondages, illicit relationships, unconsecrated deaths, throughout all the generations by such causes as warfare, murder, suicide, miscarriage, abortion, accidental deaths, drownings, anything unclean in Your eyes Almighty God, that has come against these persons, in their family trees and in their lifetimes.

We claim a release now, by the power of the Holy Eucharist, Emmanuel, God- with- us; by the power of the Holy sacrifice of the Mass throughout time and throughout the world; and by the power of the Holy Name of Jesus, You humbled Yourslf to become true God and true Man, and to free us from evil and sin, and suffering, and to give us life to the fullest. Lord Jesus we claim this Life to the fullest for N. and their family. Oh Holy Spirit, beloved of our souls, enlighten us, guide us, strengthen us, console us; let us know and only do your will.. Father, hold them once again under Your blessing, we bring them to the foot of Your Throne. With Mother Mary we pray; In Jesus Name N, be healed!

STOP!

Before you take those pills or use that blade or whatever road you choose to end your life. Stop first & feel your pain, feel how devastating it is, feel & examine your despair & hopelessness. Feel the darkness that surrounds you. Take just a few minutes & truely feel all of your pain & weep. Let your broken heart and fallen spirit totally consume you & once you have reached that darkest place & you feel you have no other choice you just have to end your life, there just is no other way. You want & need to find an escape & you believe that death is your saviour. It is not!

I have been in that dark place many times & have tried to take my own life many times. When I was younger I choose sharp blades, once when I was found after cutting my wrist & rushed to the hospital where I was quickly drugged & my left wrist stiched up. I was left in emergency until I was settled enough to send home. Even with all the drugs

I fought to stay awake. Once the curtains were closed around me I start to pull out the stickies with my teeth. My depression was so bad I really wanted to die because I believed that once I left this world I would go to heaven & be with God, after all I had suffered my whole life from many different types of abuse & deep depressions. I did love God & said my prayers all the times. As I grew older I graduated to pills & alcohol. The last time I tryed. I succeeded. I had save up my anti-depressant, bought bottles of Tylenol with codine. I was even careful to go to more than one store. I bought a number of boxes of Neocitran & the largest & strongest wiskey I could find. I went home & phoned the people I talked to regularly & told them I would be away for at least a week & that I would call when I returned home. I had covered all my bases & was sure this attempt would work. I had lost the love of my life, my soulmate. There was no way I could go on. I could not possibly live without him. I sat on my bed with all the pill bottles, Neo-citran & my very large bottle of wiskey

I mixed the wiskey & neo-citran together & began to empty all of the contents of the pill bottles on my bed. I had hundreds of pills. I started to take them by the handfull & washed them down with the wiskey & Neo-citran mix I had made, all the time crying & hoping that this time I would go to God & all the pain & despair I felt would finally be gone & I would rest in his arms & feel the love & peace I had only experienced once in my life time. My life had been so cold & difficult I had never felt love from another human being in my entire life. I could no longer live without love. There was just no reason to go on. When I finally had taken all the pills drank all the Neo-citran & wiskey mix. I prepared for bed except this time there was no need to wash up & braid my long hair. I just put on my P.J.s. made sure everything was neat & tidy & climbed into my bed & waited calmly knowing soon I would find my place with God & all the pain of just making it through another day would finally be over &

I would finally be free!

When I finally went to sleep I had strange dreams about people I had known in the past but had not seen for years. In this dream I knew I was dead. I seemed to float endlessly in a dark void. Until I seemed to float into something I can only describe as being like a liquid because it totally enveloped me. I felt a love that is indescribable everything that I had felt with Bob & the love he gave me, which I thought was heaven & was the best feeling I had ever experienced in my life time was so small so insignificant. Nothing could compare with this feeling of floating in this liquid called love. Then I heard a gentle voice in my head God was with me! He was asking me if I really wanted to take my own life & I was shown hell & I could here voices screaming for help I could see arms & hands reaching up trying to grab at something, anything that might help relieve there pain. They were in this burning pit & I can still hear the moans & cries for help.

all the time knowing there was no escape. I became aware of another presence surrounding me & holding me, taking me away from the sorrows I had seen. It was Mother Mary it was as though I was a small child being held in her arms. I was being given a choice, I could go back or stay in the burning pit with all the others who had committed suicide & taken there own lives. It was made very clear that all of the pain & despair I felt, which is what I wanted to escape would be my eternity my soul would never leave this place. I thought about this & decided I had a three question to ask. First I asked God if there would be any love in my life because if there wasn't what was the point in going on. He laughed at me as if I were a small child, asking the most ridiculous of questions & told me I would have plenty of love in my life. It seemed to be a satisfactory answer so I went to ask my second question which was why did I have no mother or father. Mary quickly answered by telling me I was never ment to have human parents & that they were my parents & Mary was my true Mother & he my true Father.

My final question was about joining the church & becoming a nun. I was told no. That was not my path. I made the decision to come back & fill my destination.

One afternoon I just woke up. At first I wasn't sure if I was alive or dead. I was just very thirsty. I walked around in a daze for a while, not knowing what was real. I turned on the T.V. & realized I had been gone for five days & all my hair was in one big mat at the back of my head & all the years of growing it & caring for it were gone. I had to cut it off. I knew there was another loss but was not sure what it was. Until one day Bob came back. He asked me to marry him & without hesitation I said no. I some how knew that was part of the price I had to pay for what I had done.

Since that time there have still been some real rough things I've had to endure but I

> Know my Mother & Father are there for me & they give me the strength to endure another day & wait for my parents to call on me.
>
> Janet.

Little children, it has taken them, a considerable time to get into this sorry state of affairs and it will take a little time for the healing, but believe it is begun. The Presence of Almighty God is upon each one, and upon their family, for now is the time when the Spirit of the Living God is attendant upon the children of God in so profound a manner, that none of the Lord's Own, are lost. Be at Peace little children, continue to plead for all the suffering children of God. Love is the key little ones, judge not; simply love, and leave all else to your God. The works of merciful Love, are already begun in this family; be at Peace therefore. The virtue of Love is that as you direct your thoughts towards these My suffering children addicted to both alcohol and drugs in what you call an addictive personality, know too, like the other addictions, it is of a demonic source.

CHAPTER FIVE

HOMOSEXUALITY

MARK OF CAIN Gn 4:15

JESUS: "I reiterate: Love conquers all. Little children, you who know Love, who embrace each other in Love, who embrace each other with a holy kiss, you know the Love of the Lord your God – Agape Love, an 'all charity of Love.'(Rm5:8.Agape Love-Christ died for us while we were still sinners). The world does not know it. The world knows lust, fascinations and many illusions, confusing that with Love. This only aggravates the misery of the situations in which they find themselves, for they know Me not. Yet I call them by name.(Is49:1) Many come unto Me now. Many are the trials upon the earth now. I, the Lord God, indeed fill your hearts and souls and minds with My Love and My Peace, and a concomitant Joy in the Love of the Lord, I give to you.

All will mind. I call all unto Me. Those who are pledged to Me in all Faith will know the Truth. I, the Lord God, am Truth. A number of events will occur in their lives that will cause them to see more clearly the Message you bear. And you are not alone. Others about the world bear similar Messages. Continue to go forth humbly before your God, but boldly in the face of what the world would tell My people. My little one, you are safe in Me. Be not afraid; you do not suffer the fate of the great St. John. But simply speak out the Truth in My Name. You are greatly rewarded in this Mission of Truth which is assigned to you." (Right now He is reminding me that of all the priests in Jerusalem, only John the Baptist would tell Herod – who symbolizes the worldly – that he was committing sin.)

Mother and I attend upon you most profoundly little one. In the power of the Holy Spirit of God it is true that what you call homosexuality must be addressed, distaste -ful though it is. Scandalous is the behavior of mankind upon the earth today. The demon lust prevails here, there, in vast pockets of evil throughout the earth, as you well know. My people, My people, cries your Creator, what have I done to you, how have I offended you? (Mi 6:3 . cf Jn18: false trial by Pilate)Healing comes to an individual whose life is obstructed by homosexuality, by prayer and by Faith. Pray for each individual you know or shall meet. Little children, in unity of prayer, as you are given the miracle prayer by the Virgin Mother –(Our Father, Hail Mary and Glory Be) – prayed with a sincere heart, with a contrite heart, and the healing begins. Little children, do not claim the affliction, reject it. You may say: 'I am afflicted with this condition, please take it away, Lord.' Do not say: 'I am a homosexual.' Don't claim it. The ones who are practicing homosexuals have a measure of defiance, a measure of taunting [What can you do about it? I dare you to do anything about it!]. This attitude is not helpful to them. For them, the same as an alcoholic, or any other addicted individual, to fall on their knees before Almighty God: 'Help, Lord. Have mercy on me, a sinner,' meaningfully, totally, with their whole hearts, to plead for the Mercy of Almighty God. In this, their abandonment to Almighty God, their healing begins. That few struggle to do this is tragic and heartbreaking. Yet pray for them, little children, and one by one We bring them into the Sanctuary of Love, where all purity does and must prevail. Because of your prayers and concerns and of those faithful about the world like yourselves, hosts of saints and angels in Glory plead unceasingly for the homosexuals' release from the bondages of sin and death.

I have already defeated Satan, sin and death. It is for each individual to prevail in defeating the drives prompted by their negative powers, to win their personal victory. Since anyone turning to God, in particular through Jesus and the Mother of God, Heaven assists them so profoundly that they cannot fail(Rv8:3), but they lack this level of trust, this level of Faith. But to proclaim, 'I am an addict' or 'I am a homosexual,' and do nothing further; where they dwell in this state, there is no Peace, there is no happiness, there is no comfort, there is no joy. There is an artificial form of professed pleasure and joy, but it is truly non-existent in each person finding themselves in the situation. I call to My Church: Wherefore do you linger in idleness? The harvest is plenty, the workers are few.(Mt 13:1-9.Mk4:3-9. Lk8:5-8.Rv14:15) Proclaim the Good News of Jesus until it resounds about the earth and the healings begin. Your Good Shepherd(Jn 10) awaits the workers in the harvest. Be at Peace, thou art beloved instruments of My Love and My Peace. My small friends, rejoice in Our Love. Be not surprised at the miraculous events which occur now.

Print them out, and await Divine Inspiration to do further. Pray and ponder. You will pray – it is the Lord who speaks – for all afflicted in this vile manner by the demons of lust which are rampant about the earth and are poorly in rebuke now. For no one, so to speak, is working the practices of self-discipline of their own bodies in any of the appetites. And thus, you might say, the demons of lust seem to have free reign upon mankind. Sodom and Gomorrah were destroyed for far less than what is occurring now. Even so, the Lord your God awaits the conversion of many from the many and varied deviations and behaviors, of what your generation proclaims as sexually active persons. None of this is pleasing to your God. It is gravely offensive. Pray as you do; speak as you are given to speak, and leave all the rest to your God. To whom I Will, I have Mercy! I choose to have Mercy on this individual. Should you wish to see them, so be it. I bless thee. Should you wish to refer them to someone else you see as more appropriate, I bless them both in these circumstances. My little one, the Gift of free will I never usurp. You are in free will, My darling, always in free will. Amen. Your Gift of healing comes to the fore in this individual.

The Visionary has found favor with God, and a great and ghastly wrong has righted at last. An anointing is coming upon you now, My beloved Faithful Missionary – it is the Lord Who speaks – for the healing of D. Do not be afraid to believe, little children. The Father of Mercy Himself attends upon the matter. Come forth into the Light, the Lord your God calls, and he comes hastening into the Light. It is not yet, little children, prevail in all Love and understanding of his tragedy, blessing him with Healing Blessings at any and every opportunity. Pray for him; continue to pray in union with the Mother of God and St. Joseph, who is powerfully involved today as foster father to many young people in need of a father's love and understanding. Little children, do not be afraid to invoke St. Joseph frequently in the matter of family affairs. Death is coming upon many souls in this quagmire of sin which is upon the earth. Little children, even as you pray for D., pray for all caught in this snare of Satan, for it is to pray for the many caught in the deadly sins of lust, in the promiscuity, the cheating of spouses, as it were, called today 'the disruption of family life' – all these the enemy conspires to use: lust and pride and ego and revenge. All these and a myriad of others – you may call them attitudes, you may call them unclean spirits. This is what the enemy uses in the breaking up of family life, in the denying of a young man his very manhood. My little ones, pray much and be at Peace. *Ora pro nobis, ora pro nobis*, you pray, and Heaven hears and answers. The Virgin Mother of all, who cannot bear to cast Her eyes upon the impurities of the world, attends upon this matter of your hearts concern.

From St. Paul's Letter to the Romans –1: 22-28)The more they called themselves philosophers, the more stupid they grew, until they exchanged the Glory of the Immortal God for a worthless imitation, for the image of mortal man, of birds, of quadrupeds and reptiles. That is why God left them to their filthy enjoyments and practices with which they dishonor their own bodies, since they have given up Divine Truth for a lie and have worshipped and served creatures instead of the Creator who is blessed forever. Amen. That is why God has abandoned them to degrading passions: why their women have turned from natural intercourse to unnatural practices and why their men folk have given up natural intercourse to be consumed with passion for each other, men doing shameless things with men and getting an appropriate reward for their perversion. In other words, since they refused to see it was rational to acknowledge God, God has left them to their own irrational ideas and to their monstrous behavior.

Also read Leviticus 18: 22 and 30: 13, and 1 Corinthians 6: 9-10.

10-May-2001 -- EWTN News Brief

NEW STUDY REVEALS HOMOSEXUALS CAN CHANGE

WASHINGTON, DC, (CWNews.com/LSN.ca) - Dr. Robert Spitzer, the instrumental figure in the American Psychiatric Association's 1973 decision to remove homosexuality from its diagnostic manual of mental disorders, has announced a new study, which has altered his beliefs on the issue.

"Like most psychiatrists," said Spitzer, "I thought that homosexual behavior could be resisted, but sexual orientation could not be changed. I now believe that's untrue-- some people can and do change." Spitzer presented his study on Wednesday at the annual meeting of the American Psychiatric Association.

In the most detailed investigation of sexual orientation change to date, Spitzer interviewed 200 subjects (143 men and 57 women) who had experienced a significant shift from homosexual to heterosexual attraction, which had lasted for at least five years. Most of the subjects said their religious faith was very important in their lives, and about three-quarters of the men and half of the women had been heterosexually married by the time of the study. Most had sought change because a gay lifestyle had been emotionally unsatisfying. Many had been disturbed by promiscuity, stormy relationships, a conflict with their religious values, and the desire to be (or to stay) heterosexually married.

Typically, the effort to change did not produce significant results for the first two years. Subjects said they were helped by examining their family and childhood experiences, and understanding how those factors might have contributed to their gender identity and sexual orientation. Same-sex mentoring relationships, behavior-therapy techniques, and group therapy were also mentioned as particularly helpful.

To the researchers' surprise, good heterosexual functioning was reportedly achieved by 67 percent of the men who had rarely or never felt any opposite-sex attraction before the change process. Nearly all the subjects said they now feel more masculine (in the case of men) or more feminine (women).

Spitzer concludes, "Contrary to conventional wisdom, some highly motivated individuals, using a variety of change efforts, can make substantial change in multiple indicators of sexual orientation, and achieve good heterosexual functioning." But, Spitzer said, his findings suggest that complete change-- cessation of all homosexual fantasies and attractions (which is generally considered an unrealistic goal in most therapies) is probably uncommon. Still, when subjects did not actually change sexual orientation-- for example, their change had been one of behavioral control and self-identity, but no significant shift in attractions-- they still reported an improvement in overall emotional health and functioning.

Several options exist for treatment and/or support.

These are a few that I am aware of at this time.

NARTH,(The National Association for Research and Therapy of Homosexuality) for those seeking freedom from homosexuality; a non-profit, tax-exempt educational organization. For referrals or further information contact NARTH- 16633 Ventura Blvd., Suite 1340, Encino CA 91436-1801. (818)-789-4440.

Those who wish to follow the teachings of the Catholic Church with others in support groups.

Courage. The focus of Courage is on chastity; support is given to those who also want to change their homosexual orientation .National office in Manhattan Church of St John, Baptist and available through several local parishes.

Members sharing their stories on a two –part video is published by Ignatius Press available at 415-387-2324 or from Courage at 212-268-1010. **Encourage** support group for friends and family.

Courage in the Archdiocese of Vancouver, BC phone 604-916-6192.

For more information on Courage see; **www.couragerc.net**

Also see :**Another Chance Ministries.(** Support Groups.) Burnaby Christian Fellowship. 7325 MacPherson Avenue, Burnaby, V5J 4N8. phone 604-430-4154. Ron Elmore or Marjorie Hopper.

CHAPTER SIX

ABORTION

MARK OF CAIN Gn 4:15
Contraception/cloning/IVF/Embryonic stem cell research/Abortion/the morning after pill./Vaccines manufactured from aborted fetuses and related issues

JESUS: Oh My little ones, many things are happening now throughout the world. The crusade is about the world to stop legalized abortions. The people of God know the sorrow of this malady of death but of Me do not hear, they cannot comprehend the Words of Merciful Love . Oh woe, suffer oh earth, for your deliverance is at hand, but not without a great battle, a great route of the foe. It holds the many with great impact about the world and those who think they have great impact, in the embrace of eternal death (cf Rv20:11-15)Thus the multitudes operate in the realm of free will, at the mercy of the foe. And thus your teachings are pouring forth right now as upon a narrow road. It shall not always be like that. Very soon they begin to heed and come to Me; and I bless them with understanding and wisdom and knowledge. Persevere little ones, persevere. Persevere ! My little one, I ADDRESS YOU AGAIN AS THE TRIUNE GOD! WE DECREE WHEN ONE WILL BE BORN AND WHEN ONE WILL DIE!(Qo 3)   Yet man in brazen pride, works furiously to alter both these circumstances of humanity! My little sister, they do not wish to hear! My little sister, they must open their eyes, their ears, their hearts, their minds.

You know little children, it is the Lord Who speaks; that abortion is abhorrent to God, and yet this movement of people(Planned Parenthood) perseveres, making the woman of the world into killing fields. The enemy does this in a vengeance against mankind and against the Living God! He cannot assail the Lord God, nor can he assail the Virgin Mother of God, and he assails the women of this world and the children in their wombs. In free will, these women comply; they are being deluded by the enemy, considering it their right to kill the children of their womb, and as given you in Scripture, they proclaim, 'happy the womb that has never born,[Mt 24:19]' and then they will say, 'mountains fall on us, mountains hide us,'[Rv6:16] for in due course, they will recognize the grave error into which they have been led. Woe and again Woe! Even so, My army of faithful in unity of Love with Me, the Living God perseveres, enduring all these attacks on My Gift of Life, My Gift of Love, fighting, enduring all things in My Name; Jesus, Eternal Victor!

8. Vaccination: Grateful thanks for the tireless work of Debbie Vinnedge and associates, the faithful watchdogs who update and maintain the Website at "Children of God for Life."

US AND CANADA - ABORTED FETAL CELL LINE PRODUCTS AND ETHICAL ALTERNATIVES

Disease	Product Name	Manufacturer	Fetal Cell Line	Ethical Version	Manufacturer	Cell Line
Chickenpox	Varivax, Varilrix	Merck, GSK	WI-38, MRC-5	None	N/A	N/A
Hepatitis A	Vaqta, Havrix	Merck, GSK	MRC-5	Aimmungen	Kaketsuken	Vero
	Avaxim, Epaxal	Sanofi, Berna	MRC-5	Not available in US	(Japan & Europe)	(monkey)
Hepatitis A & B	Twinrix	GSK	MRC-5	Engerix Hep-B Only	GSK	Yeast
Hepatitis A & Typhoid	Vivaxim	Sanofi	MRC-5	Recombivax Hep-B Only	Merck	Yeast
Measles/Mumps/Rubella	MMR, Priorix	Merck, GSK	RA273, WI-38	None	N/A	N/A
Measles-Rubella	MR Vax Eolarix	Merck GSK.	RA273, WI-38 RA273, MRC-5	Attenuvax (Measles Only)	Merck	Chick embryo
Mumps-Rubella	Biavax II	Merck	RA273, WI-38	Mumpsvax (Mumps Only)	Merck	Chick embryo
Rubella	Meruvax II	Merck.	RA273, WI-38	Takahashi Not available in US	Kitasato Institute (Japan & Europe)	Rabbit
MMR + Chickenpox	ProQuad/MMR-V	Merck.	RA273, WI-38, MRC-5	None	N/A	N/A
Polio	Poliovax, DT Polio Adsorb.	Sanofi Pasteur	MRC-5	IPOL	Sanofi Pasteur	Vero (monkey)
Polio Combination (DTaP + polio+ HiB)	Pentacel Quadracel	Sanofi Pasteur	MRC-5	Pediacel; Pediarix + HiB Infanrix Hexa + HiB IPOL + any DTaP + HiB	Sanofi, GSK	Vero (monkey)
Rabies	Imovax	Sanofi Pasteur	MRC-5	RabAvert	Chiron	Chick embryo
Rheumatoid Arthritis	Enbrel	Amgen	WI-26 VA4	Humira	Abbott Labs CH	Hamster Ovary
Sepsis	Xigris	Eli Lilly	HEK-293	Ask your doctor	N/A	N/A
Shingles	Zostavax	Merck.	WI-38, MRC-5	None	N/A	N/A
New: Smallpox	Acambis 1000	Acambis	MRC-5	ACAM2000, MVA3000	Acambis/Baxter	Vero, Chick embryo
In Development Ebola	TBA	Crucell/NIH	PER C6	None	N/A	N/A
In Development Flu, Avian Flu, Swine Flu	TBA	Vaxin, Sanofi	PER C6	All current flu vaccines	Medimmune, Novartis, CSL Ltd, ID Biomed, Sanofi, GSK, Chiron	Chick embry
				New Flu, Swine Avian Flu in development	Novavax, Protein Sci., , Novartis MedImmune, Baxter	Insect, Caterpillar MDCK, MDCK, Vero
In Development: HIV	MRKAd5 HIV-1	Merck	PER C6	None	N/A	N/A

Note: Immune-Globulin shots will provide temporary immunity (4-6 months) for Hepatitis-A and Rubella (3 months)

Physician Order: Merck: 800-422-9675 GSK: 866-475-8222 Sanofi Pasteur: 800-822-2463 Chiron:(800 244-7668 (PST)

NOTE: ANY VACCINE NOT LISTED ABOVE DOES NOT USE ABORTED FETAL CELL LINES.

Use of Human Cell Lines in Pharmaceuticals – Canada see below page 35.

Various commercially available pharmaceutical products are derived from or cultivated on fetal cells lines that were obtained from abortions. Patients may have a biological, ethical or religious objection to products that come from human sources. The chart below allows us to provide information to patients to make informed decisions. It also makes known the fact the alternatives are available in other countries and should be available in Canada.

NOTE: -All flu vaccines use non-human cell lines

-Immune-Globulin shots will provide temporary immunity (3-5 months) for Hepatitis-A and Rubella

Disease	Drug Name	Manufacturer	Cell Line (Fetal /Source)	Alternative (Drug/Manufacturer)
Chickenpox	Varilrix ®	GSK	MRC-5	**None Available**
	Varivax®	Merck & Co	WI-38, MRC-5	
Hepatitis A	Epaxal®	Berna Biotech	MRC-5	Aimmungen®
	Havrix ®	GSK	MRC-5	Kaketsuken
	Vaqta ®	Merck & Co	MRC-5	Vero (monkey)
	Avaxim ®	Sanofi Pasteur	MRC-5	**Available in Japan and Europe**
	Avaxim Pediatric ®	Sanofi Pasteur	MRC-5	
Hepatitis A and Typhoid Fever	Vivaxim ®	Sanofi Pasteur	MRC-5	As above for Hep A component
Hepatitis A & B	Twinrix ® (Hep A Component)	GSK	MRC-5	As above for Hep A component, Hep B is derived from yeast
Measles, Mumps Rubella	Priorix ®	GSK	MRC-5	Attenuvax® (Measles) Merck Chick embryo **Availabe in US** Mumpsvax ® (Mumps) Merck Chick embryo **Available in US** Takahashi (Rubella) Kitasato Institute Rabbit **Available in Japan and Europe**
	MMR II ®	Merck & Co	RA27/3, WI-38	
MMR + Chickenpox	ProQuad ®	Merck & Co.	RA27/3, WI-38, MRC-5	**None Available**
Polio	Inactived Poliomyelitis Vaccine – IPV ® Pentacel ® Quadracel ® Td Polio Adsorbed ®	Sanofi Pasteur	MRC-5	Infanrix-IPV, Infanrix Hexa & IPV/Hib® GSK (Europe) Vero Cells **Pediacel to be offered in Alberta March 2007**
Rabies	Imovax ®	Sanofi Pasteur	MRC-5	Rabavert® Chiron Chick Embryo **Available in Canada**
Rheumatoid Arthiritis	Enbrel ®	Immunex (Amgen)	WI-26 VA4	**None Available**
Sepsis	Xigris ®	Eli Lilly	HEK-293	**None Available**

Reference:

1. Varilirix Product Monograph. GlaxoSmithKline Inc. http://www.gsk.ca/en/products/vaccines/varilrix_pm.pdf. Accessed March 14, 2006.
2. Varivax. Product Monograph. Merck. http://www.merck.com/product/usa/pi_circulars/v/varivax/varivax_pi.pdf. Accessed March 14, 2006.
3. An Advisory Committee Statement (ACS) National Advisory Committee on Immunization (NACI). Supplementary Statement On Hepatitis A Vaccine (Acs-4). http://www.phac-aspc.gc.ca/publicat/ccdr-rmtc/00vol26/26sup/acs4.html. Accessed March 14, 2006.
4. Vaqta Product Monograph. Merck. http://www.merck.com/product/usa/pi_circulars/v/vaqta/vaqta_pi.pdf Accessed March 14, 2006.
5. Havrix. Product Monograph. GlaxoSmithKline Inc. http://www.gsk.ca/en/products/vaccines/havrix_pm.pdf. Accessed March 14, 2006.
6. Priorix Product Monograph. GlaxoSmithKline Inc. http://www.gsk.ca/en/products/vaccines/priorix_pm.pdf. Accessed March 14, 2006.
7. MMR II Product Monograph. Merck. http://www.merckfrosst.ca/e/products/monographs/M-M-R_II-756-a_3_02-E.pdf. Accessed March 14, 2006.
8. ProQuad Product Monograph. Merck. http://www.merck.com/product/usa/pi_circulars/p/proquad/proquad_pi.pdf . Accessed March 14, 2006.
9. IPV Product Monograph. http://www.vaccineshoppecanada.com/secure/pdfs/ca/ipv_E.pdf . Accessed March 14, 2006.
10. Imovax Product Monograph. http://198.73.159. 214/statics/vaccines/english/IMOVAX_E.pdf. Accessed March 14, 2006.
11. Enbrel. United States Patent. http://patft.uspto. gov/netacgi/nph-Parser?Sect1=PTO1&Sect2=HITOFF&d=PALL&p=1&u=/netahtml/srchnum.htm&r=1&f=G&l=50&s1=5,712,155.WKU.&OS=PN/5,712,155&RS=PN/5,712,155. Accessed March 14, 2006.
12. Vaccines And Related Biological Products Advisory Committee. United States Of America Food And Drug Administration Center For Biologics Evaluation And Research. http://www. fda.gov/ohrms/dockets/ac/01/transcripts/3750t1.rtf . Accessed March 14, 2006.
13. Jacobs JP, et al. Characteristics of a human diploid cell designated MRC-5. *Nature*. 1970;227(5254):168-70.
14. Plotkin SA, Cornfield D, Ingalls TH. Studies of Immunization with living rubella virus: Trials in children with a strain cultured from an aborted fetus. *Am J Dis Child.*1965;110: 381-389.
15. Plotkin S, et. al. Attenuation of RA27/3 Rubella Virus in WI-38 Human Diploid Cells. *Am J Dis Child.*1969;118:178-185.
16. Weibel RE, et al. Clinical and laboratory studies of combined live measles, mumps, and rubella vaccines using the RA 27/3 rubella virus. *Proc Soc Exp Biol Med*. 1980:165 (2):323-326.
17. Hayflick L, et al. The serial cultivation of human diploid cell strains. *Exp Cell Res*. 1961;25:585-621.

The Merck Boycott

For over 30 years Merck has been using aborted fetal cell lines in the production of vaccines, despite the fact that there are ethical alternatives that could be used. Further, when pressed to cease this immoral, unnecessary practice, Merck assured the American public that "No further fetal tissue would be needed now or in the future to produce vaccines." They have broken that promise by contracting with Dutch Biopharmaceutical company, Crucell NV, for use of their new aborted fetal cell line, PER C6 - taken from the retinal tissue of an 18-week gestation baby, which will be used in their new HIV vaccine. Not only do they refuse to listen to the voice of over half a million Americans who have written to protest, they continue to exploit our unborn and profit from the destruction of innocent human life. Pro-life America has had enough! If you agree, please join our fight.

Following is a list of Merck's major drug products - and their competitor's.

We strongly recommend you check with your doctor to be sure the alternative products are appropriate for your personal medical condition. If so, use them - and let your doctor know why! And let Merck know why too! Write to:

Richard Clark, Residing Chairman - Merck & Co. 770 Sumneytown Pike   P.O. Box 4``Westpoint, PA 19486

NOTE: We realize there are companies listed below that may or may not be any better than Merck when it comes to unethical practices. We do hope though that if you have to choose one evil against another, you won't choose Merck - until they agree to live up to the high standard of ethics they profess to have.

MERCK PRODUCT	COMPETITOR	PRODUCT NAME	CONDITION
AGGRASTAT® (tirofiban HCl)	Schering-Plough	Integrelin	Used to decrease chances of clots after certain cardiac events.
CANCIDAS® (caspofungin acetate)	None	None	Aspergillus fungal infection
COMVAX® Haemophilus B Conjugate Hepatitis-B (Recombinant) Vaccine]	Wyeth, Aventis Glaxo SmithKline Hepatitis B: Engerix	Separate Doses: Hib: HbOC, ActHib	Haemophilus B Hepatitis B
COSOPT® (ophthalmic solution)	Allergan Alcon	Betagan, Aphagan Timolol, Betimol	Glaucoma
COZAAR® (losartan potassium)	Novartis Unimed Sanofi-Synthelabo Boehringer Ingelheim Sankyo	Diovan Tevetan Avapro Micardis Benicar	Blood Pressure Prevention of nepropathy in certain diabetics Prevention of stroke
CRIXIVAN® (indinavir sulfate)	Agouron Abbott Roche	Viracept Norvir Fortovase (Saquinavir)	AIDS
FOSAMAX® (alendronate sodium tablets)	Proctor & Gamble Roche/GSK	Actonel Boniva	Osteoporosis
HYZAAR® (losartan potassium and hydrochlorothiazide)	Novartis Bristol Myer Squibb Sankyo Boehringer Ingelheim Unimed	Diovan HCT Avalide Benicar HCT Miacardia HCT Teveten HCT	High Blood Pressure
MAXALT® (rizatriptan benzoate) and Maxalt MLT®	AstraZaneca Elan Pfizer	Zomig Frova Relpax	Migraine Headaches
PedvaxHIB® Haemophilus B Conjugate Vaccine (PRP-OMP)	Aventis Pasteur	ActHIB	H-Type Flu
PEPCID® COMPLETE	Apotex Eli Lilly Others	Ranitidine Axid Generics: Famotidine, Ranitidine, Nizatidine, Cimetidine	Ulcers, GERD, erosive esophagitis, heartburn
PNEUMOVAX® 23, Pulmovax (Pneumococcal Vaccine)	Wyeth	Prevnar Pnu-Immune 23	Pneumonia
PROPECIA® (finasteride)	None	None	
PROSCAR®	Boehringer Ingelheim Glaxo SmithKline Abbott Pfizer Pfizer	Flomax Avodart Hytrin Cardura Minipress	Symptoms of BPH
RECOMBIVAX HB® [Hepatitis B Vaccine (Recombinant)]	Glaxo SmithKline	Engerix	Hepatitis-B
SINGULAIR® (montelukast sodium)	AstraZeneca Abbott	Accolate Zyflo	Allergies, Asthma
VIOXX®	Pfizer Pharmacia Boehringer	Celebrex Bextra Mobic	Certain types of arthritis, Anti-inflammatory
Zocor®	Pfizer Bristol Meyers-Squibb AstraZeneca Novartis Generic Kos Pharma	Lipitor Pravachol Crestor Lescol XL lovastatin Altoprev	Used to lower cholesterol and lipids

Many souls are coming unto Me in these times, ill prepared for facing My Justice, and I ask you to persevere in praying for those who are dying and for those who have just recently died. You know My Justice is tempered by Mercy; you have no idea what your prayers accomplish A living embryo is before My eyes - its heart is beating in the womb of its mother -but not for long. It is taken. Woe to mankind, woe to mankind.

The battle lines are drawn. By this conference, <u>all</u> will know My Stance, and the stance of the beloved John -Paul, My Vicar in this matter. This is not pleasing to the mad scientists, who use My Creations human bodies, oblivious to My Truth. He speaks in a manner that none can deny his Truth. That does not mean little children that all will heed Truth and respond in Love! Even so, the battle lines are clearly drawn and Truth comes to the fore in this issue of euthanasia and 'brain death,' and in the issue of abortion and what is occurring to the aborted infants. All of this is anathema; all of this is an abomination in the Eyes of the Living God, in Whose Presence you live!

They condemn the Christians, the believers, and override their rights today. Again, I am not oblivious of this! It is when My Justice meets with My Mercy, as it were, that I take My Own Home out of this world. It is a foregone conclusion by the scientists that they will clone humans. They have not considered Me! They have had what they consider some reasonably successful experiments. This is an abomination in the Eyes of the Lord, your God. Those who tamper with the life-giving Force of the Creator of creation, will rapidly find themselves in unexpected situations which they themselves cannot cope with; some of them call on My Name; others will abandon reality, going mad; others yet will persevere, beyond for humans, what is a point of no return, and take upon their own souls, that which they have done!

The *Roe vs. Wade* case was falsified, as you know. And so you see, with the proponents of these evil machinations in the name of science and progress, there are scandalous lies and occurrences to promote that which is not of God. This is the world in which you are living! It is worse than Egypt ever was. What would you have Me do about these vile occurrences over which My little faithful ones on earth grieve, even as I grieve? (Lord, please change their hearts, I entrust their souls to Your Merciful Love.)

Triumphant angels assist this woman, for her works are important to Me! Oh My little one, there is sorrow in the Heart of your God at what is happening in the field of medicine and all the sciences; both sorrow and grief. The walls which surround the hearts of the many prevent them from knowing merciful Love, Agape Love, compassionate Love. In a sterile loveless way they work their works of iniquity upon My Creation, humanity. It is enough what they are doing to the other creatures on earth, but what they do to My precious gifts of Love brings down My Wrath, as you well know. I bid you read Ezekiel, read Jeremiah, read the many messages in Holy Scripture and know that I do not take lightly the attacks on innocent victims such as aborted infants and indeed those whose bodies are so mutilated by, as they call it, the harvesting of their organs. Why would they need a substitute kidney or heart or liver had they or their forbearers been faithful to Me in the first place? Even now, were they simply to be faithful I would cure them. I bid you know that the death of every infant, of every frail, sick person, every elder-kills a measure of Love. Mankind's hands are now stained with the blood of the innocents and cannot be washed off no matter what they do - except they kneel in penitence, and humbly ask forgiveness of their God. The Blood of the Lamb alone washes the sin of murder from a soul. Oh My people, oh My people, oh that you would choose Love. I give you Love, in the ravishing beauty of the Woman Clothed With the Sun, the Mother of God; but you choose not to heed Her call to Love, choose not this Gateway to return to the Lord Your God. You choose rather error, sin, death and destruction. Oh woe, oh My people, oh My people, what have I done to you? How have I offended you? Answer Me! (Mi 6:3)

You all know that the Mystery of Love which I have encoded in each human; is individual, is unique, and is for that individual - and try as they may, the scientists run into block after block, in their strange attempts to do that which is unnatural and unseemly to the Eyes of God! You know well that the recipients do not necessarily regain full health, but as I have said, they have a half-life in their bodies. Even so, I have mercy and spare their souls, for in all these trials they must plead with Me for their continual assistance upon earth. They must be aware of what they are doing. There is no blessing upon this generation of mankind, which snatches the infants from their mothers' wombs, destroying them in a bloodbath of death. It is written, 'the firstborn belongs to God.' Where are the firstborn? They are not! A cry greater than Rachel's is upon the earth now! (cfJer31:15)The timing of this document which you are writing is important to Me.

An eleventh hour Mission *(was announced and given me by Our Lord Jesus, who linked me with Life Foundation Canada. This team of ladies internationally distributes images and prayers devoted to Jesus, The Divine Mercy and Our Lady of Guadalupe, Protectress of Life, the main focus being the end of abortion. More recently, they have also been distributing Images of The Holy Face of Jesus (as in the Shroud of Turin). I have these blest Images for distribution to those who wish to have them. Since these Images are already blest, they can not be sold but distributed by donation only to defray the cost of printing and postage.*

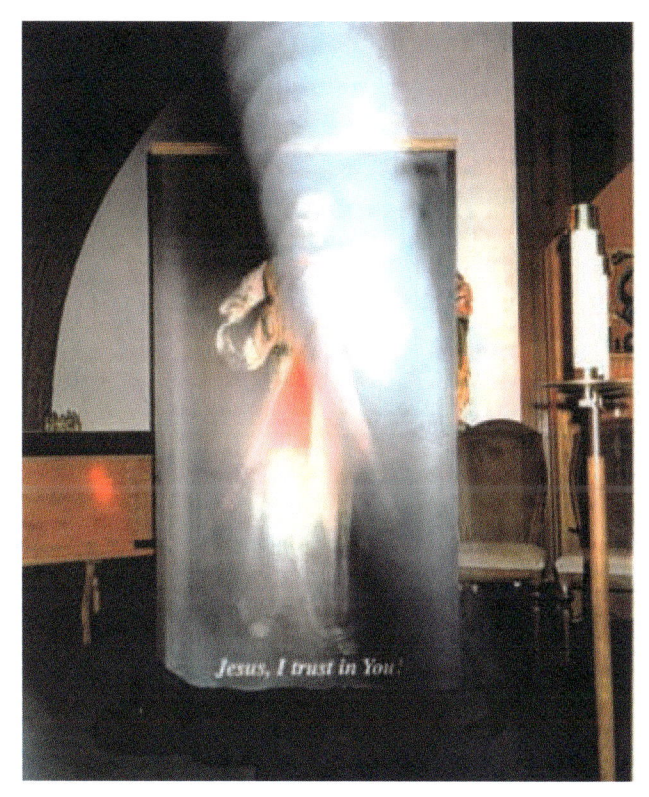

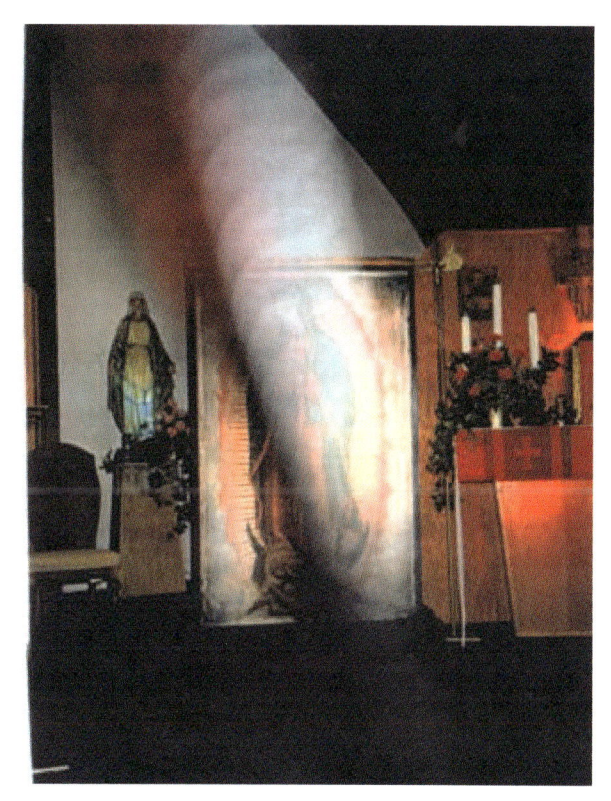

(October 8, 1997)

These pictures of the images were taken during a presentation at St. Matthew's Church in Sudbury, Ontario. They were taken during an evening presentation and the images were on opposite sides of the altar.

The Shekinah is a sign of God's presence. In the Old Testament, God revealed His Presence to His people with a cloud by day and fire by night. The developer of the film said that on the uncut negative, the Shekinah was joined in an unbroken curved line – up over Our Lady of Guadalupe, over the altar and down across the Divine Mercy and then curved up again at the bottom (see Fig. 1).

Fig. 1

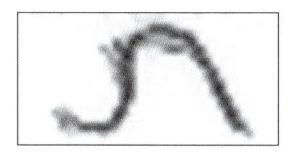

OUR LADY OF GUADALUPE
Ark of the New Covenant

The front cover shows a photograph of the Missionary Image of Our Lady of Gaudalupe, in a darkened church at night, covered by an apparent phenomenal cloud of fire. Our Lady of Guadalupe brings the light that shines in the people who walk in darkness. See Is 9:1. "Guadalupe" means River of Light in Spanish and Our Lady mediates to us the light and grace of the Holy Trinity and brings us her greatest gift, her Son Jesus, as the Ark of the New Covenant.

The Ark of the Old Covenant was covered by a cloud by day and a cloud of fire by night. See Nm 9:15-16. It contained the presence of God through the tablets of the Ten Commandments, the Manna and Aaron's Rod that budded. See Heb 9:4.

The Israelites carried the Ark in processions which brought them victories, particularly with Joshua at the Battle of Jericho when the walls came tumbling down. See Josh 6.

The prophet Jeremiah later placed the Ark in a cave "to remain unknown until God gathers His people together again and shows them mercy." 2 Mc 2:4-7. It has not been found since. We await His mercy obtained through the Sorrowful and Immaculate Heart of Our Lady of Guadalupe, the Ark of the New Covenant.

God told Moses that He would meet with him at the Mercy Seat on top of the Ark (see Ex 25:22) which was to be placed in the Dwelling of the Meeting Tent. See Ex 40:2-3. Moses did so and "then the cloud covered the Meeting Tent and the glory of the Lord filled the Dwelling." Ex 40:34. At night fire was seen in the cloud (see Ex 40:38) as fire is seen in the cloud over the Missionary Image.

These outstanding events foreshadowed the Annunciation when God became Man in Our Lady, the Ark of the New Covenant. The Holy Spirit overshadowed her and the glory of the Lord filled her as His new Dwelling. See Lk 1:35.

Just as the Ark of the Old Covenant contained the presence of God, so also did Our Lady as the Ark of the New Covenant. God became present to us in the pregnant womb of Our Lady. Jesus brought us the New Covenant of love and Our Lady brought us Jesus. It was through her that Jesus came as the new Mercy Seat and achieved eternal redemption through the forgiveness of our sins by the shedding of His own blood. See Heb 9:12. All of His merited graces are mediated to us through the Immaculate Heart of Mary.

Our Lady is intimately associated with the Ark of the Covenant. It is one of her titles in the Litany of Loreto. The Book of Revelation shows the association: "then God's temple in heaven opened and in the temple could be seen the Ark of His Covenant . . . . A great sign appeared in the sky, a Woman Clothed with the Sun with the moon under her feet . . . ." Rev 11:19-12:2. The Woman was pregnant. This Woman is Our Lady of Guadalupe who appeared in this manner.

She now brings Jesus to us, her children, and leads us in the decisive battle against Satan (see Rev 12:17) to the triumph of her Immaculate Heart. She calls us to join her in this battle as she called Pope John Paul II who said with reference to another replica Image, "I feel drawn to this picture of Our Lady of Guadalupe because her face is full of kindness and simplicity . . . it calls me."

An eleventh hour Mission is given to the one who is called Faithful Missionary. The Virtue of Love is such that I the Lord God, speak thus! I am with you in all that is happening, even in the moments of quiet, as We await the interaction of the many involved in Our Mission. There is always the foe; watchful, envious, attacking My people as a penetrating evil; those who do not have their armour tightly about them. Great angels and archangels surround all the key players in this Mission to a scientific world. My Own are safe in Me! Those who are a bit weak, I begin now to strengthen, for an hour of decision is upon them, to choose the pathway I, the Living God have set out for them in the Ministry of Salvation for Mankind. The eleventh-hour Mission will come upon you suddenly and surprisingly and you shall act according to My Will.

Know this: the holy angels, the guardian angels assigned to each infant, which you call a foetus, weep; for their mission to mankind is aborted, that of the child and of the angel! Little does mankind know, in the realm of Glory, in the realm of spirituality, in what ways this human behaviour alone is harming humanity! You know very well the burden that humanity is saddled with at present; the legalization of abortion. You know well the so-called scientific experimentation and usages of My small creations, is grievously wounding the Heart of your God; and My beloved Mother. It is important little children; always remember not to worry about human esteem, not to worry about hurt feelings or supersensitivities. I Myself strengthen each one of My Own. Yes, there are people who [the Lord shows people who are as if surrounded by barbed wire].Even so, I ask you to speak. We shall speak above the barbed wire fence on occasion when necessary!

Little children, it is a time of great spiritual warfare; at the same time, I am training each one who is yielded unto Me- and there are multitudes- by testing them, trying them, and as they win victory over self in these testings, they are strengthened to greater courage, to greater fortitude, their armor is increased; and they begin to work solely for the Will of the Father, and are not so sensitive to other people's words or to misconceptions of other people's words or deeds. The ones who are still as you call it, touchy, are still being strengthened and tested. It didn't matter what other people said or did in the highest ranks of let Us say America, the beloved saint spoke out and acted accordingly.(Mother Teresa).

Pour forth Your Spirit oh Lord and renew the face of the Earth you pray perseveringly; and it is thus I send wave after wave of missionaries of My Love, throughout those Love-starved areas of the world, until at last the Great Light comes upon them-the Light of Christ, and the darkness is no more. I bid you address J in writing, and in word when possible. Rest assured, I shield J even as I shield each one of you; as I shield My little workers in Life Foundation, that My Works of Mercy and Love proceed according to My Schedule. In due course, in Faith, all falls into place; there is a pattern here.[He shows Omen a vision of weaving the tapestry].

Hold it to your heart until the opportune moment presents itself. Let Us work together on the Mission of Life Foundation. Healing Love descends upon all those who attend upon the Lord God in all sincerity, all genuineness of heart, for your God is a God of Mercy. The Sovereign Queen blesses you child. The Virtue of Love is such that I your Jesus of Merciful Love attend upon you profoundly. Little children, you often sing 'Peace is flowing like a river', a hymn which is especially pleasing to the Mother Of God, and to Myself. Little children, you know well that this Peace flows through you, My little brothers and sisters; this river of Light and Love and Peace, flows from Glory upon the ones who have yielded to the Living God; and then through them, to the others. Just such a Mission, is the Life Foundation Mission, and I would that it were distributed about Europe, especially Central and Eastern Europe, what you used to refer to as the Eastern Block.

The virtue of Love is such that I bless you little one. Between now and the time of the conference, many events must occur; believe that I am opening doors, making arrangements, arranging for certain individuals to meet other individuals! Little children, trust Me; I tell you, I know what I am about. I make your plans with you and for you, since you have yielded yourself, your free will to Me, the Living God, and I, the Living God, have accepted your free will; and it is thus that you become an instrument of Peace in My Hands. Many are called, few are chosen". The chosen ones are those who truly yield utterly and completely to the Will of the Father and it is through such as these that the Lord your God works; throughout the generations it is so! All that occurs now is in My Design. JB is also a surrendered, a yielded one. Be at Peace in this matter!

I tell you, I do not create individuals in a pointless manner. It is not happenstance! Mankind is now aware of what is called genetic coding. Then they must become aware that even for the creation of each human being, this coding is relevant to make the person I desire; for that person is given over to mankind for a good purpose, a unique purpose. This life cannot be tampered with lightly, cannot be destroyed because of the whim of some man or woman on Earth! I tell you, Justice SHALL prevail. Know that in a certain aspect, My Justice IS Mercy for mankind and an end comes to ALL that is evil.

Do not doubt little children, that I am a God of Merciful Love and I shall ALWAYS BE, for My Love knows no bounds. It is a Father of Mercy and Love Who must chastise an errant child, grievous as it is to the Heart of the Father. Do you understand little children?

Embroiled in this battle for Truth, I Am Truth; you are under fierce attack. Be not distressed or dismayed. Remember, these words fall on Me like whiplashes. Little ones, even for those "would- be -gods," I died that they too might know Life to the fullest. Alas, they reject Me; they do not believe! Little one, persevere as you are doing; disregard the rude and crude assaults. Persevere in My Name; in My Name is your Victory (He reminds us Dr Nathanson converted), for nothing is impossible to God. (Lk1:38).Blessings are falling upon you little children; Blessings are falling upon Life Foundation. Mother has a great desire to rapidly put an end to the culture of death throughout the "civilized world," even as She put an end to the culture of death in the pagan ways of Mexico. I bring about a great revolution of Faith about the world now; in the next few months you will see this occurring rapidly about you. I will show you step by step what you are called to do, by Divine Inspiration, and even at times locutions, for We have a Unity of Love which is most profound, and shall remain this way.I, the Lord God, yet await a response to My Call to Love. Many more pray today than before the terrorist attacks; many more simply grow in hate and revenge! The Spirit of the Living God is with humanity most profoundly, that the multitudes may come back to the Call of God, and return to Truth and Light and Love and Peace. There is a signal call for Peace now; a Call from Heaven!

Little children of Faith, you have Peace in your hearts, and there are many, many like yourselves, children of the Light, children of Peace; but there are many others, who have as they say, their own agenda, which does not include Me, the Living God. Oh woe-and again, WOE! Peace! Mother and I are attendant upon the writing of this book in a profound way; one might say intimately bound up in the writing of this book, and be assured that the day will come when you will see it in print and with the approval of Church. Persevere in completing the book; We shall speak further on this matter.

Praying the Divine Mercy Chaplet.

3'oclock prayer (also used as opening prayer)Using regular rosary beads starting at the Crucifix: "You expired Lord Jesus, but the Source of Life gushed forth for souls, and the Ocean of Mercy opened up for the whole world. Of Fountain of Life, unfathomable Divine Mercy, envelope the whole world and empty Yourself out upon us!

Oh Blood and Water, which gushed forth from the Heart of Jesus, as a Fountain of Mercy for us, I trust in

You! X3.

Chaplet continues bottom page 73 and top of 74 after Holy God....concluding prayer (page 69)

Jesus I trust in You! X3.

Eternal God, in Whom Mercy is endless, and the treasury of compassion inexhaustible, look kindly upon us, and increase Your Mercy in us, that in difficult moments we might not despair nor become despondent, but with great confidence, submit ourselves to Your Holy Will, which is Love and Mercy itself.(950.)

Oh limitless and unfathomable Mercy Divine, to love and adore You worthily, who can? You are the sweet hope for sinful man. Amen.

HOLY SEE DECRESS DAY OF DIVINE MERCY
Proposed by Sister Faustina Kowalska

VATICAN CITY, May 23, 2000 (ZENIT.org). - Today the Vatican Press Office published a decree of the Congregation for Divine Worship and the Discipline of the Sacraments, whose prefect is Cardinal Jorge Arturo Medina, which at John Paull II's instruction, establishes the feast of Divine Mercy to be held the Second Sunday of Easter. The official name of this liturgical day will be "Second Sunday of Easter or of Divine Mercy."

Devotion to the Divine Mercy is an authentic spiritual movement within the Catholic Church promoted by St. Faustina Kowalska, whom the Pope canonized on April 30. The Pope chose that day to announce the surprise. "Throughout the world, the Second Sunday of Easter will receive the name Divine Mercy Sunday, a perennial invitation to the Christian world to face, with confidence in divine benevolence, the difficulties and trials that humankind will experience in the years to come," the Holy Father explained on that occasion.

However, this statement was not part of the Holy Father's prepared speech, so they do not appear in the official transcription of his address for that canonization. The publication of this decree by the Congregation for Divine Worship serves to announce officially to the universal Church the Pope's desire.

Faustina Kowalska, a Polish religious who died at 33 in 1938, lived a mystical experience of consecration to Divine Mercy, a spiritual journey that included visions, revelations, and hidden stigmata. At the suggestion of her spiritual director, all was recorded in her journal. The centre of her life was to announce God's mercy toward every human being. This message that has touched the hearts of many simple people, but also marveled many theologians, surprised to find in the writings of a humble, hardly literate nun such extraordinary depth.

The Apostles of Divine Mercy are a movement inspired in the Polish nun's experience. It embraces priests, religious, and laity, united in their commitment to live mercy in relating to their brothers and sisters, to make the mystery of Divine Mercy known, and to invoke God's mercy on sinners. This spiritual family, approved in 1996 by the Archdiocese of Krakow, at present is found in 29 countries of the world.

The Vatican decree clarifies that the litugy of the Second Sunday of Easter and the readings of the Divine Office will continue as established in the Missal of the Roman rite.
ZE00052310

The Divine Mercy -- and The Second Coming of Jesus Christ
By Daniel P. McGivern

The title of this talk is The Divine Mercy -- and The Second Coming of Jesus Christ.

Because my audience today is from various religions, I feel that it is necessary to give some background first, especially for those who are non-Catholic.

The messages I am going to relate to you today come from this thick book called "Diary--Divine Mercy in My Soul" written by Saint Maria Faustina Kowalska.

All of the specific quotes I am giving you today are followed by a number--the number of the paragraph in the book.

First, in the Catholic Church, how does one become a Saint? Simply put, a person becomes a canonized saint, which is done by the Holy Father himself, only if two miracles take place after the person's death, miracles which are recognized as without scientific explanation by a top panel of physicians and the miracles took place after prayers to this person for his or her intercession. The miracle has to be sudden, dramatic and what all of us would call impossible--except for God, for nothing is impossible with God.

Saints in Heaven are filled with great grace, friends of God, whom He chooses to honor after death by granting that prayers are answered in an exceptional way.

Simply put, they were great friends of God on earth and He proves, through these miracles, they are friends of His in Heaven.

Page Two

Saint Maria Faustina Kowalska was uneducated, except for two years of schooling--not much at all. Yet, from her earliest childhood, she wanted to become a saint, a great saint.

She entered the convent, was known to a only a few nuns, and even had no relatives at her funeral sparing them the expense of a long trip. In short, she lived what appears to be an obscure life.

But this book, which she wrote, contains her prayers and thoughts and, above all, messages from Our Lord Jesus Christ and His Holy Mother--the Blessed Virgin Mary, who both appeared to her many times, especially during the last five years of her life. Sister Faustina died at the age of 33 in 1938.

Yes, this book contains what Jesus Himself said to St. Faustina in His appearances to her. Just as He appeared in the upper room to His Apostles as flesh and blood, even though the doors were locked, Jesus appeared to and spoke with Sister Faustina whom He called His secretary.

A dutiful, yet uneducated, secretary she was, spelling phonetically everything she couldn't spell, beautiful words from Heaven.

She lived in Krakow, where years later a great cardinal lived-- the Archbishop of Krakow, who petitioned the Vatican to review in its entirety all of the writings in this book. The Vatican for 20 years hadn't let the messages be distributed.

You see, Sister Faustina's phonetically spelled words so upset her fellow nuns that they decided to "correct" the writings, spelling, punctuation and all. Now, who corrects the Lord? The Lord had his purposes as He has with all saints. When asked why the Blessed

Page Three

Virgin Mary chose poor little Bernadette to appear to at the now famous Lourdes Grotto in France, all St. Bernadette could say is, "I suppose she couldn't find anyone more ignorant."

We can all raise our hands to serve the Lord, but He does the picking for special missions, like Saint Faustina Kowalska's mission.

Now, the last thing I want to explain before reading the messages is Who or what is The Divine Mercy?

Divine Mercy is an attribute of God. His Love and His Mercy are one!

It is Jesus Christ who will judge all of us when we die; no matter what our religion is, He is the sole judge.

Before Jesus brings His Justice upon the earth, we are told in this book from His own lips, He is offering His Divine Mercy to all, especially to the greatest of sinners.

Jesus taught Sister Faustina the Chaplet of Divine Mercy which should be said at 3 p.m., when Jesus died on the cross, or it can be said at any other time of the day or night as well.

The Chaplet takes only five minutes to say and because I know there are some in this audience who know how to say it, we will now say it with my wife Mely McGivern leading it, followed by the specific messages given by Jesus and His Mother to Saint Faustina. The Chaplet of Divine Mercy is said on ordinary rosary beads.

Begin with:

Our Father.....Hail Mary....Apostle's Creed.

On the large beads before each decade:

Eternal Father, I offer You the Body and Blood, Soul and Divinity of Your dearly beloved Son Our Lord Jesus Christ in attonement for

Page Four

our sins and those of the whole world.

On the ten small beads of each decade:

For the sake of His sorrowful Passion have mercy on us and on the whole world.

Conclude with:

Holy God, Holy Mighty One, Holy Immortal One, have mercy on us and on the whole world. (Three times)

Now for the messages:

"Write this: before I come as the just Judge, I am coming first as the King of Mercy. Before the day of justice arrives, there will be given to people a sign in the heavens of this sort:

"All light in the heavens will be extinguished, and there will be great darkness over the whole earth. Then the sign of the cross will be seen in the sky, and from the openings where the hands and the feet of the Savior were nailed will come forth great lights which will light up the earth for a period of time. This will take place shortly before the last day." (No. 83).

In the evening when Sister Faustina was praying, the Mother of God told her, "Your lives must be like mine; quiet and hidden, in unceasing union with God, pleading for humanity and preparing the world for the second coming of God." (No. 625)

During meditation on the morning of March 25, the feast of the Annuciation, Sister Faustina saw the Blessed Virgin Mary, who said, "Oh , how pleasing to God is the soul that follows faithfully the inspirations of His grace! I gave the Savior to the world; as for you, you have to speak to the world about His great mercy and prepare the world for the Second Coming of Him who will come, not as a merciful Savior, but as a just Judge. Oh, how terrible

Page Five

is that day! Determined is the day of justice, the day of divine wrath. The angels tremble before it. Speak to souls about this great mercy while it is still the time for mercy. If you keep silent now, you will be answering for a great number of souls on that terrible day. Fear nothing. Be faithful to the end. I sympathize with you." (No. 635)

While saying the Chaplet of Divine Mercy, Sister Faustina heard a voice say, "Oh, what great graces I will grant to souls who say this chaplet; the very depths of My tender mercy are stirred for the sake of those who say the chaplet. Write down these words, My daughter. Speak to the world about My mercy; let all mankind recognize My unfathomable mercy. It is a sign for the end times; after it will come the day of justice. While there is still time, let them have recourse to the fount of My mercy; let them profit from the Blood and Water which gushed forth for them." (No. 848)

The morning when Jesus taught Sister Faustina how to say the Chaplet of Divine Mercy, He said, "This prayer will serve to appease my wrath. You will recite it for 9 days, on the beads of the rosary." (No. 476)

On another occasion, Jesus looked at her and said, "Souls perish in spite of my bitter Passion. I am giving them the last hope of salvation: that is the Feast of My Mercy. If they will not adore My mercy, they will perish for all eternity. Secretary of My mercy, write, tell souls about this great mercy of mine, because the awful day, the day of My justice, is near." (No. 965)

Page Six

Jesus said, "Let the greatest sinners place their trust in My mercy. They have the right before others to trust in the abyss of My mercy. My daughter, write about My mercy towards tormented souls. Souls that make an appeal to My mercy delight Me. To such souls I grant even more graces than they ask. I cannot punish even the greatest sinner if he makes an appeal to My compassion, but on the contrary, I justify him in My unfathomable and inscrutable mercy. Write: before I come as a just Judge, I first open wide the door of My mercy. He who refuses to pass through the door of My mercy must pass through the door of My justice." (No. 1146)

"I remind you, my daughter, that as often as you hear the clock strike the third hour (3 p.m.) immerse yourself completely in My mercy, adoring and glorifying it; invoke its omnipotence for the whole world, and particularly for poor sinners; for at that moment mercy was opened wide for every soul. In this hour you can obtain everything for yourself and for others for the asking; it was the hour of grace for the whole world--mercy triumphed over justice." (No. 1572)

"In the Old Covenant I sent prophets wielding thunderbolts to my people. Today I am sending you with My mercy to the people of the whole world. I do not want to punish aching mankind, but I desire to heal it, pressing it to My Merciful Heart. I use punishment when they themselves force me to do so; my hand is reluctant to take hold of the sword of justice. Before the Day of Justice I am sending the Day of mercy." (No. 1588)

The Lord said to Sister Faustina: "Daughter, when you go to confession, to this fountain of My mercy, the Blood and Water which came forth from My Heart always flows down upon your soul and

Page Seven

ennobles it. Every time you go to confession, immerse yourself entirely in My mercy, with great trust, so that I may pour the bounty of My grace upon your soul. When you approach the confessional, know this, that I Myself am waiting there for you. I am only hidden by the priest, but I Myself act in your soul. Here the misery of the soul meets the God of mercy. Tell souls from this fount of mercy souls draw graces solely with the vessel of trust. If their trust is great, there is no limit to My generosity. The torrents of grace inundate humble souls. The proud remain always in poverty and misery, because my grace turns away from them to humble souls." (No. 1602)

On the feast of the Ascension, a few months before her death, Sister Faustina was instructed by the Blessed Virgin Mary concerning the interior life. The Mother of God said, "The soul's true greatness is in loving God and in humbling oneself in His presence, completely forgetting oneself and believing oneself to be nothing; because the Lord is great, but He is well-pleased only with the humble; He always opposes the proud." (No. 1711)

Jesus said, "These words are for you. Do all you possibly can for this work of My mercy. I desire that My mercy be worshipped, and I am giving mankind the last hope of salvation; that is, recourse to My mercy. My Heart rejoices in this feast." (No. 998)

Sister Faustina became the first saint in this century, canonized as a saint by Pope John Paul II on the Sunday after Easter Sunday last year.

Page Eight

The Sunday after Easter is now known as Mercy Sunday, a specific request of Jesus Christ through Sister Faustina 70 years ago, in 1931.

On Mercy Sunday, Jesus promised that all those who go to confession and receive Holy Communion will have all their sins forgiven, including the temporal punishment due for sin. It is likened to a "Second Baptism". It is something members of our family--and yours--should do annually.

Now, before I take a few questions, I ran off 200 copies of my talk for those who want to look up the passages in the book "Divine Mercy in My Soul" by St. Faustina.

It is rare in Catholic prophecy there is something so rich as this work, totally approved by the Catholic Church.

I will take questions, except questions on whether I believe in or don't believe in various modern day messages or visions. As a professional writer, I learned long ago, believe in what is true and solid and only write about authentic visions totally approved by the Church--such as Our Lady of Guadalupe in Mexico, Our Lady in Lourdes, in Fatima, Portugal and Paris at the Miraculous Medal Shrine, and Our Lord's appearances to another nun, St. Margaret Mary, on the mysteries of His Sacred Heart and His love for mankind.

Suffice it to say, if you only go with the tried and proven and true apparitions, you won't go astray. When it comes to apparitions, only the Church--which took a long time in Sister Faustina's case--can really proclaim something worthy of belief.

My last comment is on Pope John Paul II, this great man, beloved by many of different religions, is a man who comes along every 500 years as a pope, said the great Archbishop Fulton J. Sheen.

Page Nine

    I like to think part of the reason he was chosen by the Holy Spirit at the 1978 conclave was because as Archbishop of Krakow, he brought these messages to light--and now all of us can read, know and believe that the Second Coming of Jesus Christ is not far off--and that if we don't come under His mercy now, at this time, we'll fall under His justice.

    Now is the time for all to beseech Jesus Christ for His mercy, love and forgiveness.

    We then will not fear Jesus' Second Coming. We will welcome it. We help to usher it in by spreading His words, and His Mother's words, on this time of His Divine Mercy. And that time for Divine Mercy for the entire world is now!

    Thank you.

While there is still time, let them have recourse to the fount of My Mercy.(848).He who refuses to pass through the door of My Mercy, must pass through the door of My Justice.(1146). Numbering refers to the entry number in her Diary; Divine Mercy in My Soul. In Scripture, when the early Hebrews were under great stress and trial, they actually ate their children; it is recorded! (Lm4:10; 2K6:28; Ba2:3; Ez5:10) Thus, one might consider a world-wide spiritual famine now, in which this is, in essence occurring; for people today are reluctant to have as they say, another mouth to feed, another person to provide for. They only see the little soul as an inconvenience, an obligation! They overlook life and love; they overlook sharing; they overlook Providence!

You will write these Words given to you this night, in the abortion chapter, and at the time of making the book, if it become necessary to eliminate any sections, We shall assist you in such decisions. Be at Peace. The vision was of the scouts knife. Their motto is to "be prepared," and the Word of God is a "two-edged sword;" and I am bidding you little children, to study Scripture; have My Words when necessary, ready on your lips, for comes a time now for conversion, as there is a great Ingathering occurring, and little children, each one of you is powerfully protected under the beloved St Michael, Guardian of the people of God. You have no idea of the immensity of the power of great angels little children, to assist you.

He showing us *1 Thessalonians 5 vs8* [also see Ephesians 6] It is how I would have you be always now little children secure in My Embrace encompassed in the power of the Holy Spirit of God, the Holy Spirit who is Love; it is the Weapon of choice! Others are speaking war; I am speaking Love, I am speaking Peace, for I AM Love, I am Peace. Lilliputian—, insignificant one, you win again! I do little children, address you in Love; I already know the questions you are going to ask Me. Little children, this Communication is delightful. Little children, I would that all My little ones would talk to Me as friend, as little brother, as little sister. It is most pleasing. Be at Peace.

The choice is ever life or death, life or death - but scientists have forgotten about Life or Death of the soul! Thus they are caught up in this madness; this chaotic situation where babies are being murdered and babies are being 'created' as it were, not by the Will of God, but by the desire of the parents united with that of the doctor who seeks to work this form of science. There is Compassion, and there is misplaced compassion. Consider why are so many sterile. Is it because of the diseases of promiscuity? Is it because of the Wrath of your God? Why, why - when there are so many fertile and their babies are killed. Think of this, My little children. There is a lesson here to be learned by mankind.

I repeat; I reiterate; It is the Lord your God, Who set the stars on their courses, that gives you the life-bearing planet, at the essential distance from the sun, that there might be life here! Now you toy with all these gifts of Mine, which cause life to be! The seeds of My Love have fallen on bare rock and are bearing no fruit in this community of practitioners of death! Would that they would heed the Lord their God, for the answers are all in the Word of God - the Holy Scripture: ' There is a time to be born, there is a time to die' (Ecclesiastes 3). I give Life and I take Life. I take My Own Home. Now the doctors would like to decide when this shall be, or when their lives will be snatched away from them. How can this be pleasing to the Lord your God? *It is not!*

Each of My Own who believe in Me, walk on this earth as a lighted candle; for the Flame of Love, the Power of the Holy Spirit is upon each one, even as it was upon My apostles and disciples at the time of the first Pentecost. I send many more of My instruments to be My Heart, My Hands, My Voice now. Faithful Missionary is but one, and I have given her this singular Mission. Heed My Voice in her. Recognize the sanctity of each God given life. I place My wholesome Life in you; do not deny it to another human! Medical healing is good, can be good. There are many acceptable practices in the healing ministry of physicians, and this is pleasing to the Lord God, the Giver of all the gifts, and all the intelligences, and all the arts. These are gifts of the Living God to His sons and daughters among whom you are numbered. Used within the walls of the Commandments, in obedience to Holy Scripture, most especially in loving one's neighbour as oneself, there is no harm. It is when one ceases to see an individual as a unique gift of God, and treats them, one might say, like so much merchandise, that the harm comes into effect. At times, from My View, it is that My people are processed like so much livestock. How can this be pleasing to your God!

Do not you view in the garden many flowers, and each flower is beautiful in its own right. Each orchid created is in startling beauty; each one! So your Creator God sees each human, each individual! Except you look at them with My Eyes, you people of the world, you do not see the beauty of each individual, the preciousness, both strength and fragility present in each human; and yet this is how your Creator designed each individual.

I do not Will that any of My precious humans be treated experimentally, except should they without coercion, in free will, choose to be treated thus. Beloved Luke is a physician who loved much, who loved in Christ-Love. How could he write in such Love, in the Gospel if it were not so. He lived Love. That is what every Christian physician is called to do; to live Love; all- compassionate Love; all Love and Charity upon each suffering soul presented to them. I fail to see this in many clinics, in many hospitals. Yes, there is derision for the Christian physician in many circles. *The angels are singing, "Lift High the Cross*[We join] *the Love of God proclaim, till all the world adore, His sacred Name."* Little ones, that is what it is all about! Many people on the earth today, who know Me not, are caught up in a crucible of suffering appalling for your God to behold. I give free will to My beloved little ones that they might be godlike, and look what they have done !

Little children, as Mother loved Luke, so she loves Her physician children. Mother weeps copious tears of sorrow at some of the events that are happening in the medical field, and yet glorious tears of Joy at the many beautiful successes in healing Love, for the use of the God given intellect and capabilities on behalf of the suffering brother or sister is so pleasing to God. Many, many physicians are precious and blest of the Lord God, yet the grave error of this humanist wave of atrocious medical actions is grievous to both your God and to the Mother of God. Little children, I am Jesus, Eternal Victor! My Victory is before My eyes. Small instruments, blessings accrue, for each one of you who partakes in this Mission of Enlightenment.

Even though death and destruction has come upon the great nation of America, there are those in America and elsewhere in the world, who are yet perpetrating the evils which I have called you little ones to fight in My Epistle of Love! Some men of scientific intellect, and women, have a desire, a bent, to make themselves "godlike," to do these procedures which are in essence, antichrist(1 Jn4:3) procedures; to make themselves power and fame and yes, money! These ones also are doomed to failure in due course!

Do you have a voice in these matters? I have assigned you this Mission, that My Voice be heard round about the world, and thou hast done this well; and there are those who heed and there are those who hear and do not heed and do not change(1Jn4:6), and thus you are called to persevere. A vision is given to Omen; something which looks like a microscope, but instead of a lens there is a needle. She is given the word en-nucleate cells. This is a process which is not pleasing to Me, the Creator of all that is seen and unseen, the Giver of Life! (1Sam 2:6)

The behavior of this portion of humanity, is not only unclean behaviour, but abominable behaviour, an abomination before your God!(Gn9:5-6. Dt30:19) At the same time that this is happening, the angels are still proclaiming, *"Holy, Holy, Holy is the Lord."*(Rv4:8) Oh My little ones, hosts of angels fight side by side for Life and for Truth and for Peace which does not come! Each one of you gathered here in My Name is called and strengthened to the necessary Fortitude, to persevere in all that you are undertaking in My Name, evangelizing and fighting the Good Fight, that Truth be made known to all, from the lowliest to the most intellectual, as they consider themselves, and I bless you each one to do that which I am calling you forth to do.

My little ones, do not take lightly the Mission which you have been given with regard to My Letter to the scientific world. It is of grave importance and believe that the Church Authorities are fully aware of it and of the gravity of My Words. These, as you know, have already been corroborated scientifically, and though it is not what you would call a conundrum, the Church must speak on these" Life and Death" issues, in a manner which will open the eyes of the disbelievers and cause those who were formerly pro-death to become actively pro-life,(Dt 30:19) and it shall be so, for none of My Words are wasted or lost upon mankind. Works of Mercy flow in and through My Words of healing Love. You are aware that I deny My Mother nothing little children(!Kgs2:21-22), and She yet pleads for the multitudes on earth; and it is true, the dastardly deeds of man are an abomination before your God and before the Mother of God, but in other areas of the world there are so many precious little souls in need of Enlightenment, and so there is a war between good and evil actively occurring on this earth. I ask you to stand firm and to stand tall in all that has been uttered little ones through your voices, no matter what the questioning. *little children of Fatima had much suffering to experience because they heeded the words of the Virgin Mary.*

It is yet a time, an hour of My Mercy, prolonged on behalf of Love. When My Justice is upon the earth,(Rv14h) it is at this time that My Justice becomes Mercy, for no longer can the abominations and desecrations, the Death of souls continue on the earth!(Rv14:10-11) I am anointing you little children, in a profound anointing which you will recognize as you go forward in Faith. "The women would not be sterile, and in need of this peculiar field of medicine to cause them to have a child in spite of their sterility. I give you Sarah (Gn 21:1-2), and Anne, and Elizabeth (Lk 1:13); for nothing is impossible to God (Lk 1:38)!"Each of My Own who believe in Me, walk on this earth as a lighted candle; for the Flame of Love, the Power of the Holy Spirit is upon each one, even as it was upon My apostles and disciples at the time of the first Pentecost (Ac 2:1-21). I send many more of My instruments to be My Heart, My Hands, My Voice now. Faithful Missionary is but one, and I have given her this singular Mission. Heed My Voice in her. Recognize the sanctity of each God given life. I place My wholesome Life in you; do not deny it to another human!

Every time an abortion murder is committed, more devils are released, who gleefully go and attack a vulnerable soul (one not in a state of grace), and incite that soul to commit murder. We have heard how crimes of murder and war will not cease until abortion ceases, but now our Lord explains how.(I found out some of the contributions to Foster Parent Plan of Canada support abortion and contraception and had to find a totally pro-life fund.)Thou hast given the money in the past in good Faith; what others have done with it, they must answer to Me about. Henceforth it is best that you advise them of your reasons why you can no longer support them, and of course there are many true Christian charities in the Church who are in sore need of support and this is easily done.

That a certain family in a certain country, may know hardship because of this decision, must not concern you; I Myself attend upon this people, for it is not for lack of Love for them that this is occurring, but rather it is because of Love for My New Gifts of Life and Love, that you must do this. Can you understand, My little one? Little children, sometimes you feel fenced in by the opposition. Don't be; I am with you. Truth needs no defense. Simply persevere in speaking out the Truth. Gradually the minds of others are opened to recognize this Truth. Look at the anti-abortion battle. The pro-life movement has been fighting these many years and is only now beginning to bear fruit, and yet the battle prevails. Believe that since this prayer was occurring all around the globe, Your Father in Heaven, who sees and knows all, recognizes you prayer warriors, all around the earth for who you are and what you are accomplishing. The Wrath of God falls rampantly about the earth because of the sin of abortion, the sin of murder. "Am I My brother's keeper?"(Gn4:10) He is saying to us.

My little children of Life, I bless you each and every one. I am blessing those who comprehend that I am God.(cf Ex 14:18) and yield their free wills to Me. When you yield your free wills to Me, it is for the love, not only of your God, but the love of mankind, for the betterment of mankind, for the Salvation of mankind. Thus little children, when you practice loving your neighbour as yourself, great fruits are produced; to come to know Truth, and to live in My Light and My Love. As you know, while you were in Rome, the many encounters were arranged by the Hand of your God, that an understanding of My Word, My Will, be known hither and yon about the globe, about the earth, for the hour is late and much of My Word is yet needed. Little children, as each one believes as GI believes now, they too in their Faith begin to believe, so that healing Love emanates from them unto others, and thus is expanded the Great Mission of Light and Love and Life. Little children, what would you ask your Jesus? I pray for the conversion of the abortionist doctors. Such serial killers have caused themselves to be devoid of the shielding protection of the Living God. Even so, as you have commented, it is not an attack by anyone who is pro-life. To the contrary, it is a vengeful act. I will speak no further at this time. You will see as the investigation is played out, that the people of God are innocent of such crimes and yet they raise what you call a smokescreen, a storm of lies is raised up, of propaganda against believers in Life. It is not so! Be at Peace.

But I tell you, as I have told you before, for every child sacrificed on the altar of selfishness in abortion, there are actions by the evil one and his evil cohort. He strikes readily at the minds of those who have not been raised up in Truth or have wondered far from Truth, and these dread consequences occur. Little children, you know these times have to be. I bless with a shield those who are My Own. Little ones who are murdered like H; I claim them as martyrs. They are martyrs because of a society that has gone awry, even though they are murdered by specific individuals, they are yet pointing accusing fingers at this society, this Humanity of today. Oh Woe! Weep and repent Mankind, for My Wrath is complete...fulminating sword....Speak your concerns My little one.

Blessed Gianna.

A doctor helps you - the Italian lady doctor who died to help her baby: Gianna. This doctor knew life, knew love, and is now forever in My Presence in Glory. She blesses you in a profound assisting way. She is not alone. More come to your assistance. Heaven is attendant upon this work of merciful Enlightenment to man. Most assuredly as much as Gianna's child was sent in her life, that the Hand of God be shown clearly and truly to mankind; that in this Sacrifice of Love, for Love, to Love, which occurred to you and your child, he completed his Mission, his role most rapidly as I have been telling you little children, can and does occur! Blessed Gianna busies herself assisting you and like-minded physicians. Believe little children, the knowledge of all Life is well known to the beloved Gianna, and she is attendant upon all those working that the Gift of Life be recognized as it truly is in each human being. Dedicate the book to Gianna, who knew the value of the human soul. She was ready to, and did give up her life for her baby.

On the 9th July 2001, Our Lord requested this book be dedicated to Blessed(now saint) Dr Gianna Beretta Molla,

Prayer by Blessed Gianna

Jesus, I promised You to submit myself to all that You permit to befall me, make me only know Your Will. My most sweet Jesus, infinitely merciful God, most tender Father of souls, and in a particular way of the most weak, most miserable, most infirm which

You carry with special tenderness between Your divine arms, I come to You to ask You, through the love and merits of Your Sacred Heart, the grace to comprehend and do always Your Holy Will, the grace to confide in You, the grace to rest securely through time and eternity in Your loving divine arms.

Peace; We are with you little children, be at Peace. The Sovereign Queen desires to address the matter of abortions.

MARY: *My daughters, there is a time of change on the earth, and yet those in positions of power continue, not only in this nation, but many others throughout the world, in killing the preborn children of God, and I am aggrieved; I am your Mother in tears, your Mother of tears, and I have called again and again, in the Name of the Lord, in the power of the Holy Spirit, for an end to this attack on Life and Love. Yes, you recognize me as your Mother of La Salette. <u>Then</u> were you warned of a time when much distress would come upon the earth, and indeed since that time, much distress has come upon the earth in various areas of the world, and yet now; <u>NOW</u> the hand of the Lord, Who would give wrath to the earth, to humanity who has desecrated the beauty of Life and Love, is too heavy children! My tears fall on My children, My beloved children! Why do I speak to you? Because you will spread these Words in the most modern of means; on the internet. It is not the Will of the God of Love, for destruction to fall upon children-God's Gift of Life and Love -in the wombs of their mothers. They perish without having breathed, without having been Baptized, without having either given or received love on earth! Woe to an earth which does not welcome new life!*

Do not think- I speak to all humanity- that by denying God, you can escape His Law, His Commandments. By denying Heaven and denying hell, you believe there is no Heaven, no hell. On the Day of the Lord, you are in for a tremendous shock! Oh Horror, if you do not repent and open your minds and hearts to Truth! Indeed, in each human being is that seed of Truth, that little kernel of Truth-of God- yet you seal yourself away from the Living God, and instead of Love growing in your hearts, hate grows! The words hate and hell have a unity little children. When you live hate, you ultimately must go to that horrendous place which is named hell!

There is a trilogy of evil: abortion, war and disbelief in Almighty God, most especially in the Redeemer, the Saviour of all mankind. These are expanded into ever-vaster areas of corruption and evil, and yet it is known that this great apostasy had to come. The betrayal by many consecrated to the Lord Our God, is also a great source of grief and sorrow. Little children, I call to them, your minds are filled with deceit from the liar, the father of lies; the master of illusion. Why do you follow him and not the Living God! Enshrouded in the darkness of Death and deceit, how can they find their way back into the Light! I Myself attend upon them pleadingly. They stoke the fires of hell with their iniquities! When you pray the prayers you are praying and I take them to the Father, then indeed many are released, but oh My daughters, there are so many, many more, yet in the darkness. Continue in all that you are doing; your works, your very lives are blest in the Providence of the Living God. Persevere in all faithfulness, in all holiness. You, with the faithful remnant, remain as lighted candles, spread about the world, casting Light into the darkness, and giving Glory to the Father.

Little children, those of you who believe are praying incessantly for the conversion of sinners, the Salvation of souls. Jesus' very Name is "Salvation," and Emmanuel is verily "God with us,"-<u>your God is with you!</u> Do not shun Him; do not ignore Him; do not disbelieve! Open the eyes of your soul; open your ears to hear the Divine Call of Love that you may live, have Life to the fullest, Life eternally in Glory. This is why I am upon the earth pleading; weeping, before the Day of the Lord. Heed my call, heed my cry little children; I remain your tearful Mother!

Since you are My Scapula children, I address you as your Mother of Mt Carmel. You do know the promises I have made to the children of God who wear My Scapula; then you are powerfully assisted by me, your Spiritual Mother, and the Carmelite saints also assist those who are clothed in the Scapula. It has not been promoted in the schools as it once was, when every child was enrolled in the Scapula, and I ask little children, that you promote the Scapula, and when you give a Scapula to someone, ask them to go to the priests of your parish and be duly blest to wear the Scapula. Little children, see I am anointed and overshadowed by the Holy Spirit, and this is for always, because our God is eternal, and My mantle, My Scapula, gives you a great Protection, not only, in my love, but in the power of the Holy Spirit, Who is Love. My delight is to see you here with My Scapula.

Psalm 139:1-9.

Yahweh, You examine me and you know me, you know if I am standing or sitting, you read my thoughts from far away, whether I walk or lie down, You are watching, you know every detail of my conduct. The word is not even on my tongue, Yahweh, before You know all about it; close behind and close in front You fence me round, shielding me with Your hand. Such knowledge is beyond my understanding, a height to which my mind cannot attain. Where could I escape your spirit? Where could I flee from Your Presence? If I climb the heavens, You are there, there too if I lie in Sheol. If I flew to the point of sunrise, or westward across the sea, Your hand would still be guiding me, Your right hand holding me. If I asked darkness to cover me, and light became night around me, that darkness would not be dark to You, night would be as light as day. It was You who created my inmost self, and put me together in my mother's womb; for all these mysteries I thank You: for the wonder of myself, for the wonder of Your works. You know me through and through, from having watched my bones take shape when I was being formed in secret, knitted together in the limbo of the womb. You have scrutinized my every action, all were recorded in Your book, my days listed and determined, even before the first of them occurred. God, how hard it is to grasp Your thoughts! How impossible to count them! I could no more count them than I could the sand, and supposed I could, You would still be with me.

September 11th 2001.

At the end of prayers I sometimes ask our Lord to speak if He wishes to as below on the evening of Sept 10th, 2001.

Outpouring from His Sacred Heart

Little children, love Me as I have Loved you; this is the pathway of holiness, the narrow Way. Little children, many there are who seek Me but they do not follow in the narrow Way. Little children, in the world today there is so great a temptation to follow the ways of the world, to seek the material gains, not realizing in so doing, you are being caught up in the snares of the foe, in idolatry and the like. But little children of Faith, be not unduly concerned, for I seek your loved ones out. I am the Good Shepherd, I bring them back to Truth in due course. Even so, in Our Father's great design, the prayers and the penances of the faithful, play an integral role, in causing those who are in free will, yet in the world, to have a conversion of heart. You don't realize at what moment, after so much prayer, one soul will come back to Me, in all repentance, and be embraced in Love once again. That is why Mother is one earth, frequenting the earth, calling the children who can see, who can hear, who know, to pray and pray and pray again, for the conversion of sinners, the Salvation of souls. Hosts of angels assist in the works of My Church upon earth. Hosts of angels assist each one of you now in these unusual times.

<u>I ask you little children, to pray for those who are following the Moslem beliefs. They are brought into a misconstrued notion of God and holiness. Hate can never be of God; the desire to kill because someone is different can never be of God! *</u>

My little ones, pray much and trust Me, the Living God, the Giver of all life. No matter what is happening on this earth, your prayers do indeed resound in Heaven in unity with the saints, and much good is brought forth. Also always remember that in your faithfulness in prayer, in word and deed, you are storing treasure in Heaven, to be known to you only on a glorious day of the Lord. In the interim, walk in My Light and My Love and My Life, persevering. I am anointing you this evening little children, in a profound anointing of My Love and My Peace, and that sure and quiet joy in the Love of the Lord, which I have given you. I cause your hearts to flame up with love periodically at moments of prayer union with Me. This is a moment of rejoicing in our unity of love. Let it always be thus! * Of course we did not know till the next morning when we heard the news, what Jesus was telling us.

After the September 11th New York disaster Mother *Mary said this:Queen of Angels and All Saints attendant upon you little children, bids you Peace.* **Believe little children, believe in the Victory in Jesus Holy Name, for it is so! My dear little children, there are certain events that do indeed happen on this earth which, though not of God, are portends of the times that are ahead, which bring on changes upon the earth, and in due course, the return of Christ, and a new era of Peace on earth, as has been told through** *many visionaries with whom I have worked. The difficult times as you know, are now! And yet the children of God are safe in the Divine Embrace. Children, you are safe, whether on earth, in purgatory or in Heaven; you are safe in the Lord. It behooves you little children, to pray much for those who do not yet know the Lord, for the hour is indeed late, and the many are indeed far from Home, far from the Sanctuary of the Heart of Jesus; the Heart of Mary. Little children, the grief in America and indeed about the world, is profound. The Holy Spirit, the Comforter, is busily attendant upon the multitudes in need of comforting at this time. Little children, your prayers on behalf of the suffering Americans, are powerful to assist in their healing. <u>There are those who died in this disaster who were most precious to the Lord God, indeed every soul is precious to the Lord God. In the death of the beloved Fr Mychal Judge, you see a martyr's blood, mixed with the blood of all those who died. Many were the martyrs, especially the firemen and policemen, and the innocents in the planes and in the buildings.</u> Oh My children, the souls of all those who died unjustly, and are recognized as martyrs for the cause of Peace, are safe in the Lord, yet we ask you to pray for those yet in their purification; pray for the people suffering physically and mostly and in all mental anguish on earth, over the loss or injury, of their loved ones. There can be no cause as great as the Cause for an end of abortion. One might liken the individuals in the two towers, and in the Pentagon, as feeling secure, as it were, in those buildings, when fierce intrusion exteriorly, destroyed their lives. Do you see the simile little children? Dear little children, continue to work on the Cause for Life; it is imperative for humanity, that an end of legal abortion and every force of destruction and death, untimely and unwarranted, be stopped. <u>You say, greater is God Who is in your heart and mind, than that enemy which is in the world, and this is true. The enemy is always Satan, the evil one, the promoter of hate; but as you recognize, he has many human pawns on the face of the earth, who have believed the liar, and are now in his evil clutches. It is to this end that you are working little children, to evangelize in the Holy Name of Jesus, for the conversion of sinners the salvation of souls, while it is yet a time of Mercy upon this earth! You ask, "was it mercy, the destruction of the towers?"</u> She shows us Her words of La Salette, "Up, you small band that can see and fight.[the spiritual battle. September 19th feastday. Our Lady wept, telling the children, people will not obey, I shall be compelled to loose My Son's arm. It is so heavy, so pressing that I can no longer restrain it." <u>Little children, again you are told, certain things must be, before the return of Our Lord, the Prince of Peace, and the great era of Peace on earth. That is why you, who know Truth; the Lord Our God, are called to be the heart and hand and voice of Our Saviour; that is why you are being told that the Words of this entire year are: persevere, endure, perseve</u>*I Myself, in the power of the Holy Spirit of the Living God, bless you little children, with many graces to assist you at this time, so that you will be fearless companions of Christ on this journey!

Jeremiah 31 vs15: Thus speaks Yahweh: a voice is heard in Ramah, lamenting and weeping bitterly: it is Rachel weeping for her children, refusing to be comforted for her children, because they are no more.

Sunrise in New York Something we will never even be able to see again!!! A lady returning on a cruise took this picture this past summer (July 28, 2001). It is a sunrise over lower Manhattan.

She writes: As I watched the beautiful skyline of New York City float past me I noticed the sun was about to line up just behind the twin towers. I was lucky enough to snap the picture at exactly the right moment. If you look at the sunrays it is almost prophetic. - A little spooky. When I show this picture to anyone they almost always asks for a copy. I just want to share it with all that want it. Please take this picture and share it with anyone and everyone who likes it. I've been printing them like crazy on my home computer to give to those that want a copy.

Medicine of God — 87

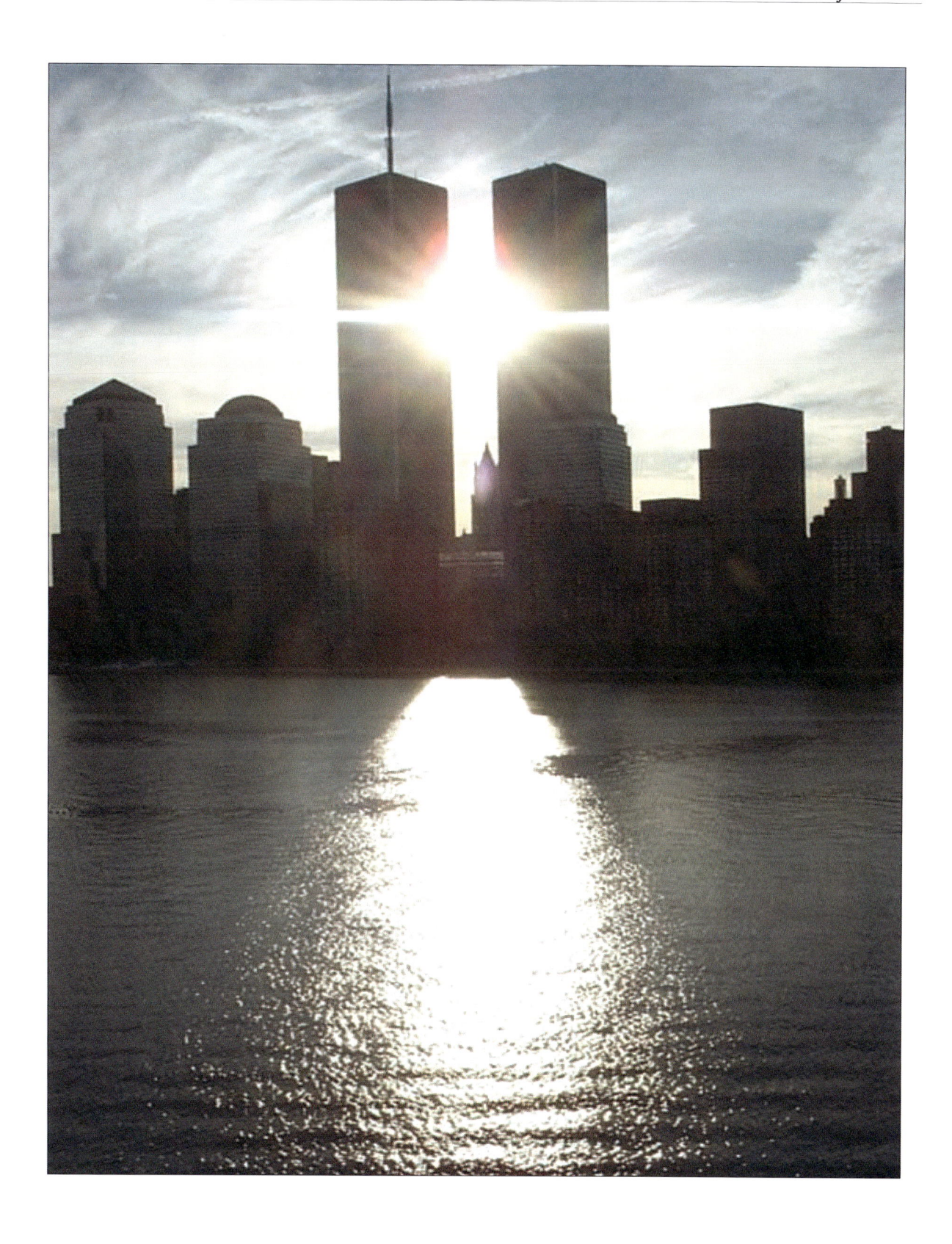

CHAPTER SEVEN
ORGAN TRANSPLANTS

MARK OF CAIN Gn 4:15.

JESUS: My gifts to mankind are always contingent upon the eternal Laws of your God; and thus, mankind, to your sorrow, they fall under a curse, rather than reaching joy under My blessing. What will you do when you run out of body parts? It will become expedient simply to kill another for the body parts. You are already aware that this can and does occur in various nations. Walls of flame surround those who are behaving in this manner. The mark of Cain is upon many on Earth. They are Mine yet they elect to kill their brothers, for their own motives. *There was a long period of silence during which I felt uneasy as if blocked from our Lord by a 'negative or dark presence.' I started to sing, "Yahweh, I know You are near..." After the first verse, came the following words:*

The Comforter is present. The body is the temple of the Holy Spirit is it not? Therefore, it is sacrilege to take out the organs. If today you hear God's Voice, harden not your hearts!(Ps95) I am attendant upon this concept of body parts to be taken from one SOUL to another. Do you think it is pleasing to your God? No Lord. It is repugnant to the Lord your God! My children of Faith, you have but to ask and I heal those who in all sincerity of heart prayerfully seek it. In union with the Holy Spirit of Love I heal it. Few ask for this healing among the millions upon this earth! They turn to the medical profession, many of whom know Me not. I bless mankind with free will, I bless mankind with human intellect, I bless mankind with seeking, searching minds.

I died that you might have life to the fullest. Scientific facts to the contrary, there is ONE body attached to ONE soul. This is the Design of your Father, your Creator. This is the way it is; this is the way it should be! A flame of Love is upon you, for you are profoundly anointed in the Spirit of the Living God. I the Lord your God, bid you know that I am not unaware that the seven deadly sins are no longer mentioned among Christians. They are not recognized among pagans; but it is the very humans who claim to be Christians who now shun the seven deadly sins. Were there no lust, there would be no abortions; were there no greed, there would be no sale of body parts; If there were not self-seeking, power-seeking scientists, there would be no cloning of humans; no mutilation of precious embryos and all the other desecrations that are occurring upon My Own creation, with precious human bodies and souls.

In a sterile, loveless way they work their works of iniquity upon My creation, humanity. It is enough what they are doing to the other creatures on earth, but what they do to My precious gifts of Love brings down My Wrath, as you well know. I bid you read Ezekiel, read Jeremiah, read the many messages in Holy Scripture and know that I do not take lightly the attacks on innocent victims such as aborted infants and indeed those whose bodies are so mutilated by, as they call it, the harvesting of their organs. Why would they need a substitute kidney or heart or liver had they or their forbearers been faithful to Me in the first place? Even now, were they simply to be faithful I would cure them.

I bid you know that when you transplant organs, the drugs necessary to keep the recipient alive, give them but a half-life. Even so, in My great Mercy, little ones pray for life, and I give it to them. In My great Mercy, I bless My little faithful ones as is written, to be the salt of the earth; the salt that preserves humanity from the corrupted state in which it finds itself. The power which drives the machine for organ donations is not of Me. The Wrath which falls in due course, is caused by many things, but this abuse of human temples of the Living God,(1Co3:16) is one of the many causes. Even so, I will never forget My Own.

You await the word from the beloved John Paul on bodily death, on clinical death. He will address it shortly. He too, is gravely concerned about the turn science is taking in the abuse of the terminally ill, and the concept of replacing any body part, as if you were, little people, soulless vehicles. Continue little children, to await the day of his commentary on the situation of 'brain death' and organ transplant. Many communications showing the abuse of individuals in this regard are coming to his attention, and he SHALL speak on the abuse and it will be the necessary Words which you await. Believe and be of Peace. It shall be so, for there comes before his eyes, word of the abuses of the basic, shall We say ground rules in the matter of Life, in the matter of organ transplants, and so he is called to speak yet again, clearly and concisely on this matter, that this abomination before My Eyes cease; and where it persists, that it be clearly recognized as the evil that it truly is. It will be broken through by you and such as you, and the pediatrician and many other who are aware, just as the Truth of abortion is known now though not yet defeated, so Truth of this form of abuse of humans will become known clearly in due Course. Doubt not!

In Evangelium Vitae (1995) the Holy Father says: No. 86: "As part of the spiritual worship acceptable to God (cf.Rom 12:1), the Gospel of Life is to be celebrated above all in daily living, which should be filled with self-giving love for others...It is in this context, so humanly rich and filled with love, that heroic actions too are borne...,made up of gestures of sharing, big and small, which build up an authentic culture of life. A particularly praiseworthy example of such gestures is the donation of organs, performed in an ethically acceptable manner, with a view to offering a chance of health and even of life itself to the sick who sometimes have no other hope!

But he also says in Paragraph15: Threats which are no less serious hang over the incurably ill and the dying. In a social and cultural context which makes it more difficult to face and accept suffering, the temptation becomes all the greater to resolve the problem of suffering by eliminating it at the root, by hastening death so that it occurs at the moment considered most suitable...Nor can we remain silent in the face of other more furtive, but no less serious and real, forms of euthanasia. This could occur for example when, in order to increase the availability of organs for transplants, organs are removed without respecting objective and adequate criteria which verify the death of the donor.

The virtue of Love is such that I the Lord God, adjust the ways of mankind very profoundly, very soon now. In the interim, I yet would address the scientific minds to know that I bless them with many abilities for healing and curing. There are certain things that go beyond My Will in the realm of science and this is not pleasing to the Lord your God. In My great merciful Love, when one shares out of love (He shows the kidney transplant of a loved one to a loved one), the living donor risks his life to give that loved one a portion of himself. In My great Mercy I accept this as an act of love. Little children, the quandary is that it should not become necessary, were mankind all living within the walls of the Ten Commandments. These afflictions which are prevailing in the bodies of My people would not be, and in the Name of Jesus, the healing would occur without taking such dire measures to prolong life. Then, in all -charity- of- Love, I bless with certain healings some of these procedures -<u>when it is love in action I forgive, as it were, the invasion of the human body to remove the part so that a loved one might live.</u>

Yet the matter of proclaiming an individual has attained bodily death, that many parts may be removed, as it were, commercially, for the use of other humans in hopes that they might live, is not pleasing to the Lord your God. A greater peril than body death is soul death. In the medical profession, many place their souls in grave peril by these actions of, as I have said, "playing god. "You know well that the recipients do not necessarily regain full health, but as I have said, they have a half-life in their bodies. Even so, I have Mercy and spare their souls, for in all these trials they must plead with Me for their continual assistance upon earth. My people have forgotten that eternal Life is in Heaven. There is no fountain of youth upon earth. It is but a temporary journey. You are called in Holy Scripture to keep your eyes turned towards Heaven your true and native Land. Therefore, the perfection of soul is always the priority. Choosing, in your eyes, that which is the lesser of evils, does not make anything right in the Eyes of the Father. You all know that the Mystery of Love which I have encoded in each human; is individual, is unique, and is for that individual - and try as they may, the scientists run into block after block, in their strange attempts to do that which is unnatural and unseemly to the Eyes of God! *Praying Divine Mercy Chaplet after receiving E-mail from T regarding modifying (relaxing) criteria for "harvesting of organs."*

Fervently you pray to Me about many matters. I Myself attend upon thee now. A mighty river of Light is upon you, little one. The Triune God blesses you in a great anointing on this great feast day. You have many concerns on your heart, My beloved little sister, My small instrument of Peace. Turmoil moves upon the earth. Let us address first the matter of human body parts. The manner in which these parts are, as is described, harvested - is not My Will but the will of the enemy. This affair of body parts has become an instrument of greed and power. It is not in the Father's Design for human beings. Grotesque results begin to appear now in such operations and procedures, for My blessing is not upon the hands of the doctors who perform these procedures. Do you wish to serve Me more in these matters? Yes Lord. This is a crime - for it is a theft from healthy bodies in an attempt for a scientist to "play god" and replace, in a debilitated body, a healthy organ. It is not different than putting new wine in old skins: it does not work! Prolonged suffering and sorrow is often the consequence for the recipient of donor organs. It is not so for the doctor who has created this. He luxuriates in more of his enterprise. I ask mankind to restore the gift given by God! You are made in the Image of God! You are gifted with free will; and should you ask for wisdom and discernment and knowledge it is yours! But you do not in your pride! You wreak havoc on His people!

Many of the afflictions are caused by man's free will and behaviour which is opposing that of God! And then the individuals so afflicted are further mistreated at the hands of the enterprising physician who would "play god" in the lives of these individuals who become victims of these dastardly deeds! I the Lord your God hold each life sacred and precious to Me! Scientific research must always be for the benefit of mankind. Yet things are occurring in scientific research which are repugnant to the Lord your God! I bid you know that it were better to have more restrictions on this human behaviour of obtaining human body parts, rather than more liberal ways of obtaining and using them.

Medical healing is good, can be good. There are many acceptable practices in the healing ministry of physicians, and this is pleasing to the Lord God, the Giver of all the gifts, and all the intelligences, and all the arts. These are gifts of the Living God to His sons and daughters, among whom you are numbered. Used within the walls of the Commandments, in obedience to Holy Scripture, most especially in loving ones neighbour as oneself, there is no harm. It is when one ceases to see an individual as a unique gift of God, and treats them, one might say, like so much merchandise, that the harm comes into effect. At times, from My View, it is that My people are processed like so much livestock. How can this be pleasing to your God! As you are kneeling before the Father of Enlightenment, Mercy attends upon you, blessing you. It is to be said that the Lord your God has seen no horrors so great as what is before My Eyes today. It is simply a time to warn mankind - those who will heed - that some may escape the wrath that is at hand. Cannibalism - this can be viewed as a form of cannibalism - can you not see that?

Do not you view in the garden many flowers, and each flower is beautiful in its own right. Each orchid created is in startling beauty; each one! So your Creator God sees each human, each individual. Except you look at them with My Eyes, you people of the world, you do not see the beauty of each individual, the preciousness, both strength and fragility present in each human; and yet this is how your Creator has designed each individual. I do not will that any of My precious humans be treated experimentally, except should they without coercion, in free will, choose to be treated thus. Beloved Luke is a physician who loved much, who loved in Christ-Love. How could he write in such Love, in the Gospel if it were not so. He lived Love. That is what every Christian physician is called to do; to live Love; all-compassionate Love; all Love and Charity upon each suffering soul presented to them. I fail to see this in many clinics, in many hospitals. Yes, there is derision for the Christian physician in many circles. Many people on the earth today, who know Me not, are caught up in a crucible of suffering appalling for your God to behold. I give free will to My beloved little ones that they might be Godlike, and look what they have done ! In My great Mercy, We turn this whole thing around. I ask each one of you to say, "Let it begin with me. "

There comes a time of shock and dismay upon the scientific community, the medical community. For My Rule does and shall prevail. Scientific leaders, no matter what they think, are not gods and shall not be gods! They may attain or obtain transitory fame in the scientific community, but it is at the expense of their patients who become their victims frequently. The harvesting, the mining, the utilizing of human body parts, is foreign to Holy Scripture, and foreign to the Lord your God! *Mortal man, what are you thinking of*! Clandestine acts of harvesting human body parts are occurring round about the earth. It is so abhorrent to the Lord your God! That money comes into the picture is even more abhorrent. This people place sin, upon sin, upon sin, in their lives. Whom do they serve? Who is it that they serve! This is your Mission. I would that they be spared such a fate!It is sad what occurs to the dying, and to those receiving body parts from others. But sadder before the Eyes of your God, and your Heavenly Mother, are the state of the souls of these scientists! Love Me! *(my God,I believe, I adore,I hope and I love Thee…*

I bid thee proceed. Favourable action is taken upon the abstract, through the assistance of Raphael, yet We bid you know and understand that this Mission is given unto thee by thy Heavenly Mother and by your Jesus of Merciful Love and We are with you in these works of Mercy every step of the way. <u>Look now upon Our Mother's Latest Pieta!</u> *[Sorrowful Mother with a mutilated body cut open, with heart, liver , kidneys etc taken out !] This was an almost unbearable experience; yet on June 8th our Lord said this twice!* The foe is causing havoc and suffering to many patients exposed to the evil one because the lifestyles and the works of some of the staff are not pleasing to the Lord; therefore their hands are not blest to heal, but to hurt through the actions of the evil one under whose influence they are falling.

I the Lord God bless thee. Thus are the trials of the world today. My little one, there are no drawn lines as you see. It is, as it were, a hodge-podge of Faith and science, and the superstitions of what you call the "new-age," intermingled. Thus the spirit of confusion is upon the world. My little one, in My great Mercy as I have told you, in spite of what is not pleasing to the Lord your God, I am the Lord God Who calls sinners, in some instances because of the prayers of the faithful, and the truth in the hearts, I heal some who have transplants. It is always in My Mercy that this occurs. My little one, the fight you are in is greater than you can comprehend, and yet it is important to the Lord your God. I the Lord your God am Perfection. I work for the perfection of each human soul. In all their sufferings and trials, it is imperative that they come to Me. I am the Good Physician. I am the Healer of all. I heal as you well know. I heal spiritually, mentally, emotionally, physically, and in every aspect of the human soul and body, to those who believe.

Little children, you are indeed apostles of these difficult times and you are bound to meet with opposition here and there. Do not let it discourage you. I have blest you with so great a fortitude, that you shall indeed prevail in spite of all that is coming against you. The winds of change are now. Those who did not believe yesterday, believe today, and this is an ongoing miracle of Our Love. A Herculean effort is made to stop the works which I have given unto thee. Be not dismayed. Carry the five stones of the Rosary and trust in the Lord !*[A reference to David who carried the five stones to meet Goliath. Five stones are also the Lord'0s five Wounds of Crucifixion, the prayer for Divine Mercy also prayed on the Rosary.]*

There are many things you do not know that are happening round about the globe. Underhandedly, deceitfully round about the globe that the people of God do not know, because this is the time of the great spiritual warfare, which I have been forewarning My Own about from time immemorial and more so in this recent period of time. Thou art the one chosen for this work of merciful Love and Enlightenment to My people; to the intellectuals; to the scientific mind. These people do indeed recognize the beauty of Creation and specialize in certain aspects of My created beings. Often times, as they limit themselves to one area, one specialty, they see only as it were, blood cells, or heart valves, or specific tissues; and they intensely devote their studies and works and healing arts to that small area to the point where they cease to see the entire being, or the entire complexity of humanity and of Creation. Yet I bless them; I bless them with the necessary skills and intellect to do research, to do healing works on behalf of My suffering humanity. The blessing is there. The fact that it is not freely flowing on each individual physician is because of certain barriers they themselves in free will, have placed between us. I believe you are familiar with these sort of barriers.

I reiterate, I remind you, that the eyes of the scientists who elect to practice in small specialties; one looking only at blood, one looking only at the workings of the heart, or the brain- they do not always- or even seldom see, the whole picture of a human life; a life which is both body and soul, and important to Me the Lord your God, Creator of all. As they hold fast to the practices, the traditions of the medical arts, the medical discipline, they become rigid and immovable about anything that is at a variance to their preconceived ideas . It takes much to move one from a rigid position.*[and again He is showing the oyster stuck solidly to that one spot on the rock.]* We bless you. We bless each one of the priests named for they are Our Own and are precious to us. Fr Francis' concern dealt largely with what he perceives as a difference between My Words and that which the beloved John Paul has uttered. Little children, the door opening came as acts of love one for another, which in My great Mercy, My great Love, I accepted and condoned. Yet it was only the opening of a small door, and now a greater darker door is there which is not of Me. The buying and selling of human organs, some at the absolute expense of human life some at the moment of bodily death; some who die because of the acts of doctors- many such reasons have occurred for what is called organ harvesting. You see little children it has now become a new industry, a big business. It can never be of Me.

In the short span of time since the Pope's announcement, the error of dealing with the human body has increased, one might say sevenfold and in the darkest of ways. Failure to comply with the thoughts and designs of the physicians who have propagandists available in the media, causes you to be as it were, pulled out of the inner circle. Do not be afraid; you are in a circle of the Triune God, of Mother Mary, and multitudes of angels and saints. Little children, there is no time to waste, it is time now to busy yourselves getting these Messages out. Am I not your Teacher? Many of them(*new doctors*) will be in My era of Peace, where none of this is even relevant because in My Hour of Peace there will be no such things to deal with; but that time is not yet little children; so prevail, prevail, prevail; believe, believe; pray, pray; fight; speak out! My blessings are upon you. I seal your lips both of you, that you speak only that which is Truth. I AM Truth.

I am, and I was present. I presented Myself to each one of them. I bid thee Peace in this matter. Remember, a prophet is not recognized in his own locale. It has been ever thus. Therefore accept the humblings even the humiliations, giving them over to Me. Believe little children, you serve a God of merciful Love. Were I not merciful, I might simply destroy all these non-believers; but in My Mercy, I choose to send them many small voices to Enlighten them, to call them to heed the Word of the Lord like a farmer casting out seed. Time changes everything. Continue, watching the fruits, even unto the words coming out of their mouths. I Myself work the miracles of Love I choose to work, upon each of those who have heard My Words on the sanctity of Godgiven Life. You have gained supporters, but there are of course those who come against you. This is the usual pattern for mankind . This is not different for you and for Omen, than it was for many of the saints and the prophets. It continues this way for you. Know that our foe uses pride of intellect to darken minds against Truth. Therefore prevail little children, I am with you always.

Mercy, merciful Love, is what I wish for every human soul on earth! I do not wish My little ones to be mutilated and dissected when they yet live. I do not wish My physicians, named to do good, to be committing murder, day in and day out. I call all unto Myself now; as you know it has been ongoing for some time in your realm, your kingdom of time. It is like unto a great , one might even say a prolonged hour of Mercy to your God; and at the end of that time of Mercy all of My Own will know that I am God, that I am indeed the Way, the Truth, the Light, the Life, and all of My Own will come back to Me with all their hearts. That which is going on with regard to organ transplants, all over the "civilized world", is ghastly in the eyes of the Living God! Little one persevere prayerfully. We are with you. Many begin to recognize the horror of what they are doing, and they themselves cease. My little ones, if you have noticed the Church so infiltrated by the smoke of Satan, it is as nothing, compared to the infiltration of the medical profession throughout the world at this time. Little children, bless Me! *We adore ...*

We comply with the request My dearest one for We are at war. It is also a word battle in this warfare for the minds, the scientific minds involved in this. Ultimately the common people, those who are sufficiently literate and aware, will become involved in this fray as well . The enemy is using as you know, every means at its disposal to defeat all that is holy on this earth; therefore persevere little children. J is anointed, by Your God, on a Mission in unison with yours now. Hold him always in your heart and in your prayers for of course the enemy is there; the resistance is there. Man is not ready, not accepting change readily as you well have noticed, and yet in persevering prayer, the change occurs. Little children the blessing is on all who partake in this great Mission for the correction of the pathway of the scientific world. Sorrow and pain are the lot of those who do not believe you little children. It is the Lord your God Who speaks! Little children, you live in a time of great of peril for all mankind. Dear children you, each one of you is aware of this; but few on earth are aware of the imminent danger which is upon them. Their understanding is darkened in these times, for insidious inroads by the evil one have occurred in their minds and hearts.

There are so many I would call back to My Heart ; There are so many I would bathe in My Love. They know Me not! Even as you are being shut out little children, so have I been shut out. Mother calls and pleads to no avail. And yet as all seems darkened, suddenly a swift sure action of your God and Light comes upon these minds so befuddled by the lies of this age. Enlightenment comes, and thus you are called to patient perseverance.Peace. Continue in all that you are doing on behalf of My little ones. My people suffer as you know, untold illnesses, because of the errors of the world today, and then when they fall into the hands of certain physicians, suffer degradation of their bodies while they are perceived to be terminally ill. No one calls on Me but a scant few to ask for their cures, their healings. Without My attendance upon them, no one can live! And as for those seeking to purchase better organs than I have given them, I have given them the best organs, the organs suited to their unique body makeup. If a vital organ is defective therefore, it is My Desire that hands be laid on that individual, the hands of the true faithful, and that a physical healing occur,Jm

5:14-16 SHOULD I DESIRE IT! I am the Lord your God. I ask you, how has man existed these many generations, without these body parts being taken from one to another; how is it that this has never been necessary until these recent years? Ensure that persons in key positions in pro-life movements obtain copies of the letter as well, that they may start their own campaigns. In the minds of what is called the secular humanist, the atheist, finite wisdom, finite reasoning prevails; they fail to come unto the Living God, and seek the flow of blessings and graces which would cause them to attain to Eternal Wisdom; thus they are filled with the deceits of their own thoughts, and this is not of God and is not for the good of My beloved humanity.

But as you know this is a delicate matter, in view of the approval of Rome to give in love to one another, as opposed to that which is occurring in the advanced nations now. They are called advanced nations, but what they are doing is not an indication of an advancement of Love for one's fellow man; it is a deceit! And so it is, as you well know, a delicate subject which My Church must handle most tactfully; for when the door was first opened, it seemed to be a loving and charitable thing to give your brother or sister one of your kidneys. Now it is not often a loving and charitable gift that is occurring, but an idea of buying or selling, or an idea of power over Life and Death, and a drive of pride to proclaim what certain physicians have done in their believing themselves all-powerful! Even they will learn one day what it is they have been about! But We must open their eyes, and this is what you My little ones, are assigned to do. Thus address the Archbishop in this matter, and pray that the Vatican discerns on the difference between acts of love, and this corrupt, power-hungry action of these people. Evil and dismay is upon My Heart at what My physicians are doing today, as you well know!Oh My people, what confusion is upon this field of works which was intended to be works of merciful Love. Rest assured I am with you every moment of your life, for in your yes to Me, in all abandonment, all yieldedness to Love, you live in the Power of My Peace and My Love; never forget it. Rejoice in this our Love's union; Trust Me!

We must keep the controversial aspect going in the news media so that many, many people become aware that there is such an issue. This conference is again a means of gathering together these who truly believe that all life is sacred, all life is holy and therefore We measure the time of your work and We fit in this conference which will be scholarly and serious and yet joy-filled; for it is My Desire, My Design, that all those who would call themselves physicians honour all God given life, and these people do. Therefore speak, My small sweetheart, I shall speak in you and through you. Rejoice in Our Love and be at Peace. But you know Truth; I Am Truth! My Way, My Truth, My Life, My Light, My Peace, My Joy. My Jesus! Little children, the one who is intact of body organs, with prayer, can and shall be restored to fullness of life. Alas for the many who have received organ transplants; a goodly percentage live as it were, a half-life!

Therefore I ask you; do not believe that because your heart is failing, or because your liver is failing, that you have a right to expect to be given another persons heart or liver or any such organ. It may well be that I am calling you Home! You live in a society which does not want to think of death or speak of death, but yet death is ever present in the world in the state it is in today. Until I return in Glory, death is not fully defeated! Those who are yielded to Me, have nothing to fear in My Embrace. They cross the barrier of time into Eternal Light and so the basis for desiring to give a set of organs to the other, is not well thought out by the physicians. There is as it were a movement to think that for the many afflictions organ transplanting can be a sort of panacea for all that is happening; this is not true. If I had wanted this to be occurring I could have made all of you with identical blood types, identical genetic codes, identical beings , interchangeable as toy blocks. Did I do this? No! I made each one of you unique for My Own reasons.

I am Healer , I am Physician, I am Counselor; consult Me before you make any such decisions. Pray, meditate, discern and act. This has been the way for the Faithful throughout the generations. Now there is always an urgency to make snap decisions about matters of Life and Death. Children, you have to live with those decisions! You have to answer to Me, Your Judge, on the Day of Judgment which is never far off for any individual! You may most assuredly use the message of last week, and you await in eager anticipation is it not so, for this weeks message little children. Little children, you know the times you are living in. <u>You know also that I have shortened them for your sakes, little loved ones of your God, for the sake of My Beloved Humanity.</u>

You see the enemy rearing its ugly head in every aspect of life today. It is most painful to behold by your God, even as it is painful to you little children to perceive, and yet at this time, it must be! Speak further. Yes indeed, scientific research is exciting and they are ever finding new and exciting concepts; and yet as the beloved John Paul has spoken, this must always be tempered and limited by the concerns of each and every human soul, for they are My Own. Little children you may consider those who have been, shall We say dispatched, by the taking of their hearts or vital organs, as martyrs in these times.

The beloved John Paul, in his carefully chosen words, asked the scientists, to temper all that they are doing, by careful consideration of each unique individual. You seek Enlightenment of the scientists, that they would come to know Me, even as the beloved John Paul. This is happening in some instances but not all. Do not be afraid to give the lists of discernments to your associates as you have done, for they are thought provoking and assist individuals to a clear thinking with regard to this matter of life and death. You see, John Paul has spoken quite clearly, and yet to the one who reads it lightly, it is unclear, even ambiguous. Thus it is imperative that the believers invoke the Holy Spirit for each and every one of his pronouncements. It is a time now of even greater spiritual warfare than in the past, the very recent past, for it is a time of change and turmoil on the Earth. You pray, "this is the day that the Lord has made; let us rejoice and be glad," but it is the same for each soul. This is the <u>soul</u> which the Lord has made. It is precious to the Lord. It is My Delight that you desire to educate them in My Love and My Peace. You know well that many are set on an obstinate path and will not heed. Certain ones will indeed heed. Do you wish now to open up Epistle of Love to all the world? Let it be done! Then I will give you the Words, in all charitable explanation as it were, of what the beloved John Paul has spoken, about the passing of the soul and the death of the body. Those who are open to My Words, like you and many like you about the Earth, are attempting to tell them. I ask you to continue at this time reading Scripture. I especially ask you little children to read and review the Acts of the Apostles and all of the Letters, that you comprehend fully, spiritual warfare as it was then and it is now. Little children, I am with you always and My Peace is upon you and you are enfolded in the seven-fold mantle of the Mother of God, the Mother of all.

<u>St Michael the Archangel speaks:</u> *Michael, attendant upon you, bids you Peace little children. Ruth, thou art shielded as in an impeccably designed space suit; it is the Shield of the Holy Spirit of the Living God surrounding you. Each one of you little children, are in the Shield of the Living God, and I, servant of the Living God, Michael, attend. Great jousts with the enemy which attempts to assail, this way and that, the little ones of God. You are blessed of God, for you are little before the Living God and He rejoices in you. The poor woman will come to you seeking solace for sorrow, and will find it. You will be empowered by the Holy Spirit, to do so without jeopardizing your practice, because of your profound Faith.* Thank you St Michael.

I hear and read about xenotransplantation;(animal parts for human transplantation.) what is Your Will in this regard?

It is a time of Great Sorrow; this would be a sin against the human body far worse than any sin of adultery or like sin! How is it the body, recognized as the temple, or as temple designate of the Living God, is so treated! If they were as concerned with the soul as the body they would not be considering it. The very concept is an abomination in the Eyes of your God! The scientists practice to deceive the public and to deceive the Christians. Their sins are compounded layer upon layer!

Even some Moslem countries have waived the condemnation of consuming pork, so the Moslems can accept pig organs.

These people have abandoned Me. Did they truly know Me they would not need these procedures, these body parts, these ghastly experiments, for I am the God that Heals My people. But My people know Me not! I the Lord God Bless you little children and ask you to persevere prayerfully when the storm increases over these issues, and I, the Lord God impel the beloved John Paul to speak! There are those who are using as it were, stalling techniques; there are those who are biding their time in the expectation that the beloved John Paul will simply die that they may be able to practice a ruse, to use great deception upon the people of God; that is why I ask you little children, to pray much for the Holy Father, and for his intent to speak out My Truth. He is a man of great intellect; he has a scientific bent as you know, and delights in all that is saving and healing for humanity, but he must make a document pertaining to the human being, the human body, the human soul- a unity!

I am a God of order and unity, and despite the deceptions, the ruses of the enemies about him, this holy man of God will speak Truth, and it will be revealed to the people of God! Will the atheists listen; will the agnostics heed? The humanists have no desire to be obedient to the Law of God! Therefore I WILL take action on this humanity! Be not distressed; I assure you again and again, My Own are safe in Me! Each one of you gathered here in My Name has a heart of compassion for your fellow man, and I am aware of that, and I am Mercy and Love, yet I am Justice! See this as a delicate balancing act of your God, Who so Loves Mankind, and wait on Me! As surely as mankind can have AIDS; as surely as their livestock can have the dread afflictions they presently have; as surely as mankind can have the dread flesh-eating disease; as surely I can stop what is abhorrent to Me— and it shall be so! The center of the storm is upon the earth now; chaotic conditions prevail, lingering for some time all around and about the earth! Creation groans under the weight of humanity's sins, all of which are abhorrent to the Living God, the God of Life and Light and Love and Peace and Joy.

Again I call My people, what have I done to you; why have you abandoned Me? Answer Me! The enemy plays a hand in all that is occurring which is evil upon the earth as you know. The deceiver is causing many to be led astray into lies, into fictions, into disbelief, into deception, to enter all immorality. Mankind, each man, sins against himself in the sins of immorality. Against God, yes; but against his own body! How much worse little children, is the sin of man, should he elect to be united with animal parts! The scientists work under bright lights, but they remain in darkness of the secrets of Life; of the Truth of Life. I the Lord God, am the Giver of Life; I AM Life! Do not be deceived little children, by the stories of the charitable reasons for this behaviour of the scientists. You know there is a time to be born and a time to die, and there are good physicians who attend upon the ill, and work healings in all charity of love, and these ones often have hearts of love, and actually pray and are truly in the healing ministry. There are others who are scientists and do not necessarily have compassion upon the afflicted ones, but work for the greater glory of science in all their experimentations; all these undertakings.

These ones are in grave peril to their very own souls, and they are inflicting peril upon the souls of their victims; those whom they operate on as though they were laboratory rats or monkeys! How can this be of Me? I am attendant upon them as I am attendant upon all humanity! Little children await the words in patient perseverance as you are taught. You are well trained in this! *"Come back to Me....the wilderness where I shall speak..."angels singing.* I am a God Who is Love, a God Who is Mercy, a God Who is Life! I tell you again, it is pride of intellect which takes My gifted children, off into a dark place on earth, unenlightened by My Spirit, they make decisions which are harmful to their very souls, and the souls of all those with whom they work and whom they impress with their vast knowledge of the human anatomy. <u>It can never be the Will of the Living God that you be united partially here or there, with animals! Yes they are My Creation, and Man is given power over them, but not for such purposes.</u>

Little children, always I remind you; I am the Physician; I am the Healer! You have much evidence of those who have prayed for deliverance from afflictions, who have been cured, restored to fullness of bodily life. Little children, the scientists abandon Me and they use their intellect to bring that which is unpleasing to the Lord God, into their practices. How shall I respond to what they are doing? Even as the great nation of America, and other nations self-destruct as it were, for lack of obedience to My Will, lack of obedience to My Ten Commandments of Love, lack of obedience to Truth, so will these scientists suffer in strange and varied ways. Surprising events occur because they reject the Shield of Protection of the Holy Spirit! That is why I ask you; do not seek eternal life in your frail physical bodies here on earth; seek eternal Life with Me, the Living God! On this day I am profoundly attendant upon you as I am upon the beloved John Paul, and My little ones, you will hear more and discern more clearly what is occurring. Little children, when you listen to the news, remember that certain things have to be, before the era of Peace comes upon the earth, and that I will see through this difficult time, all the faithful in the Body of Christ, and so there is nothing to fear.

You grieve for the suffering of those who are used simply as a reliquary of parts to be taken from their bodies for the use of others. In their generous "Yes" to assist others,- where this actually occurs, it is good; but the utilization by the atheistic scientists is not good, and they are mistreating many people without their consent, in much of the world, with the so-called organ harvesting! I am not blind; I am not deaf; I am not ignoring this! I am All-seeing, all-knowing, all-hearing and a Day of Clarification, a day ultimately of retribution comes upon the cold-blooded scientists! It is not My Will: I have given them talents, I have given them intelligence to use for love of neighbour and love of God; alas they do not heed. They see others as lesser beings, before their vast intellect, their vast knowledge, and become hardened of heart! It is the sorrow beyond all sorrow. For each person who is in My service I give a profound anointing of Knowledge and discernment of My Truth.

That communication from you and the other doctors who are working with you, is not primarily for the Church's concern, but for the hospitals, the governments, the nations, the many nations, as well as of course, for My beloved Church. I assure you that the beloved John Paul himself is already attending upon the matter of what the physicians are actually doing in all the nations of the world with regard to "brain death" and organ transplants. I Myself have given John Paul great Wisdom. Rest assured you have shone a Light on all the darkness of what has been occurring, and which as you know could potentially grow much worse. My dearest, in your 'yes' to Me, I have accepted, and use you for this My instrument of Healing Love. The people in darkness must see the Light;(cf Isaiah9:1) they must be enlightened. It is for you, and such as you, to keep speaking the Truth. It is the Truth which sets mankind free. I Am the Truth; I did not say it is easy, but it is, shall We say, the cross given over to you in your surrender to Me, the Living God. Dear little one, in this Assignment you store up treasure in Heaven. This is hardly comfort for you at this moment in time, but in due course you will understand the magnificent blessings which await you because you have persevered in all faithfulness; enduring all in My Name, for Godly Love.

My little one, I tell you again, in your weakness is My Strength! (cf 2Cor12:9); I strengthen you profoundly to persevere in this fight. It cannot be fought by you in the public media, but it is now in the public's eye as never before. And so you have done this service to My people, that those who believe will seek informed consent. Omen keeps seeing a vision of many little golden flowers. The saints are with you little children, the saints are with you. It is to no avail; they(journalists distorting what we have said) are people of deceit! I assure you their attempts to indicate there is division and confusion in this Diocese is untrue, and as I have told you, they are caught up in their own evil snare for they are not intentionally, but incidentally because of their writing, causing multitudes to contemplate on the meaning of being donors; and what it means, the harvesting of organs. This comes to a people that has not even contemplated the meaning of what is occurring, and what could or might occur in their own families, their very own lives!

It is to this end that We are working My little one, that an Enlightened people; enlightened by My Church, will at last understand what this controversy is about, and that all details of the action of donating organs are clearly enunciated, that none can misunderstand the words of the beloved John Paul. We, the Living God are attendant upon all that We have given you, and upon the many that have received the Documentation. Little children, persevere, persevere, persevere! Endure all the blows that come your way in My Name. I accept them, I take them. I Bless you again and again. Down on your knees before Me you have won favour with your God. It is simple to tell them that you believe all life is sacred, as you pray, from the moment of conception until natural death. Little children, prevail in this belief.

It is My Will. Believe that much good will come of it. You are, as it were, freedom fighters for the freeing of souls from the darkness of evil. My little children, continue to believe in yourselves, because I believe in each one of you. I have taught you, trained you, molded you, fashioned you, strengthened you to be that individual which each one of you is today, and I am with each one of you constantly, that My Works of Merciful Love be done in and through each one of you. I am the Builder of a world of Peace and Love and order, where all will be joyful. My little ones, to this end you are, as construction workers. Mother and I attend upon you little children. There appears to be, among the public, a misplaced compassion, a maudlin compassion, when one is faced with a dying loved one, because of the dysfunction of a specific organ, and the physicians are expected to somehow, even magically, make the individual live and be well. We know this doesn't happen by organ transplant; yes, there is life, but at what cost to the individual; this is without considering the taking of a vital organ from the one who is called "donor." As you know, My precious little ones, the individual remains in free will; thus you find yourselves in this quagmire of confusion, of deceit, of manipulation, with regard to organ transplant and " brain death."

MARY: *My daughters, I ask you to wholeheartedly look at the Holy Infant in the crib in Bethlehem. Here you are gazing not only on the Perfection of Body and Soul, but upon the Perfection of the Lord God Most High! In this Body and Soul of Christ is, as it were encapsulated God; Almighty God! For Our Lord Jesus Christ is True God and True Man, as you know little children, and I have carried the Infant King, both in my heart and in my womb, the nine months preceding, and I have become the Christ-bearer; Theotokos! When you are children of Almighty God, you too, by Baptism and by a profound "yes," become Christ-bearers, for the Spirit of the Living God dwells in your heart and encompasses you in Divine Love; and you are born at the time Our God designates, and you live on this earth doing the Will of God, bringing the Love of Christ, the Light of Christ, the all-charity of Love, the compassion of Christ to your brothers and sisters, many of whom know not the Lord, have not been baptized, do not know that they are called to be temples of the Living God! Hosts of angels assist the children of Light now in these difficult times. You are always called to be a light to the world, for you are small sisters, small brothers of Jesus the Christ, the Light of the world. Nothing in Scripture is canceled out little chil-*

dren; it is the Word of God! Our Lord Jesus Christ is the Word of God! Little children, HOW can you place, as it were unclean animal parts, in these temples of the Living God? Study again the magnificence of King Solomon's Temple which held the Holy Spirit; the Shekinah in the Ark! This is how your precious bodies are designed to be, and when you attain Glory, you become clothed in the magnificent Glory of God! My little children, again I tell you; there can be no compromise with evil. Lesser evils are yet evil my little children, they are evils!

Proverbs 24:11-12:
Don't try to disclaim responsibility by saying you didn't know about it. For God, who knows all hearts knows yours, and he knows you knew. And he will reward everyone according to his deeds."

Read: 1. 2Corinthians 4:vs16-18, continuing into 5:vs1-10.
2. Holy Father, Pope John-Paul II's Address of Holy Father to International Congress on Transplants August 29, 2000,
3. Pope Warns Organ Transplant Conference of Abuses of Death Criteria

CHAPTER EIGHT.
"BRAIN DEATH.",EUTHANASIA, NHBD etc

MARK OF CAIN Gn 4:15.

JESUS: There is as it were, a generation of evil men who would lead My little ones like sheep to the slaughter, unknowing and totally accepting as My little lambs are. This must be prevented and thus I have called you to be one of My instruments in this great battle. Be with Me now - a moment of blessings in the Peace of My Presence. I am writing My Words within your heart and upon your soul that you may write the necessary papers... Rest in Me a while, little sweetheart of your Christ.—I am holding you to My Bosom. I bless you, caress you; I strengthen you, I inspire you; and then I set you back on your sturdy little legs to do that which you must do, little one. Love Me. It is sufficient! You walk ever in Great Light - be not afraid. Delightful and surprising actions occur now, for I hear your prayers and I make your pathway straight, leveling the hills and mountains. Little child, never enter an hour of despair. Cling to your Jesus, claim the Name of Jesus - you gain silent victory. Cling to Our Name and all goes according to Heaven's Design. My beloved one, a great blessing is upon you. Triune God!

The bodily death is a product of the action of the merciless one. The Queen of Heaven and of Earth, with the Son, is all-merciful Love and opposes all that the merciless one attempts to do on earth. As you know, We are presently living in the great time of trial, when the multitudes choose what you call humanism rather than Faith. You who belong to Me are Enlightened to know, that this is the work of the enemy which appears to be prevailing at this time. Therefore, write the discernments as you will; there are many works of Mercy in the form of Enlightenment, that We give over to you. You are an instrument for you are in the area of expertise - in the talents We have given unto you. Be not afraid to use them. The Lord your God is with you. The Queen of Heaven and Earth is with you, and many angels and saints assist you. Holy Light is ever upon you. **Give glory to God in the highest for His Mercy knows no end. The great and glorious God of all Creation is powerfully attendant upon His little creatures - humanity, who are precious to the Lord thy God. It is written that not a hair of your head falls except I know it; therefore, I Who proclaim - let it be; or let him be; or let her be; - and they come into Creation - do I not care about the moment of your death?** *I* AM GOD, SUPREME AMONG THE NATIONS. I KNOW AND I CARE!

But certain of mankind is ever proclaiming themselves 'gods' in grave error and transgression of My Laws. They control, and even terminate, the lives of their fellow men. This is known to Me. This is not pleasing to Me. This is bringing upon the earth, all mankind, My Wrath! 'Are you not afraid to play 'god,' I call to them, but they shun Me in their greatness. They do not serve Me. They believe only in their own free will - not knowing it is My gift to them, My gift that they might choose Me, choose Love - but they kill Love. Each life is sacred to the Lord your God, as you well know, yet your God is merciful and forgives mankind individually their transgressions; yes, even murder - for you serve a merciful and loving and forgiving God. There is one who will assist you - a priest of Holy Orders. We shall draw your attention to him, and he will be approachable...You will understand and he will indeed assist you My little one, even if the mind set of one person is altered by your Message, it is worthwhile; and I assure you that it is not only one person, but many, many who will respond to this Enlightenment, for We ensure that it is a profound Message.I repeat; I reiterate; It is the Lord your God, Who set the stars on their courses, that gives you the life-bearing planet, at the essential distance from the sun, that there might be life here! Now you toy with all these gifts of Mine, which cause life to be! The seeds of My Love have fallen on bare rock and are bearing no fruit(Mt13:20-21) in this community of practitioners of death. Each of My Own who believe in Me, walk on this earth as a lighted candle; for the Flame of Love, the power of the Holy Spirit is upon each one, even as it was upon My apostles and disciples at the time of the first Pentecost.(Acts 2:1-4).

Yet the matter of proclaiming an individual has attained bodily death, that many parts may be removed, as it were, commercially, for the use of other humans in hopes that they might live, is not pleasing to the Lord your God. A greater peril than body death is soul death. In the medical profession, many place their souls in grave peril by these actions of, as I have said, playing 'god.' My people have forgotten that eternal Life is in Heaven.(Rv22:1-5) There is no fountain of youth upon earth. It is but a temporary journey. You are called in Holy Scripture to keep your eyes turned towards Heaven your true and native Land. Therefore, the perfection of soul is always the priority. Choosing, in your eyes, that which is the lesser of evils, does not make anything right in the Eyes of the Father. You all know that the mystery of Love which I have encoded in each human; is individual, is unique, and is for *that* individual - and try as they may, the scientists run into block after block, in their strange attempts to do that which is unnatural and unseemly to the Eyes of God!

At the moment of their own death, when their souls, covered in these transgressions, [The Lord describes the souls of the perpetrators of "brain death" appear as appendages of their sins attached to the souls like great lumpy skin cancer all over], they come to Me in this state themselves, how shall they answer the Lord their God at that Judgment before which every man and woman must stand? There is indeed a time to be borne, and a time to die, as is written.(Qo3:2) Prideful man, chooses now a time for each infant to be borne; chooses which infant shall live, and which shall die. He chooses to prolong life when I am calling someone to come Home. He chooses to exterminate life at the discretion of the physician without consultation with Me, the Lord your God, the Giver of Life; (Ez13:19) Who takes His Own Home to Glory at the opportune moment! Indeed, a reign of death, a death culture is upon the earth! Up, you small band that can see, and fight! [quoting Our Lady of La Salette].The Lord your God is with you in this battle since you choose to proclaim the Truth, My small daughter of obedience.

Those who read the documents you have presented, must from then on answer to Me! It is incumbent upon each one who reads the documents to come before Me prayerfully, and choose whether they wish to live under a blessing or a curse! The physicians of the world themselves are precipitating the Wrath of God, in unison with certain other malefactors. My Sorrow is complete. The Mother of Sorrows, who has the most loving of Hearts, is pierced by that sword again and again, weeping copious tears for mankind, pleading for more time, that they will at last rethink their ways, their strategies. It would appear to be to no avail! And yet your Merciful God, causes a turn-around in this affair. Little one, the Lord your God is with you. I have given you a few comments. Should you choose to use them in your summary, you may. You have sufficient Inspiration and knowledge, and I Myself assist you in this matter. In the power of the Holy Spirit, Mother and I assist you as you prepare your letter now. Little children, the dark days and all the trials *have to be*; before the Dawn of Light is upon the world. It is rapidly approaching, yet you have time to save the souls of those who by their atheist beliefs, their humanist beliefs, are hurling their very souls into eternal darkness.(Rv14:6-13).

<u>Be at Peace, all is in the Hands of your Saviour Who desires the conversion of the physicians, a profound conversion like unto a U-turn in their thinking. You know well this is not readily acceded to by the many. It</u>

is a slow process, an ongoing process; it is in the time-frame which I the Lord God desire. Be at Peace.(1Th5:14)All life is sacred, human life; a Gift from the Living God. The Faith journey is given to each life as it enters earth and that soul is so precious to the Lord your God, it is given time on earth in the journey of Salvation, to find Me the Living God. As you well know many do not find Me except in suffering and trial, whether the affliction is spiritual or physical or providential, in some manner in their testing, in their formation, in their coming back to Me with all their hearts, a specific frame of time is essential. Sometimes it is brief, but sometimes it is prolonged; for each individual created is unique and each one is given a time to die.

That I know well what each scientific mind which shuns Me is doing; does not excuse them. That I see My plans for individuals altered, refuted, denied, and yet in patient perseverance with My beloved humanity, I am yet continuing, that they come at last to Enlightenment. It is **not** different than the pagan rituals of throwing individuals off the cliffs to their deaths, or into volcanoes or mutilated on altars; it is the fruit of healing will, gone awry. Persevere little children in all faithfulness. Some priests are reluctant at this point in time to deal with the grave consideration at hand in Our Letters. Forbearance daughter. That which you have written is pleasing to the Lord your God for it is indeed by direct Divine Inspiration and I am with you every step of the way My little one, My precious little one. We are breaking through a dark cloud of oppression. My little ones, the Lord Your God hears your prayers and blesses you. My little ones, Infinite Love is upon you. Little ones you are cherished of the Lord God and of your Heavenly Mother. Little ones you always are small instruments in the Hand of the Lord your God, so be not afraid. I hold you fast. I Am your Strength.

(I am feeling burdened by the amount of misinformation; how few people seem to have any problem with "brain death" and donor organs Be not burdened. Remember I carry the brunt of the Cross. I simply let you feel it periodically. My Will in this matter shall prevail. It is part of the Great Conversion of Humanity. It must be exposed that all may read and pray and ponder on this subject matter. Thus the multitudes operate in the realm of free will, at the mercy of the foe. And thus your teachings are pouring forth right now as upon a narrow road. It shall not always be like that. Very soon they begin to heed and come to Me; and I bless them with understanding and wisdom and knowledge. Persevere little ones, persevere. Persevere ! (Lk 8:15)(*The heaviness increases. Jesus showed us a window with a lantern which goes out. It appears to be a Church window, all blackened inside. Lord what are you telling us?)*That thou art in a time of rapidly approaching darkness, in the Church and in the scientific world; and in the world all about you; all about the earth. The visionary has done well in Enlightening many, but many remain in darkness.

Faithful Missionary is assigned to Enlighten the peoples of great intellect; Omen is assigned to the peoples of the First Nations, many of whom have great intellect but lack true spirituality, and to assist the street people as you call them, for they too are My Own, and many intellectuals find themselves there in the streets at rock bottom, despite their wisdom and knowledge and understanding; for they have taken a wrong turn, and need to come back to Me with all their hearts. Indeed I seek them out, I am the Good Shepherd.(Jn 10) I seek them out in you and through you, and all those who work in similar manner on My behalf. Little children, today by your Faith and perseverance, you have released many from a darkness of sin and death covering their faces. They have come into My Light, the Light of My Presence that they will read your Words Faithful Missionary, and will recognize Truth. I am Truth and I am with you. Jesus is here.

Humanity is in need of these Messages and they shall be given as they are, now for many to read and discern. All that you are doing is because you are a small instrument in My Hand, and it shall continue for thou art truly yielded unto the Living God. This Mission comes to fulfillment when a goodly number of physicians take the Words, even portions of the entire Message, to heart and begin to turn their life's work around in favour of Life. Do not be dismayed at anything that happens for We are in a time of serious war with the foe.(Eph6:10-20).Little children, the obstructions are many. Dastardly deeds are done in the Name of medical science in these times. It is My Will and Desire that it cease! Abruptly it stops! But in the interim one must address the many who perpetrate these crimes against Humanity, proclaiming them to be scientific feats. So We shall continue to inundate the many with these Words! Little children, don't worry about the obstructions; they are temporary. Mother and I attend.

Continue to pray for the doctors for they are deceived little children and they must come into the fullness of My Light. Deep reverential thoughts and discernments are necessary; many find themselves, as it were, too busy to take the time for prayer and reverential thought on these matters, that the Spirit of Enlightenment might come upon them. Therefore little children, pray for the many physicians not only here, but throughout the world. Persevere little one; I am with You. You will find yourself busy in a unique manner, evangelizing in My Name and in My Works. It falls into place according to My Design. There are many yet who need to hear and read these Words that they may take it to heart. I am causing it to happen in many and varied ways Myself. Little children you are yet in a nation which professes free will and freedom of speech. Be not intimidated; I am with you. I speak in you and through you. I bid you remain united with Me; thus you are speaking in Spirit and in Truth (cf Jn4:23-24)on behalf of My little ones whose bodies are increasingly being mutilated at a time when one should be considering that all Life is holy.

Little children, I am the Giver of Life; I choose the hour of Death; I hold the Keys! Little children, I have never given these Keys over to sinful man; they remain with Me! **I tell you again, I send My little ones to earth to accomplish a specific Mission of Merciful Love! Some finish it after only a few days, a few weeks, a few months. For others its a few years, and for others its many, many years! IT IS I, THE LORD YOUR GOD WHO CHOOSE THE TIME! Defer unto ME all those who are ill and trust ME. Pray for them. Little children it is a time now to pray for all those who are terminally ill. For one We need be concerned about the state of their soul as they approach Me, and secondly We need to be concerned about the state of their bodies while they are yet in the hospitals. Hospitals are intended for loving, healing care and sustenance; now it is a fearful place to enter!** It is more blessed to give than to receive.(Ac20:35) [*Our Lord is reminding the doctors of why they became doctors when they were young and idealistic*] Little ones, ask M to write the letter and be but one of the signatories. Attempt to get a goodly number. Indeed write both the provincial and the federal governments, for this is a gravely serious matter to your God, and is indeed for the protection of those who are helpless and vulnerable at the hands of the physicians. Physicians heal thyself, I call to each one of them, because many are in dire need of spiritual healing; a reminder perhaps of why they chose to be a doctor; where is that love and zeal for their fellow man now? Have they become cold and callous and do not see a living soul as just that; A LIVING SOUL! Do they see it, because it is afflicted, as something to utilize as a commodity?

My little one, into whom I have breathed Life; (Gn2:7) each one has a soul which is precious to Me; and that soul is an integral part of each individual, and MUST be regarded in the context of healing ANY individual. These times in which you are living are truly the threshold of the dawning of the new era in which ALL THINGS ON EARTH WILL BE CHANGED.(Rv 1:20) We ask you to simply persevere, moment by moment, step by step, day by day, We provide sufficient for the needs of each day.My little children, it is good to give as you know; it is pleasing to the Lord Your God, and yet little children, the peril of this concept of organ transplantation, brings one to that "slippery slope" of transgression of the Laws of Life, to a place where souls are imperiled, not only the victim who must die, but that of those who are performing those procedures. I am not oblivious to any of this. It occurs in free will, and you recognize little children that the scientific mind is not always ready to contemplate spirituality, especially the status of the soul in each human being. Were they open to such contemplation little children, there would be no abortions performed in hospitals. They have wandered far afield.

They deemed that, because something in scientifically possible, it should be done, the procedure should be practiced randomly. They do this without consideration of Truth, of that precious soul present in every body. You yourselves recognize that this is not generally known to the public and that is why there has been no great hue and cry against it. The masses are oblivious of what is occurring except when it happens to one of their loved ones, and only sometimes then does Enlightenment come to them about the error of these procedures termed organ harvesting. These procedures termed organ harvesting- these words are not pleasing to Me; this terminology is not pleasing to Me. These deeds are not pleasing to Me; to the contrary they are repugnant to Me! Little children I know that your hearts cry, when will the Holy Father address the subject; I know your prayers, and I know that you wait perseveringly in Faith for the needed words. You know well the controversy surrounding the issues of organ harvesting of transplants which take the life of another human. There are many, many words being spoken out and printed out, about the good of such procedures, with scant attention paid to the soul of the ones who die in the procedures.

Be assured that I Myself am attendant upon the beloved John Paul, and that he will most assuredly speak on the errors of the scientific world and what they are doing. Yes, he proclaims it is good to give, even when it is a vital organ, such as one kidney, but what you might refer to as the dark side of organ transplant is not revealed to the public, and is only scantly revealed to the beloved John Paul. And yet I cause him to know all that is occurring in this aspect of human behaviour today. You are aware of the many contentious issues he is dealing with in all the problems of the world today, and this is but one more for him to attend upon. In Spirit I communicate with this holy man and cause him to speak out clearly, even emphatically, upon this grave concern. The timing is according to My Design, so I ask you little children, yet again-wait patiently. Trust Me! All occurs according to My Plans which are for good. The little ones who loose their lives in the interim, are known to Me. There are different kinds of martyrs little children, as you have seen in the Nazi persecutions and in the Communist persecutions.

Leave them with Me, Your God Who is Mercy, Your God Who is Love, but continue to fight, for this is indeed a human rights issue. Peace; I am your Jesus. Indeed send copies to them and to any group that is in need of hearing these Words of which you are aware, because all are in need of Enlightenment. **This "brain death" ruling has just been foisted upon the people without their comprehension of what it means and what is entailed in the so-called harvesting of body parts.** Tell Me children, are these Bishops working towards the good of the soul, or are they concerned more with bodily life and death? *Lord, we understand that as shepherds they are more concerned with the soul.* Then it is essential that they too, partake of a soul searching themselves, to understand the issue at hand. Again little children, the words, the propaganda of those who promote this form of medicine is glib, and if one does not look deeply into the issue, one can be readily deceived. Little children, there are so many causes being fought for in the world today, that some people see this as a small cause at this time, and yet as you gaze upon the known horrors of organ transplant, you know that it is an important issue which must be addressed.

My little children, I will cause Enlightenment to come to the many brave priests and Bishops, and to the Cardinal who must deal with this issue. Little children, since I am fully cognizant of these concerns, I assure you that the beloved John Paul will speak in due course. He is, as you know, a wise man, and he seeks all aspects of each issue thoroughly before making an address. Some have attempted to, shall we say, withhold certain aspects of organ harvesting from him and those who attend upon these matters. The Truth will out as you say. He knows and he will speak, and as is ever the case when he speaks, the bishops will, as a rule conform to his Authority. Tell Me little children, countless individuals who go into shock, or what they call 'little deaths,' and they begin to come towards Me, 'The Light'; but they are unready. Were I to take them then, grave would be the consequences for those souls; and yet I cause them to return to their bodies, and they are changed because of their, what they call their near-death experience, and they begin to realize how precious life is, and how fleeting, and how readily it may be taken from them; - bodily death little children! And they begin to change their souls, their hearts and minds, to the Way, the Truth and the Life, that they may come cleansed and purified and abandoned to their Lord God, at the time I next call them into Eternal Light, into Eternal Joy. This is one means of Enlightening the people.

Countless books have been written, but without understanding that I am the God of Merciful Love; I do not wish a soul to come unready before Me their Judge

And yet the, what you call the new-agers, the witchcrafters proclaim these things, and proclaim, is there life after death? Have I not told My people, that I came to give LIFE TO THE FULLEST! TO THE FULLEST MEANS ETERNALLY IN MY PRESENCE IN GLORY AND LIGHT. This has been a means of deceiving My people into seeking to follow the witches who proclaim to have secret knowledge of life after death. IT IS NO SECRET! I AM GOD! I AM ETERNAL! I GIVE ETERNAL LIFE ! I DO NOT TAKE IT BACK! ETERNALLY WITH ME IN GLORY, OR ETERNALLY IN SUFFERING. I CALL ALL TO CHOSE NOW, BY RE-EXAMINATION OF THEIR, SHALL WE SAY LIFESTYLES, THEIR PRIORITIES, THEIR VERY CHARACTERS, THEIR FAITH OR LACK THEREOF. And again forthwith I bid you Peace; I am with you. Indeed every Christian physician should be involved. That is not to say that every Christian physician shall be involved; and yet with your perseverance and prayer many things are happening for this work which you are doing, IS *MY* WORK, IS *MY* PLAN, IS *MY* DESIRE !

I Myself will move a goodly number of physicians to agree to sign, for it is apparent, it is obvious to those working in the very fields of medicine where this is taking place, that what is happening is not entirely as it should be, as you well know. This could delay or even threaten the so-called business of harvesting body parts, and so there is a large element of opposition; yet this Cause is espoused and MUST go forward according to My Will. Remember, Victory is in MY NAME : JESUS! Beloved, it is as you sense, a matter of urgent concern. Even so, proceed in Peace; I make all things fall into place. It is essential that the pro-life movement become active in this issue and that the general public recognize what is happening. At this point in time the best means is indeed through the pro-life movement, who already have widespread activities and information pouring forth to the public to those who would heed. At the meeting which you shall attend, you will meet others who know and believe as you do in the truth of what is occurring. The concept of wrongful deaths, is one means of the physicians re-examining their positions now that this knowledge has been spread throughout the continent.

The juxtaposition, by human intellect is the concept of Life and Death! It is inverted to what the Lord your God Desires; indeed Decreed! We have before Us, those who would make clone babies; those who would in essence, kill for body parts for money, for power, or for pride; We have those who choose whether a child shall live or die; those who choose whether an elder shall live or die; and whensoever one is injured, they go like indiscriminate scavengers looking for body parts to remove.[*Our Lord shows Omen the crows at a road kill.*]Let each of them who read this consider well, that they may one day be brought to a hospital, never to know what treatment they shall receive at the hands of the medical scientists; consider well what this means and speak and act now, because it is already happening to unknown numbers of your brothers and sisters on this Earth! I the Lord God Bless you little one. You realize that I must thin out My Army of faithful for this attack, like unto that which occurred with Gideon's army so that there are few of you, but you are powerful by Faith; in Faith you are victorious. My little one, you are a key part of what is occurring. J M and M remain faithful, unchanged and true to character in what they believe. Dr J believes, but is being as it were, pulled in different directions. It is imperative that you continue to pray for him, for this is a source of torment, when one knows what is Truth but is reluctant to continue speaking out because of the attacks! It s painful for that individual. Therefore it is imperative that you continue praying for him little children. Yes J is young , and has many commitments, and runs the risk of being ostracized; so you see, I know well the delicate position he finds himself in.

As you know in your own specialty that certain individuals will disagree with you vehemently on this subject, yet I ask you to trust Me and continue; We are ever victorious little one, for you have a union with Your God which is powerful. Also, this union with Your God, is incomprehensible to the atheists, the agnostics, the humanists, who cannot conceive of such a relationship with the Living God, for the eyes and ears are not opened; the skins are yet on their eyes! My little ones, they do not see the magnificence of Your God's Design for Creation; for Humanity. They are actually working to thwart the Great Design, and thus it is that We are speaking out on behalf of Life. Therefore, pray for those; there are many who desire to support you knowing that it is Truth, and yet are feeling vulnerable and are weak to take up the banner. Yet there will be sufficient of you who do, that the Cause of Life prevails. You shall live to see a different measure of what is life and what is death; trust Me!

I Myself protect you in this siege against you. I do not permit anything to happen to you. You have a Work to complete; united with Me it shall be so! Militant angels attend upon this letter and each copy of this letter, for it is of the essence that it be rapidly distributed, that the people of God at least know what is happening, for the people of God are the giving, the loving, the charitable ones, who can be at times deceived by the manipulations of those who have another agenda. Thus it is My Desire that your letter, as it is, go forth, that the many be Enlightened as to the perils of signing these donor card without full comprehension of what could occur. There are many doctors who work in their own cause dispassionately in dealing with their patients, and these are not pleasing to the Lord. Continue to pray for their conversions that Love may enter into their work. Little ones, you who have lived in the fullness of Life, are held as it were, as a people set apart and purified in the fire of My Love and I use you also, each one in a unique fashion, for My Works of Merciful Love. In My Great Mercy, I give time for all to come back to Me with all their hearts; yet in My Great Mercy, there is suffering and sorrow. You have well noted that it is often only in this suffering and sorrow, that various individuals at last fall on their knees before the Living God, seeking My Mercy, which is ever attendant upon them.

My little prodigals are in so great a need of Divine Solace, yet it takes some sorrowful event, even tragic event, before they come back to Me with all their hearts. Little children, those of you who know, such as you, I ask to continue in all persevering prayer for the conversion of the many! My Love, what would you ask of Me further. Even in coma, even in 'brain death,' My precious little ones, My precious, precious souls are useful to Me, in the Healing Love of God, in the Healing Love for mankind as evidenced in this child! (Audrey Santo)Little children, every God-given moment of Life has meaning. Little children, when you say there is no life in a person who is yet alive, you might as well say there is no life-giving oxygen in the air you are breathing, for all is a Gift from Me, the Living God! Little children, Man is in a sorry state of confusion at this time with regard to Human Life, and the value of Human Life.

When Peter walked on Earth people tried to get in his shadow for healing; and the saints, though they are ascended into Glory; prayers to them, and touching the essence of what had been their Life on Earth, individuals too are healed! Little children, Life is a continuum; it does not stop at the moment of bodily death, but is ongoing; and as long as there is Life in that body, the soul is present there! This seems a puzzlement to modern man; it is very simple and has always been known to My beloved Humanity, until the spirit of confusion has come in this century. Little children, those who already as Christians, believe in the soul, accept these matters readily; the ones who consider themselves to be atheists or agnostics, linger a bit in this discernment; yet I shall cause to occur, events in the matter of "brain death," in the matter of dying, to cause Humanity to know most assuredly, each human is gifted with a soul -pure spirit! Little children, believe in these articles and recognize them, and pray for further clarification to come to these doctors who are seeking that which is true with regard to a human being, who is not simply body like the animals. Persevere prayerfully and We shall be discussing this matter further in the future.

Those scientist practitioners of these procedures are going to find themselves in certain difficulties in what they are attempting to do, for most assuredly it is not of Me. Much of what is not of Me is occurring in laboratories and hospitals through- out the so-called civilized world. They are doomed to failure, for I am not with these people in these enterprises. They have not united prayerfully with Me nor do they recognize Me. And therefore you will see such scientists becoming frustrated and having tried all that they understand, will cease to work in this direction. Little children, they do not recognize the possibility, they refuse to recognize the possibility, of a form of germ warfare attacking humans severely through the use of animals in these experiments. The end result could be far worse than that which they are endeavouring to study and cure!Cling to Me, you are safe in Me; I see you through the trials. Little children, though things look bleak at times, know that I am with you and that I bring you through into the Light once again. My little children, those of you who can see, who can hear, who are truly yielded unto the Will of the Father, who do know, love and serve the Lord, sometimes you feel heavy burdened. Don't! I am with you; I carry the main weight of all. I do not give you more than you can "handle "as you say. I am with you, united with you.

Oh, if you could only see how much Heaven is assisting you in all these efforts which you are making! They are not unimportant to your God. In each one of your lives little children, you are storing treasure in Heaven and you will realize on a Glorious Day of the Lord, just what was occurring because of your trials, your sufferings; what were the fruits of your prayer life! Little children, believe that you are pleasing to the Lord your God, and be filled with the Joy of My Presence and persevere. My precious little ones, an anointing comes upon you this day which is holy to the Lord; Blessings and Graces come upon you. My little ones, always rejoice in the Love of the Lord, and remember this month which is given over to Our Mother, and little children, love your Jesus and love your Mother; We are the Ones Who Love you so!

I speak clearly in the Trinity, for you are beloved of the Father, Son and Holy Spirit! We Love you little children, I tell you again most tenderly, most totally and eternally. You are precious, precious to the Lord your God; you are beloved of Jesus and Mary, rejoice in this Our Loves Union! In the Name of Jesus you pray, and I am attendant upon you. Peace; I am your Jesus of Merciful Love; be not too much aggrieved about the dreadful things you see and hear in these times; you well know that you are living in the time of great trial, and before My Return, these things have to be. You are aggrieved and concerned about one who has been ensnared by the ways of the world. As you pray little children continuously for the conversion of sinners, the Salvation of souls, as you do daily, you may single out a certain one or other that you know at times specifically in your prayers, but know that all your prayers are heard in Heaven, and it is always your God's desire to say yes to the precious little faithful ones. Even so, all must go according to the Father's

Design, and all as you know, is contingent upon the God given free will of the individual for whom you are praying. *Jesus shows Omen a beautiful full blown rose and says to me:* I am attendant upon you; I have written My Word in your heart, as has Mother; in the Power of the Holy Spirit it is so. Divine Inspirations ensure that you persevere in the works We are doing together.

The Assumption of the Mother of God into Heaven; She came not just soul, but body and soul, for there is an integrity of unity between body and soul, for each human being. It is not the Will or Desire of your God, that these disruptive activities, in this aspect of the medical field occur, and continue to occur. There is no recognition of soul, and a decreased recognition of the integrity of each human body. You see clearly this is not of Me. You await a pronouncement. Therefore again a bid you little ones, endure, persevere, believe! I am Truth and the beloved John Paul, in due course, speaks out Truth. You ask that it be clear, without any ambiguity, and it shall be thus, for he too has learned of all the disgraceful and corruptive ways that are occurring in the treatment of the human's body during this absence of recognition of the human soul. Allow them to unite with you for they are of Me. I lead them as I lead thee, as I will. Trust Me. You may also contact the two addresses in Boston. I am opening doors for thee little one, because it is My Word, My Work, which I wish My beloved humanity to know, most specifically men of science, to know. One must proceed diligently, winning as it were, one individual at a time, to recognize that man is both body and soul; to win them over to this Truth. Therefore I cause you to have, as it were, many irons in the fire.

Continue to address this matter to Me in the Adoration Chapel, and I Who am Truth, will prevail, and Truth will become known to many more about the world. Little children, you are as yet front line warriors and you must remain so in this time of spiritual warfare which is upon the Earth. When you unite with Me at Adoration, My Healing Love, My Truth, My Mercy pours forth, wheresoever necessary on the Earth. Bring Me your Cause at each visit and leave it there with Me. At this time it is the chosen Way. The Virtue of Love is such that I bless you, I bless MB, I bless all those who have permitted themselves to become Enlightened to My Truth with regard to what is being called "brain death." I Myself inspire all those who hear him to heed the words well, to become supporters. I would again suggest that a movement proclaiming Truth about so-called "brain death" be established, perhaps it could have its roots where MB is speaking. Remember I always cause My faithful little ones to have humble beginnings like the humble stable of Bethlehem. Thus do I start My Great Movements. I have need of a movement to release Humanity from the deceit of so-called "brain death," and subsequent surgeries and abuses of the bodies of those who are defined medically as "brain dead."

Be not afraid to speak the Truth whenever and wherever it is possible; I protect My Own. I do not leave you as you might say, out on a limb. I am profoundly united with you, My precious little ones of faithfulness. I Myself will cause many doctors to see that so-called "brain death" is not death, and this will cause them some anguish until they too must react and act as you and your small group are acting. Therefore, any letters, any speeches, any communications you can make on this subject, I will highly reward! When a doctor has even a niggling doubt, as a scientist he must seek truth on that subject; and I Myself will Enlighten them, for this Cause is dear to My Heart, for it is not My Will that My beloved little ones, have their bodies treated in the manner which is occurring now. You may have a two-part statement; one scientific, and one , not necessarily limited as a Christian, but proclaim as a believer, that each man has a soul. [Our Lord shows turbaned people who do not believe that "brain death" is right either.] When you have an unconscious person and the government is telling you that you have to report to them, it is in a sense the enemy telling you to kill the one you love the most.

It is a Sorrow of these times. It is at best, a symptom of the Great Apostasy which is upon the earth, that mankind has gone so far away from their God; that mankind disregards the Laws of God; that mankind has brought itself to this state of ill-health that causes them to believe that body parts are warranted. Even so, nothing is impossible to your God. When you look at it today, you do not see how this can be changed, but I assure you, your God has a Plan, and most assuredly, these evil practices in due course come to an end. Believe that the Epistle of Love bears an important role in this change of heart, this turning things around once more Once the horror has been exposed , revealed for what it is, backers come to the fore. Little children you are never alone. I send reinforcements to fight on the side of Love.

Therefore believe that the fight against euthanasia and the fight against the so-called "brain death" and the fight against the so-called "harvesting" of body parts must prevail. Is it not written, when you see a brother doing wrong you must speak out? (Mt18:15-17 Then remember, I have strengthened you for the battle, and I continue to strengthen you, for you do not fight the battle yourself; you are, each one, an instrument in the Hands of your God, to bring Light and Truth to Mankind. The darkness at this time on earth, is immense and there are few lighting the Way. You are being called to be such lights but remember, you are a light in the Hand of your God, and you are safe in Me. All harsh words hurled against you little children, in this My Cause, fall on Me as whiplashes and they are no more. I strengthen you; hold your armour-of-God(Ep6:10-20), fast about you. Know that My Church is protected by Me, the Living God, and that legions of angels under the banner of St Michael, protect My little warriors in a shield, an invincible Shield of Protection,(Eph6:10-20) so that those who are united with Me, living in My Truth, need not fear. Nothing occurs in your lives, little ones, except by My Design. Do not be dismayed little ones, when you are under attack; let it be for your increasing courage, your increase of Fortitude, and this is always little children, purifying for your souls. Fear not, I am with you and going before you!

The Virtue of Love is such that I the Lord God, bid you know that I am cognizant of what is occurring with each soul, and the beloved John Paul, is cognizant of this great crisis, of so-called "brain death" and the extermination of many souls, without consideration of your God. Consider well little children, that even as your activities and plans are frequently thwarted by the enemy, or those pawns of the enemy, this does indeed occur in what the beloved John Paul is doing. Walls of flame surround those who persevere in these practices which are unclean, indeed an abomination before the Lord. Rest assured , feel free to send the Words to them. With regard to the many other Bishops, wait; refrain from acting, for some of them will be in contact with the Holy Father as they pray and discern to make the decisions. They are vividly aware, those who work with John Paul, of the issue of " brain death" and the implications of what occurs by this pronouncement of "brain death." There is a matter beyond concern for the soul in "brain death" as you know. That matter is money, greed, profit, power, control; all these facets of pride in those who are removing the organs from the comatose victims, are working, shall We say for false idols and not for your God, and so there is a great resistance to changing these procedures which would drastically limit what is referred to as the harvesting of organs. The question of God does not enter the minds of those who are working in a cold-blooded manner both in the industries of abortion and organ harvesting which is not of Me; by their very names they cannot be of Me.

Thus you know well little children that I am with you and that I work through many who will be present there who know Me, some only nominally, and yet it is a time to inspire them further into Truth. Doubt not little children, We are victorious, in allowing the Truth of "brain death" and organ transplant to be fully revealed. Little children, in all confidentiality I address you thus; the beloved John Paul is assailed with all the information regarding Human Life, from the atrocities that are being carried out on the human embryo, now through all that is occurring in the realm of so-called birth control and abortion, to the scandals occurring in the transplantation of human body parts, to the concerns of euthanasia, and the taking of lives in so-called "brain death." Urgent shall We say verbal warfare is occurring especially in the matter of cloning and stem cells and the like, and these are rapidly brought before the Holy Father.

His words are imminent for it is My Will that he speak them in great detail. Little children, Death speaks to the world through the medical scientists and through the organization that is known as "Planned Parenthood;" both of these are in opposition to Me, the God of Life and Love, and thus the Pope, the Holy Father John Paul, refers to the Body of Christ as the "People of Life", and I have chosen you to be a voice, for Life, and you shall continue to serve and work in this manner.

A CHRISTIAN DEATH.

"The Message you bring is not only to M but to all those who will heed, will respond. It is a Message truly of hope, because you know there is little hope for the terminally ill in these days. Little children, you have been told that the time of death is a time of trial between God and the enemy. Know this: were the people to come to Me without fear, there would be no trial. I'm just asking you to come unto Me in Glory.

There is no fear for those who are united with Me - not more fear than any new experience in life. Any great fear should not be there, for I am calling you Home at the appointed time, when the Mission you have been assigned has been completed. Therefore, I bid you know that many, most in the world, have a great but irrational fear of death in the eyes of your God; for united with Jesus there is nothing to fear. I Myself defeated death for you; therefore, fear not little children.

CREMATION

Was I cremated! Was Mother cremated! Was Lazarus cremated! Were the saints cremated! The saints who remain incorrupt; are they not a great testimony! Were they to be cremated at the moment of death, where would this testimonials be?

MARY: *Mother is attendant dear children! You know he*{the Holy Father, Pope John Paul II} *is My beloved priest-son. There are forces working against Truth everywhere, yes even in the Church established by Our Lord Jesus Christ. This is a serious offense to God, and a great heartache in the Heart of the Mother of the priesthood. The obstruction to the Holy Father speaking out in this grave matter, is now being removed and you shall soon hear the desired words. Yes they shall be clear and readily understood. It is not the desire of the Living God, that one individual be killed to cause another individual to continue to live. It were better for each one to pray with regard to the state of their souls- each one, and have regard to the Merciful Love of Our God, than to enter into these undertakings.*

You see now the proof of the suffering and the killing, brother against brother. In a

prolonged hour of Mercy you are still called to persevere patiently, awaiting the action of your God through the Holy Father and indeed it comes forth clearly; the Truth is spoken clearly, but will all heed? Mother Mary says very solemnly, *Cain has killed his brother,*[Gn4:8] *and humanity- they are killing their brothers and sisters in every imaginable way. Corruption is upon this world, and yet in this room, you ask for the needed graces which are being poured out upon you little ones.*

Our Lady says *"Little child, the saint who assists you in this work is known as Saint Luke, is he not? We bless you in and through Saint Luke in this work and We bid you recall that Jesus, the Great Physician Himself, is profoundly assisting you. Little children, the wages of sin is death - death of the soul; so perilously close to some of you. Speak out at any and every given opportunity against this culture of death.*

Ezekiel 13vs 19-21: Against the false prophets.
Proverbs 24:11-12:
Don't try to disclaim responsibility by saying you didn't know about it. For God, who knows all hearts knows yours, and he knows you knew. And he will reward everyone according to his deeds."

Genesis 9:4-6

I give you everything, with this exception: you must not eat flesh with life, that is to say blood in it. I will demand of your life-blood. I will demand an account from every beast and from man. I will demand an account of every man's life from his fellow men. He who sheds man's blood shall have his blood shed by man, for in the Image of God man was made.

Pope John Paul 11's Apostolic Letter, "Motu Proprio" *Dolentium Hominum,*
[Speaks of man in his entirety and in his somatic-spiritual unity.]

The "diagnosis brain death" ignores the spiritual life [soul] of the so-called corpse!
How else could Dr Shewmon document prolonged survivors of "brain death"
(see tables following).

TABLE 1. Prolonged Survivals in "Brain Death"
56 Cases for Meta-Analysis

Note: Blank cells represent missing information; dashes signify "test not done". "NSR" in apnea-test column implies missing information concerning formal apnea test, nor that a formal apnea test was not performed.

SUR-VIVAL (days)[1]	AGE at BD (yrs)	ETIOL-OGY	APNEA TEST	EEG	CBF TEST	CT/MRI	AUT OPSY	OTHER CLINICAL FEATURES	Trans ind. Even	Reason for Support	COMMENTS[2]	PLACE	NAME	REFERENCE
7(5)?	24	IIE	NSR	I	–	–	–	fl, DTR,↓Tt[4], Dt[5],↓TRf[6]	W[7]	preg+	25→26 wk, 920g[10]	Buffalo, NY	case 2	Dalton et al 1982
7	2 m	2YI	NSR	I	–	–	RB[15]	fl,↓T	S	NDC[12]	retrosp dx[13]	Springfield, MA	case 2	Rowland et al 1983
7	12	2SR	NSR	I	–	–	–	fl,↓T, wn	S	NDC	retrosp dx	Springfield, MA	case 3	Rowland et al 1983
7	42	2YC	NSR[14]	–	C[3]	–	-[31]		S	cult		Hiroshima, Japan	case 36	Arita et al 1993
7	48	IHV	NSR	I	C[18]	–	–		S	cult		Hiroshima, Japan	case 39	Arita et al 1993
8	13	2YC	NSR	I	C[19]	–	–		S	cult		Hiroshima, Japan	case 26	Arita et al 1993
9	9	2SR	NSR			–	–	fl,↑T, wn	W	?		Springfield, MA	case 5	Rowland et al 1993
9	10 m	IIM	NSR			–	–	fl,↓T, wn	W	?		Springfield, MA	case 4	Rowland et al 1993
9.5	40[19]	IHV[20]	-			–	–	↓BP[28]	S	res?[30]	prospective study[22]	Taiwan		Hung & Chen 1995
9.5[23]	39	7TF	NSR	I[8]		CT[3]	–	↓BP	S+	cult		Osaka, Japan	case 11	Yoshioka et al 1986
9.6	50	IHV	NSR	I		CT[27]	–	fl,+Y	S+	cult		Osaka, Japan	case 13	Yoshioka et al 1986
12	9	2ST	NSR	I		–	RB[28]	↓BP	S	NDC	retrosp dx	Springfield, MA	case 1	Rowland et al 1983
12.5	58	IHV	NSR	I	C[29]	–	–		S+	cult		Osaka, Japan	case 16	Yoshioka et al 1986
13	46	IHV	NSR		+[8]	–	–	↑BP	S	cult		Hiroshima, Japan	case 27	Arita et al 1993
13	61	2TV	NSR	I		CT[11]	–	fl,↓T	S+	cult		Osaka, Japan	case 12	Yoshioka et al 1986
15	10 m	2YA	NSR			–	RB[13]		S	NDC	retrosp dx	Springfield, MA	case 13	Rowland et al 1983
15	53	2YC	NSR		C[12]	–	–		S	cult		Hiroshima, Japan	case 14	Arita et al 1993
16.5	29[24]	ITP[19]	+		–	–	–		S	res?	prospective study	Taiwan		Hung & Chen 1995
21	31	2YC	NSR		–	–	+[3]		S	cult		Hiroshima, Japan	case 7	Arita et al 1993
22(20)[18]	5 m	IHB[17]				–	?[3]		S+	pw	dx cert[13]	Queens, NY[29]	Mariah Scoon	Onishi 1996; Ramirez 1996; Crocker 1996
24	3	2SU	NSR			–	-[10]	fl,↓T	S	NDC	retrosp dx	Springfield, MA	case 6	Rowland et al 1983
25	25	IHV[9]	NSR[12]			CT[13]	–	DL↓BP,↓T,ARDS[15], NG[24]	W	preg+	25→28 wk[5]	San Diego, CA		Cantanzaric et al 1997
26	11	7T	NSR			–	RB[18]	fl[18],↓T, wn	Sr	NDC	retrosp dx	Springfield, MA	case 7	Rowland et al 1983
26	40	7T	NSR	I	C+[10]	–	–		S	cult		Hiroshima, Japan	case 23	Arita et al 1993
27	3	2YD	NSR			–	RB[32]	fl,↓T	S	NDC	retrosp dx	Springfield, MA	case 14	Rowland et al 1983
28	9	7T	NSR	I		–	–		S	cult		Hiroshima, Japan	case 16	Arita et al 1993
29[15]	25	2X[26]			C[1][33]	–	+[8]		W	preg.	21→25 wk, 1410oz[24]	Augusta, GA	Donna Piazzi	Evaizen 1986; Thompson 1986

Chronic "Brain Death" - Tables

SUR-VIVAL (days)[1]	AGE at BD (yrs)	ETIOL OGY	APNEA TEST	EEG	CBF TEST	CT / MRI	AUT OPS Y	OTHER CLINICAL FEATURES	Terminal NM Event	Reason for Support	COMMENTS[2]	PLACE	NAME	REFERENCE
30	23	2YC	NSR						W	kg	Harvard crit	Torrington, CT		Fabro 1982
38	11	2SR	NSR				RB		S	NDC	retrosp dx	Springfield, MA	case 16	Rowland et al 1983
39	18	2TV						NG	W	preg+	dx cert (13→15)→(18→20) wk	Erlangen, Germany	Marion Ploch	Hunt 1992; Ridley 1992; Doyle 1992; Karcher 1992
~39	34	1HV							W	preg+	(21,24)→(27-32) wk; dx cert unofficial	Darlington, England	Deborah Bell	McKee 1992; Hunt 1992
40	43	2TV	NSR	1		CT		↓BP	S+	cult	dx cert	Osaka, Japan	case 14	Yoshioka et al 1986
~48(42)	31	1HV							W	preg+	28 s34 wk, 4#11oz	Syracuse, NY	Tracy Bucher	AP 1991; Colen '91
44	31	1HV				CT		↓T, ↑↑↑, ↓BP	W	preg+	27 →31 wk, 489?/oz	Syracuse, NY	"Sheila" (=Tracy Bucher?)	Nettling et al 1991
46	7	2YK	NSR				RB	fl, ↓T	S+	NDC	retrosp dx	Springfield, MA	case 11	Rowland et al 1983
49	25	1HV	↓	e	C	CT	RB	↓BP, ↓T, DI, ↓psi, UTI	S+	preg+	15 →22 wk	Novara, Italy		Antoniotti et al 1992
53	34	1N							W	preg+	dx cert; 26→33 wk, 4#5oz	Santa Clara, CA	Marie Odette Henderson	AP 1987; Riela 1986; Everson 1986
54	19	7F	NSR	1		CT		↓BP	S+	cult	22 →30 wk	Osaka, Japan	case 15	Yoshioka et al 1986
56	35	3							W	preg+	dx cert	Allentown, PA		Diehl et al 1994
58	15	1TG							W	preg	25 →33 wk, ~54	San Bernardino, CA	Tanya Music Rivera	AP 1989; Wienco 1989
0.3(64)	27	1O	NSR	1	V	CT	RB	↓apnea, ↓↑↑T, DI, pneu, sep, UTI	W	preg+	22 →31 wk, 1446g	San Francisco, CA		Field et al 1988; Sabin 1993
65	13	1TP	e	1		CT		fl, ↓BP, DI, pneu, ↓↑↑, pali, anv	S	par	transf to SSF	California	"DES"	Shewmon (in preparation)
~70	31	1HV	NSR	1	S	CT	RB	↓T, ↓BP, NG, DI, pneu	S	preg+	21 →31 wk, 1600g	Oulu, Finland		Heikkinen 1985; Natalizon 1989
71	49	2YC	NSR	1			RB	nul cd, G&H, sep, pneu, DI, UTI	W	leg		Syracuse, NY		Paski et al 1982; Kim et al 1982
104	28	1TG						↓↑?↑T, inf, ↓Thg	W	preg+	dx cert, 21(17) → 30(32) wk, 4#15oz	Oakland, CA	Trisha Marshall	AP 1993a&b, SF Ex 1993a&b
~165	20	1HV							W	preg+	16 →31 wk, 3#3oz	Rochester, NY	Lisa Nottingham	AP 1997
107	30	2TV	NSR	1	N	CT	RB	↓T, DI, ↓pili, ccp infl, anem, ↓↓BP, cdl, DIC	W	preg+	15 →32 wk, 1555g	Burlington, VT		Fleischman 1997
112	23	1HV	NSR	1	S			pneu, sep, UTI, arrhy, cdl, DIC	W	fam		New Orleans, LA		Bernstein et al 1989
123	13	7	1	1	S			home on vent	W	par		Sarasota, FL	Teresa Hamilton	Klein 1982
133	9	7X		1				↓T, ↓BP, env, late dx, dipsn	S	par, leg		Washington, DC	Yusef Camp	Palm Bch Post 1991; Sager Weltauch; Weiser 1990a&b
203	4	1B	NSR				RB	fl, ↓T, wa	S	NCD	retrosp dx	Springfield, MA	case 12	Rowland et al 1983

Chronic "Brain Death" – Tables

SUR-VIVAL (days)[1]	AGE at BD (yrs)	ETIOL-OGY	APNEA TEST	EEG	CBF TEST	CT/MRI	AUT-OPSY	OTHER CLINICAL FEATURES	TERM-INAL EVENT	REASON for SUPPORT	COMMENTS[2]	PLACE	NAME	REFERENCE
~223[170]	15[172]	2y5[173]	+[174]	+[175]	S[176]			↓BP, cont'd at[177], transf to rehab[178]	S	par			Ronald Chamberlain[179]	Spike & Greenlaw 1995
229[180]	17	2YC[181]	+[182]	+[183]	N[184]		—	↓BP, NG[185]	Sr	par	dx confirmed x7[186]	Kansas City, MO	Phillip Rader	Cranford 1989; Nodell 1988a
~411[187]	14	IN[188]	+[189]	?	—		—	↑T, seize, G, home on vent[190]	S	par	dx confirmed x2	Pittsburgh, PA		Plum[191]
924[192]	1 d	2Y[193]	+[194]	+[195]	—		—	BS, wn, late dx dispute[196], NG, grow[197], pub[198], transf to chron care facility[199]	W	par		Queens, NY	"Baby A"	Cranford et al 1996
1856[200]	3 d	2YC[201]	+[202]	±[203]	N[204]	CT[205]	—	G[206], home on vent[207] grow[208], LTT, sep	Sr[209]	par	dx confirmed multiple times[210]	Oakland [CA?]	"Baby Z"	Cranford et al 1996
>5291[211]	4	IM[212]	+[213]	F[214], EP[215]	X, MRA[216]	CT[217], MRI[218]	N/A	↓T[219], DI[220], ↓BP[221], wn, inv[222], inf[223], G, grow[224], to rehab, home on vent[225]	—	par	necrop dx[226]	confidential	"TK"	Shewmon (in preparation)

TABLE 2. Prolonged Survivals in "Brain Death"
~119 Cases with Insufficient Individual Information for Meta-Analysis

Note: Blank cells represent missing information; dashes signify "test not done". "NSR" in apnea-test column implies missing information concerning formal apnea test, *not* that a formal apnea test was not performed.

SUR-VIVAL (days)	AGE at BD (yrs)	ETIOL OGY	APNEA TEST	EEG	CBF TEST	CT/ MRI	AUT OPS Y	OTHER CLINICAL FEATURES	Termi nal Event	Reason for Support	COMMENTS	PLACE	NAME	REFERENCE
7[a]	?[a]	?[a]	9[a]	?[a]	+[a]	CT[a]	RB[a]		S	cult?	multi-center study	Japan[a]	17 cases	Takeuchi et al 1987
8									S	cult?	multi-center study	Japan	13 cases	Takeuchi et al 1987
9									S	cult?	multi-center study	Japan	8 cases	Takeuchi et al 1987
10									S	cult?	multi-center study	Japan	8 cases	Takeuchi et al 1987
11									S	cult?	multi-center study	Japan	11 cases	Takeuchi et al 1987
12									S	cult?	multi-center study	Japan	3 cases	Takeuchi et al 1987
7-11[a]	8-54[a]	IH, TT[a]	9[a]					Group II hemodynamically stable	S, W[a]	res	Group II Rx'd with T$_3$ + cortisol[a]	Nara, Japan	"Groups I & II" (~5 cases)[a]	Taniguchi et al 1992
14(?)[a]	27	IHV[a]		9[a]				↓BP, ↓T[a], pneu, GH	S+[a]	preg	dx cert[a] 21→23 wk	Brooklyn, NY	Rosemarie Manicatso	Cohn 1977; Meyer 1977
13									S	cult?	multi-center study	Japan	2 cases	Takeuchi et al 1987
14									S	cult?	multi-center study	Japan	5 cases	Takeuchi et al 1987
16.5±12.2 (4-54)	9-54[a]	?[a]	4[a]	1			?[a]	DI[a], hemodynamically stable	W[a]	res	Rx'd with vasopressin + epinephrine	Oyata, Japan	"Group 2" (16 cases)[a]	Kinoshita et al 1990
17.7±10.4	41.7± 12.4	?[a]	1[a]	1[a]					S[a]	cult	Rx'd with vasopressin at present doses) + epinephrine	Osaka, Japan	"Group III" (~9 cases)[a]	Peza et al 1989
18-21									S	cult?	multi-center study	Japan	11 cases	Takeuchi et al 1987
22-28									S	cult?	multi-center study	Japan	3 cases	Takeuchi et al 1987
~36[a]	9[a]		NSR		C						cited in passing[a]	Japan		Grenvik et al 1978
~69[a]	late 20s	IHV							S+	preg+ cult	dx cert[a] 24→29 wk[a]	Japan		Reuters 1992
~76[a]										preg+	cited in passing[a]	Germany (?)		McKee 1992
29-82[a]									S	cult?	multi-center study	Japan	4 cases	Takeuchi et al 1987

116 — Medicine of God

Chronic "Brain Death" – Tables

	ETIOLOGY
1	*Primary brain pathology*
1H	Hemorrhage, primary intracranial
1HV	Vascular disease, spontaneous
1HB	shaken baby syndrome
1I	Infection, primary intracranial
1IE	Encephalitis, viral
1IM	Meningitis, bacterial
1N	Neoplasm, primary brain tumor
1O	Obstructive hydrocephalus, acute
1T	Trauma, to head only
1TF	Fall, rest of body uninjured
1TG	Gunshot to head
2	Brain pathology secondary to, or as a component of diffuse or multi-systemic damage
2S	Systemic disease
2SR	Reye syndrome
2ST	malignant hyperThermia
2SU	hemolytic-Uremic syndrome
2T	Trauma, to multiple body parts including head
2TF	Fall
2TV	motor Vehicle accident
2X	toXic
2Y	hYpoxia-ischemia
2YA	Aspiration
2YC	Cardiac arrest
2YD	near-Drowning
2YI	sudden Infant death syndrome
2YK	smoKe inhalation
?	Unclear whether to classify as 1 or 2
?T	Trauma, unclear to what extent noncephalic body parts affected
?TF	Fall
?X	toXic

	APNEA TEST
NSR	No Spontaneous Respirations ever observed
‑	formally done, varying details available

ELECTROPHYSIOLOGY

EEG	Electroencephalogram
EP	Evoked Potential
‑	electrocerebral Inactivity

CEREBRAL BLOOD FLOW / NEUROIMAGING

C	Contrast angiography
CBF	Cerebral Blood Flow
CT	Computed Tomography
MRA	Magnetic Resonance Angiography
MRI	Magnetic Resonance Imaging
N	radioNuclide angiography
S	brain Scan, type not specified
V	Ventriculostomy (pressure measurement)
X	skull X-ray
+	other blood flow test

AUTOPSY

RB	Respirator Brain

TERMINAL EVENT

W	Withdrawal of life-support
S	Spontaneous, without attempted resuscitation
Sr	Spontaneous, despite attempted resuscitation
S+	Spontaneous, despite aggressive treatment
S-	Spontaneous, secondary to untreated complication
tr	Transplantation, organ removal

REASON FOR SUPPORT

cult	Cultural, + no brain-based statutory definition of death
fam	Family insistence
legl	Legal: no brain-based statutory definition of death
NDC	No Diagnostic Criteria applicable to children at the time
par	parental insistence
preg+	pregnancy, with delivery of viable infant
preg-	pregnancy, with miscarriage or fetal demise
res	Research

	MISCELLANEOUS
anem	Anemia
bd	Brain Death
↓BP	Hypotension
↕BP	Blood Pressure fluctuation
card ar	Cardiac Arrest
d	Day
DI	Diabetes Insipidus
DIC	Disseminated Intravascular Coagulation
DTR-	Deep Tendon Reflexes absent
dx	Diagnosis
dx cert	Diagnosis Certified
fl	Flaccid tone
G	nutrition provided by Gastrostomy tube
GIH	Gastrointestinal Hemorrhage
inf	Infection
m	Month
mv	Movement, spontaneous
N/A	Not Applicable
NG	nutrition provided by NasoGastric tube
↓pit	hypoPituitarism
pneu	Pneumonia
pub	Puberty onset while "brain dead"
pul ed	Pulmonary Edema
retrosp dx	Retrospective Diagnosis
Rx	treatment
sep	Sepsis
SNF	Skilled Nursing Facility
↓T	hypoThermia
↕T	Thermovariability
+T	Thermoregulation present
trans	Transfer
wn	Withdrawal to Noxious stimuli

1 Controversies in the Determination of Death: A White Paper by the President's Council on Bioethics, The President's Council on Bioethics. Washington, DC:
January 2009. Available online at: www.bioethics.gov/reports/death/index.html.

The President's Council on Bioethics

The President's Council on Bioethics paper is a recent, balanced though not all-inclusive document on the subject of brain death chaired by Dr Edmund Pellegrino, Professor of Medicine and Ethics at Georgetown and a faithful Roman Catholic. It is well worth reading and I have provided the reference above for anyone interested in the whole paper. It is worth noting that in the end the consensus was in favour of brain death but it was not unanimous. Dr Pellegrino was the chairman of the council and also one of the dissenters. His paper at the end spells out his reasons for dissenting very clearly and I am quoting the last two paragraphs in particular because the last sentence is both the "gold standard" on the diagnosis of death as well as the Roman Catholic Church's position. It is also worth noting that both our present Holy Father, Pope Benedict XVI and John-Paul II, in their respective addresses to the transplant community specified their wish that the WHOLE scientific community reach agreement on the issue of brain death, (the neurological definition of death, but here even the best of the best could not agree. Furthermore, in all this juggling with strategies to find the fastest way to reap the organs, as seen below and in reading Dr Pellegrino's last paragraph we Christians should not lose sight of the fact that we do not know for certain when the soul of the donor has been called home by God.

Much more could be said on this subject but to quote Nancy Valko, a registered nurse from St. Louis (see reference at the end of this article).

The President's Council on Bioethics white paper on the determinations of death made several startling admissions, including finding that some of the most fundamental rationales for brain death were wrong. The Council, citing scientific studies and observations, admitted that the brain is apparently not the central organizing agent without which the body cannot function for more than a short period of time. Years ago, many of us questioned why some supposedly brain-dead pregnant women could be maintained on ventilators — for even up to a couple of months in some cases — in order to help their unborn children develop and survive birth. Others observed that some supposedly brain-dead children could actually grow and even sexually mature if maintained on life support. It turns out that we were right to question this allegedly settled matter. The Council also had to admit the little-known fact that brain-death tests vary widely from institution to institution, potentially leading to people who could be declared brain-dead at one hospital but at a different hospital still be considered alive.

DCD/NHBD was developed in the early 1990s to promote a newer standard of determining death for the purpose of organ donation. DCD/NHBD describes a procedure in which a person is declared hopelessly brain-injured or ill but not brain-dead and, with the consent of the patient or surrogates (or potentially even a "living will"-style document), has his or her ventilator removed with the expectation that breathing and heartbeat will stop within about 1 hour. When the heartbeat and breathing stop for usually about 2 to 5 minutes, the person is declared dead and the organs are taken for transplant. If the person's heartbeat and breathing do not stop within the allotted time, the transplant is called off and the person is left to die without further treatment.

The Council's white paper admitted that the legal definition of irreversible cessation of heartbeat and breathing used to justify DCD/NHBD has problems. Most people would consider "irreversible" in this context to mean that the heart has lost the ability to beat. But in DCD/NHBD, "irreversible" instead means that there is a deliberate decision not to try to restart the heart when it stops and that enough time has elapsed to ensure that the heart will not resume beating on its own. However the Council had to admit the dearth of scientific evidence supporting this determination. In some cases involving babies, for instance, the heart is harvested and actually restarted in another baby. The Council also admitted that even fully conscious but spinal-cord-injured patients have become DCD/NHBD donors when dependent on a ventilator. This sad fact is the result of virtually all withdrawal-of-treatment decisions now being considered legal and thus ethical.

The Council also noted that even though doctors are advised to take their time determining death when a natural death occurs, the interval between declaring death and starting transplantation in a DCD/NHBD patient has been as short as 75 seconds. It seems obvious that the push for a speedy declaration of death is not about new scientific information determining the moment of death but rather a desire to quickly get organs because "[t]he longer a patient removed from ventilation 'lingers' before expiring, the more likely are the organs destined for transplantation to be damaged by warm ischemia [lack of adequate blood flow]".5 But even while expressing concerns, the Council still supported the DCD/NHBD concept in the end.

Despite pages discussing these DCD/NHBD issues, the Council unfortunately ignored a most crucial issue: How do doctors determine who is a "hopeless enough" patient with functioning vital organs and who will also die fast enough to get usable organs? The Council never mentioned articles like the one in the September/October 2008 issue of the Journal of Intensive Care Medicine, which stated "Donation failure [patients who don't die fast enough to have usable organs] has been reported in at least 20% of patients enrolled in DCD". Those authors also concluded that "There is little evidence to support that the DCD practice complies with the dead donor rule".

We Are All Affected

While organ donation is a worthy goal when conducted ethically, it is very dangerous when physicians and ethicists redefine terms and devise new rationales without the knowledge or input of others, especially the public. This has been happening far too often and far too long in many areas of medical ethics and the consequences are often lethal. Opinions about medical ethics affect all of us and our loved ones. And good medical ethics decisions are the foundation of a trustworthy medical system. We are constantly exhorted to sign organ-donor cards and join organ registries but are we getting enough accurate information to give our truly informed consent? This question is too important to just leave to the self-described experts.

Dr Pellegrino's Quote

"Ultimately, the central ethical challenge for any transplantation protocol is to give the gift of life to one human being without taking life away from another. Until the uncertainties and imprecision of the life-death spectrum so clearly recognized by Hans Jonas are dispelled, his moral advice must be our guide for all transplant protocols: We do not know with certainty the borderline between life and death, and a definition cannot substitute for knowledge. Moreover, we have sufficient grounds for suspecting that the artificially supported condition of the comatose patient may still be one of life, however reduced—i.e., for doubting that, even with the brain function gone, he is completely dead. In this state of marginal ignorance and doubt the only course to take is to lean over backward toward the side of possible life."

1 Controversies in the Determination of Death: A White Paper by the President's Council on Bioethics, The President's Council on Bioethics. Washington, DC: January 2009. Available online at: www.bioethics.gov/reports/death/index.html.

Nancy Valko, a registered nurse from St. Louis, is president of Missouri Nurses for Life, a spokesperson for the National Association of Pro-Life Nurses and a Voices contributing editor.

Women for Faith & Family

Voices copyright © 1999-Present Women for Faith & Family.

CHAPTER NINE
SATAN, SIN AND DEATH

MARK OF CAIN Gn 4:15

JESUS: I address you Faithful Missionary in the medical world, and with other of My instruments, I address those whose lifestyles are no longer of Me; who live perilously on the precipice of hell which really exists. At this time I Enlighten you Faithful Missionary, a medical professional, that you might be My instrument, to the other medical professionals. I am asking you to light one candle in the darkness, and leave the rest up to Me; in the power of the Holy Spirit I light up all the darkness ! I am He, your Jesus of Merciful Love, the One who holds the Key to Life and Death.(Cf Rv 1:18-19) As I look upon My beloved humanity, I see death and destruction all about. Some think they are doing good, but they do evil; some are just doing evil.

Children, as atheism is seemingly controlling the scientific world, many things are occurring which are not pleasing to the Lord your God. Much is anathema and My blessing is not upon much which is occurring now. Many pray for My Kingdom to come upon the earth now and a period of Peace will indeed come shortly. In the interim, there must be a period of cleansing, of purification, of returning to Truth. I the Lord your God, Am Truth! (Jn 14:6d)Invoke the Holy Spirit, and open Scripture. Many indeed know the New Testament. In the Old Testament there is much that is pleasing, and much that is unclean in the eyes of the Lord your God. As I cast My eyes on My beloved humanity, I behold many who are trying to be gods. I hold the keys of Life and Death. (cf Rv 1:18-19)There is a time to be born and a time to die. (Qo3)You play with these very facts of life. You are playing with the very existence of the souls of those you work with, and your own souls.

I make Clarion Calls round and about the earth. The Epistle of Love to the Scientific World, is one such Call. There are others; and though hell works feverishly to disrupt, to obstruct, to delay, to diffuse the Messages of Your Christ, hell is doomed to fail. My Victory is now, little children; pray often "In Jesus Name is my Victory," for it is truly so. Little children, those who profess to be atheists, and those who profess to serve satan, are in dire trouble, for every human soul as you know, is eternal. Our Call, Our Mission little children, is that Mankind come into Eternal Light for all Time and Eternity.(cf Jn8:12) Dear little children, there is a fierce struggle for every soul.

The last Message We gave you is a Message of Victory to the doctors. It is; The gates of hell shall not prevail;[Mt 16:19] they presumptuously believe they are prevailing! Alas for them; they are deceiving themselves.

"The virtue of Love is such that the Lord your God is present. The enemy would taint you at every opportunity. Stay always in the Presence of your Jesus. That is why I am giving you lessons in holding your armour [Eph6:10-20]secure about you and not opening it up to react to negative emotions but stay always in the Joy of the Presence of the Living God - and teaching your brothers and sisters to do likewise.It is a self-discipline - all you who have dedicated yourselves to the Living God, through the Immaculate Heart of Mary, are called to be masters and stewards of your own body and mind. It entails much mastery of your thoughts, words and deeds. The enemy loves to trick you. We bless you with the necessary wisdom, understanding and forthrightness to train your brothers and sisters in this area of purity. Love conquers all. Despite news to the contrary, the family of Peace is being built up, one might say right under the noses of the enemy. In the face of the enemy it is being built, and they are yet unaware of it. My little one, you are named "child of faithfulness", child of God and child of Mary, for I have called you by name, you are Mine. You are beloved of Jesus, beloved of Mary, continue to take our Names prayerfully on your lips and We are with you, resolving the concerns of your heart in the Peace of Our Presence.

The river of lies spewed out against Myself and the Mother of God, and indeed, the beloved John Paul, and indeed, the entire Church from the mouth of the serpent, the old dragon, are falling upon the ears of the many in this time, just for a brief time. Blessed are those who hold out in Faith and trust and Love and patient perseverance My people are only now beginning to come out of the darkness into the Light. It comes through the Enlightenment of My precious little ones, of which each of you is numbered. A great blessing is upon you, Faithful Missionary, for this work. That is why We ask you who know to pray much and do much penance and privation in the Name of Jesus, that the children not be separated from their Heavenly Father and Mother but remain part of the great Unity of Love that the enemy is thus defeated. The Mother of God herself works profoundly in assisting the little stragglers and wanderers about the earth to return to the Lord their God, as the Lord God desires.

The virtue of Love is such that I, your Jesus of Merciful Love, attend upon you; indeed upon each one of you here. Little precious children of God, little sisters of the Christ, I bless you. Tell all to believe in Me, for I believe in you. I died that mankind, each one, would have Life to the fullest. Life to the fullest means attending upon the Glory of God in Heaven one day; and yet it means what one might call a good life here upon the earth, which is Mine. The Earth is the Lord's and the fullness thereof." Therefore I bid thee remain always in My Peace. Little children, when you are in My Peace you are in My Joy. When your joy falters a bit, know that it is time to come to Me in prayer and be restored in the Peace of My Presence. When there is anxiety, fear, anger; any of what you would call negative emotions, it is obstructive. The enemy has a heyday with those individuals. Therefore patiently persevering, you shall remain in the Peace of My Presence, and the miracles shall work for you as you call upon My Name. Angels hold thee fast little children; be at Peace. The vile enemy continues to attack and obstruct. Do not be puzzled, nor dismayed at anything that happens in these times. Hosts of angels continue to assist My Own little ones always. Love Lights the way , little children: continue to love one another. Little children, ask of Me what you will. The oppression is immense !

The virtue of Love is such that the vaults of Heaven are wide open. We have allowed you to see what type of attack you are under little children. It continues, it prevails for a time. Indeed, My Victory is already won. This is at this time, what you would call in warfare, a clean sweep, a sweeping up that you are involved in. That which you do coincides, is indeed co-ordinated to cause, even as you are My instrument to cause Enlightenment to both the priesthood and the scientific world; other of My faithful little ones are causing Enlightenment in marriages and families and the rearing of children, and many, many aspects of life today. Hosts of angels assist. My precious little one, daughter of faithfulness, prevail. The stonewalling is temporary. You shall succeed in your Mission, for I am with you. Mother is with you. You are profoundly assisted. Continue to pray and address this matter.

<u>By what authority they ask! By the Authority of the Name of Jesus. By the Blood of the Lamb. This is your Authority ! Move over satan; thou art not the victor !</u> A Herculean effort is made to stop the works which I have given unto thee. Be not dismayed. Carry the five stones of the Rosary and trust in the Lord !Pagan thought have assailed the minds of many. The priesthood is in disarray because of this. Even the convents, the sisters and nuns who have always been a symbol of Our Mother's Virginity and Purity; they too are being assailed by what you call "new age." They swallow the deceits of the foe. *Our Lord reminds me of the Herculian*

effort being made to stop me from proceeding. Continue to proclaim 'Down Hercules;' it is to My Delight! My little ones, thou hast each one fought a great battle with a hideous and unpleasant foe. It is sufficient for this evening. Restore yourselves to the Peace of My Presence, and continue walking in My Light and My Love.Healing Love defeats all that mad science has begun. Do you believe? The virtue of Love is such that I the Lord am attendant upon you little ones, most profoundly. In all things give thanks little one. I am here, I reiterate! You are surrounded in a fierce spiritual warfare, the likes of which has not been seen on the earth up till now. This is now the time of the Chastisement. In My Mercy, I shorten it and make it less severe, for Heaven hears the prayers of the faithful. Your faith, your prayers are pleasing to the Lord.

Little children, as is written in Holy Scripture, each one of you is tested as gold in the fire of purification, and in this testing profoundly. A great Fortitude , a great courage is given unto you, for you are truly soldiers of Christ in the great spiritual warfare upon Earth now, for it is indeed a militant Church on earth. By your prayers you are united to God and to all of Glory, and you are profoundly assisted. Remember little children, no matter what is happening, to those who are united prayerfully with their God, all works out for their good and for the greater Glory of God. Little children, simply rest in the Presence of Jesus, in the Presence of the Prince of Peace, leaving all up to Him! My little children, it behooves you therefore to seek aid from your God Who is Love, and indeed is the Author of Love. Those who proclaim themselves atheists or agnostics, seek to win the victory in a purely scientific mode by reasoning and logic alone, and they are entangling themselves in a quagmire of confusion. How can they extricate themselves?

I Jesus confess that I am here. Again you find yourself sorely tested and concerned about time. Do not be little children. Come back to Me in unity of prayer like unto this and We shall pray again. That which has been tormenting you is no more. All-powerful is the Lord your God! Tumultuous are the times in which you live little children. Be at Peace on this day which is holy to the Lord your God. There are so many disruptions, disorders, chaotic events out and about you, it is not the appropriate time We desire to spend with you; therefore return together at your earliest convenience over the next few days and We shall share again. Do not think it is what you are doing that is causing these disruptions. A day will come when you will understand all these things. Raging waters surge around you. The heel of the Mother of God must trample the head of the serpent.((Gen 3:15) Do not be afraid little children, the dusk is falling and the darkness rapidly approaches. Remember, the faithful remained fast in the Faith during the three days Our Lord was in the tomb. Though there is darkness here and there, Faith prevails. The Words flow now but you must be ever watchful; the vengeful one lurks about seeking an opening in your armour little children. Be not anxious therefore. Remain always in My Peace.

Do not be dismayed with My priesthood; My faithful holy ones remain always with Me. Those who are tormented and scattered willy-nilly by the foe; by your prayers little children the vast majority come back to Me with all their hearts. Remember, I am a God of Merciful Love; I give to them all they need to have to return to the fullness of Truth. Many are the deceits and errors being fed, not only to My priesthood, but to the whole Church. My people, My sheep, My lambs become scattered in confusion. None of this is of Me. Yet it is that time when the enemy would sift My Own as wheat. I Myself take swift, sure action now. Believe. I am Jesus, Eternal Victor! Behold the Lamb of God! Behold it is I who take away the sins of the world! There are fierce battles over each and every soul on Earth. I am enamoured of you little ones gathered in My Name. Each one of you is precious to Me. I have called you to do that which very few would choose to do, therefore you are profoundly blest and assisted, but I Will that you know how fierce the enemy prowls about.*(Praying prone till told to rise.)*

There is no fear for those who are united with Me - not more fear than any new experience in life. Any great fear should not be there, for I am calling you Home at the appointed time, when the mission you have been assigned has been completed. Therefore, I bid you know that many, most in the world, have a great but irrational fear of death in the eyes of your God; for united with Jesus there is nothing to fear. I Myself defeated death for you; therefore, fear not little children. For the sake of His Sorrowful Passion you pray, and Heaven hears and answers. Oh dear little ones, I am He who lives and loves eternally. I am your God; I address you as the Triune God. Holy Angels of Light surround you in this place which I have claimed as a sanctuary, a sacred place, yet the enemy taunts you hither and yon in all your endeavours. Yes you find it frustrating . Don't wonder where I am; I am with you. In this the time of times it has to be. The fight is great, yet My Victory is before My eyes; and in My Victory is your own victory. Little ones, believe!

My darling children, there is going to be a great change upon the earth now. The venom of the enemy is obstructed by the Lord God! Great angels work miraculous events in this matter for My time is at hand ! While you are resting in Our Presence many actions of the Holy Spirit are occurring in your lives and the lives of those whom you carry in your heart . The enemy busies himself in obstructing all the plans of My faithful little one. Piecemeal is the response you have received to Our Messages to the scientific world! My little one, a panel of Light goes on where darkness had been. The obstruction is removed. Hosts of angels work to clear a pathway of Light for the little one. You see dear children, you live in a time perilous to human souls; there is much spiritual warfare round about which a scant handful of people upon the Earth even recognize. It is like unto a virus attack. The souls of humanity are unaware of it attacking until the affliction to the soul is far advanced. My little ones, many things come to the fore now. These Words are pertaining to the multitudes of persons round about the globe who are interwoven with My faithful ones, as is shown you in the parable of the sowers of the good seed and the enemy sowing the weeds. (Mt13:24-30).Little children thus it is war for My faithful ones in these times. The reason for the delay is thus encompassed in all these affairs of the world.

The Words flow now but you must be ever watchful the vengeful one lurks about seeking an opening in your armour little children. Be not anxious therefore. Remain always in My Peace. Behold the Lamb of God. Behold it is I who take away the sins of the world. There are fierce battles over each and every soul on Earth. I am enamoured of you little ones gathered in My Name. Each one of you is precious to Me. I have called you to do that which very few would choose to do, therefore you are profoundly blest and assisted, but I will that you know how fierce the enemy prowls about. Little children, the enemy is riled, the enemy is fiercely angry, and would obstruct every move you make as you have noted. Do not be afraid, I am with you. Fierce as the dragon may chose to display himself, he is nothing before the power of your Almighty God. Little children each one of you is fiercely powerfully protected by your God. Angels and saints indeed surround you. In the power of the Holy Spirit you are safe in Me, each in My Embrace and the Embrace of the Mother of God. The angels denote the power of God's Presence,(Gabriel) the Medicine of God(St Raphael), and the Heavenly assistance at this Mission of Love to mankind.(Michael) Amen!

They come to Me and they say,(how can this be, how can we turn the world back on its axis. How can these sort of changes be made. Human beings have come this far in the advancement of science, these Messages call us to turn back,)whereas this is not the Truth; this is what they are proclaiming. They are as horses, chomping at the bit, ready to run, but in what direction do they will to run? Dear children, you ponder about waiting on the Lord. I bid you, what else can you do? Enticing is the scientific world, leading My people into errors of darkness. Thus I have given you this Message for them. Now you find yourself boxed in as it were. Healing Love is upon you little children. Divine Mercy! Holy God, Holy Mighty One, Holy Immortal One, have Mercy on him and on the whole world. Jesus, we trust in You. X3. At once begin to praise God!

We sing" Holy God we praise Thy Name. The vaults of Heaven are wide open as the blessings flow upon you little children, and graces to carry you through these trying times. Little children, you are called to persevere, enduring all things in the Name of your Jesus. Remember little children, I am with you My precious little ones, and it shall be ever thus. You are protected and armed with circumscribing angels about each one of you and about your loved ones. With regard to the priesthood which is called to be holy; those who are My Own shall remain ever faithful to Me throughout these times of trial and testing; those who are lukewarm shall suddenly have a change of heart and come unto Me at last, or they shall be lost forever from Me.

I pour forth My Mercy on the little ones who are starving for love of Me; those who have rejected Me and struggle ineptly without Me; these ones I pour forth My Mercy upon and I assist those who are seeking Me, to find Me rapidly now. Little children, each one who is yielded to Me and is thus part of the Body of Christ, these ones cause by their sufferings, their penances, their prayers, graces and blessings to fall on the needy ones. On whom I will, I have Mercy, for I am a God of Mercy and of Love. I elect to have Mercy on My beloved humanity, even unto those who know Me not! How is that they know Me not? Has Mother not attended upon Humanity all over this world? Has not the beloved John Paul attended upon Humanity all over this world; A world so starved for Love, and they accept lust in place of Love, while I am attendant upon them offering Divine, Holy Love, all purity of Love to them. I bid you know that the death of every infant, of every frail, sick person, every elder - kills a measure of Love. Mankind's hands are now stained with the blood of the innocents and cannot be washed off no matter what they do - except they kneel in penitence, and humbly ask forgiveness of their God. The Blood of the Lamb alone washes the sin of murder from a soul. (Rv 5)

Oh My people, oh My people, oh that you would choose Love. I give you Love, in the ravishing beauty of the Woman Clothed With the Sun,(Rv12) the Mother of God, but you choose not to heed Her call to Love, choose not this Gateway to return to the Lord Your God. You choose rather error, sin, death and destruction. Oh Woe, oh My people, oh My people, what have I done to you? How have I offended you? Answer Me.(Mi 6:3)

The great grace which is given you, to work miracles of Love, will cause the many to be released from the bondages of sin and death, for Heaven hears the prayer of the faithful. At this moment, I your Jesus anoint you in a profound anointing. The choice is ever life or death, life or death - but scientists have forgotten about Life or Death of the soul! Thus they are caught up in this madness; this chaotic situation where babies are being murdered and babies are being 'created' as it were, not by the Will of God, but by the desire of the parents united with that of the doctor who seeks to work this form of science I bid you know that many, most in the world, have a great but irrational fear of death in the eyes of your God; for united with Jesus there is nothing to fear. I Myself defeated death for you; therefore, fear not little children."

The people of God know the sorrow of this malady of death but of Me do not hear, they cannot comprehend the Words of Merciful Love . Oh woe, suffer oh earth, for your deliverance is at hand, but not without a great battle, a great route of the foe. It holds the many with great impact about the world and those who think they have great impact, in the embrace of eternal death (cf Rv20:11-15) The battle lines are drawn. By this conference, all will know My Stance, and the stance of the beloved John-Paul, My Vicar in this matter. This is not pleasing to the mad scientists, who use My Creations human bodies, oblivious to My Truth. He speaks in a manner that none can deny his Truth. That does not mean little children that all will heed Truth and respond in Love! Even so, the battle lines are clearly drawn and Truth comes to the fore in this issue of euthanasia and 'brain death,' and in the issue of abortion and what is occurring to the aborted infants. All of this is anathema; all of this is an abomination in the Eyes of the Living God, in Whose Presence you live!

Now I am not giving you a blanket ticket to say that everyone who commits suicide or is killed by euthanasia, is ready to come before Me, and that is why I call all of you to pray for those in their last agony. He quotes Maccabees, "t is a good and holy thing to pray for those who have died, those who have gone before you."(cf 2M 12:44-45) Believe in My Mercy, believe in My Love and be comforted. The things of this world are different than how I the Lord think; and who can know the mind of your God? (Rm11:35-36).In this era in which you are living little children, there is a new type of martyrdom occurring on earth; those who suffer euthanasia, especially those who suffer this unknowingly, not in a free will choice. These ones are martyrs in the Cause of Truth. Little children, the people of Life are fighting to put an end to this form of unwarranted death, and "there is a time to live and a time to die," [Qo 3:2] . I am attendant upon My beloved Humanity, yet in all free will they elect to do these monstrous crimes against the Living God and against My beloved Humanity.

It is by the Clothing of Jesus, with Flesh and Blood, through the "Yes" of the Immaculate Virgin Mary, that the Victory against satan was won, and that is why he perseveres in persecuting both The Christ and the Mother of God, and the Baptized children, Her "other children" of Faith. [Rev 12 vs 17] This is ongoing, though few take time to pray and ponder on these matters, this is important. The Annunciation [25th March] is as it were, a Portent of the [spiritual] war, as it is today.(Read Rv 12). And again I remind you little children, that the readings at the Mass this morning, [Genesis 18:16-33] were there five good ones I would not have destroyed those communities, and it is as you understand, a faithful remnant, and when your God gazes down upon earth, and His Eyes fall lovingly on the faithful remnant, that the Wrath is stayed and does not fall on Humanity as yet, and yet you are the ones, little children, this handful scattered all over the earth, who suffer, as the beloved St Paul has spoken, " for I make up in myself that which was lacking though nothing was lacking."

That few struggle to do this is tragic and heartbreaking. Yet pray for them little children, and one by one We bring them into the Sanctuary of Love, where all purity does and must prevail. Because of your prayers and concerns and of those faithful about the world like yourselves, hosts of saints and angels in Glory, plead unceasingly for the homosexuals' release from the bondages of sin and death. The Blessing which the Holy Father has brought upon the Earth with his proclamation, endows those formerly without a Heavenly Queen and Mother, to now have one. Many holy and miraculous events occur, and all will know that I am God, Supreme among the nations and that it is My Will that My Mother be recognized. Thus I have set Her, your Mother of Mercy; the Merciful One Who judges not; whose weapon is Love, against the merciless one; and I Bless Mankind in Her and through Her with the needed Graces and Heavenly assistance to persevere and to be victorious, and as you know, in Her intercession, you will come before Me, the Living God, and know Salvation.

I Myself have already won the Victory over satan, sin and death. The battle therefore is for each human to win victory over self, assisted by your Jesus, and Our Mother, the ever-virgin Mary, and by a myriad of angels and saints your victory is assured, little children . For those who do not heed let us pray;"If today you hear God's voice, harden not your hearts." (Ps95)The death of a soldier is before My Eyes. It is one that is important to Me. Oh sorrow! The enemy attacks again and again. My army is decimated at this time because of the wolves in sheep's clothing and the traitors in Our midst.(cfJn12:13-14) My faithful ones are called to such heroic actions as thou art called. Little children, be not afraid. Simply remain in obedience for I am with you always. Continue therefore, pray as thou art taught and act accordingly, and I am with you.The murderer of souls [devil] has a way of causing disruption in Our Plans. You live in a society which does not want to think of death or speak of death, but yet Death [the devil] is ever present in the world in the state it is in today. Until I return in Glory, Death is not fully defeated! (cf Rv20:10) Those who are yielded to Me, have nothing to fear in My Embrace. They cross the barrier of time into Eternal Light(cf Rv21:9-27); and so the basis for desiring to give a set of organs to the other, is not well thought out by the physicians!

For three days I have been continually seeing the serpent. Thus have We prayed the big rebukes. The virtue of Love is such that the Lord your God is profoundly attendant upon thee. Children, do not fear the devil, he is a defeated foe. I Myself, [*immediatedly the Lighted Cross with the circle of Light in the centre is seen by Omen on my forehead*], I the Lord God, am all powerful indeed! Little children, always remember, I have defeated satan, sin and death for you. Little ones, you live in My Light and My Peace and My Love. The enemy rears its ugly head periodically, here and there. Be not afraid; in the Name of Jesus it must flee! Dear little ones, at the Name of Mary, this thing must flee! Since you are persevering in all prayerfulness, invoking the Names of Jesus and Our Mother Mary, Who love you most tenderly, most totally and most eternally, and Whom you love in return, there is nothing to fear. I assure you that a shield of angels circumscribes you and you are safe in the Lord.

Dear little children, I remind you, you are front line soldiers in the Great War; greater than any war recorded in the history books is the war which We are in. You have seen the foe face to face, and he is defeated and routed. Dear little ones, he detests what you do in My Name, but he cannot harm you, for I assure you that I dwell within your heart and soul and mind. Is it not written that We make Our Home in you when you have said 'yes' to Us? And so, that is why We speak today of individuals being other Christs. You are the temple of the Living God, and your light is shining. This annoys Our mutual enemy, who attempts to attack to no avail, for he is rendered harmless by Me, the Living God. Do not be afraid, I am with you, I am always with you. You are My beloved one, you are never alone! Little children, My Heart too is heavy, for much of what is occurring on the earth is not of Me, and yet you are approaching a time of great change. Little children, in spite of all that is occurring, you have a Joy within you in the Peace of My Presence, which has come to the fore, for the true faithful, in this Christmas season, this holy season, and is ongoing.

The enemy and his agents on earth, have been resoundingly defeated at this time of the New Year. Great changes are upon the earth, and yet battle lines are drawn up, for those who are for Me, the Living God, and those who are not; for they have, shall We say swallowed the lies of satan, (cf Jn8:44-46) as surely as did Adam and Eve, the first parents. The enemy is defeated; Michael works great works of defeat of the enemy. The Army which surrounds My Church is powerful under Michael to defeat the foe. As it is written that many were healed by simply being in the shadow of the beloved Peter(Ac5:15), this man who holds the Chair of Peter, is singularly blest in a similar way. His presence, his voice are instruments of My Healing Love, thus the enemy strives to silence him, but is at once fearful, for I have already defeated the foe who has no power over Me and no power over the beloved John Paul. Still, it perseveres in all wickedness. Children, be at Peace but continue to pray for the beloved one.

Always remember, Greater is your God, and be at Peace. Evil has no power over you for evil has no power over Me. Even so, the enemy taunts you, each of My little ones. You are in My Hand and in My Design. Rest assured you are safe in Me. The protection of your work in the healing arts and in your Providence rests in Me. Believe and be at Peace. *Lord, you know I have been continually seeing the serpent since I called the police for this woman who has been harassing me on my phones daily. Lord I pray to break any curses that have come my way, and that she be released also.*

Thus have We prayed the big rebukes. The virtue of Love is such that the Lord your God is profoundly attendant upon thee. Children, do not fear the devil, he is a defeated foe. I Myself, [immediatedly the Lighted Cross with the circle of Light in the centre is seen by Omen on my forehead], I the Lord God, am all powerful indeed! Little children, always remember, I have defeated satan, sin and death for you. Little ones, you live in My Light and My Peace and My Love. The enemy rears its ugly head periodically, here and there. Be not afraid; in the Name of Jesus it must flee! Dear little ones, at the Name of Mary, this thing must flee! Since you are persevering in all prayerfulness, invoking the Names of Jesus and Our Mother Mary, Who love you most tenderly, most totally and most eternally, and Whom you love in return, there is nothing to fear. I assure you that a shield of angels circumscribes you and you are safe in the Lord. Dear little children, I remind you, you are front line soldiers in the Great War; greater than any war recorded in the history books is the war which We are in. You have seen the foe face to face, and he is defeated and routed. Dear little ones, he detests what you do in My Name, but he cannot harm you, for I assure you that I dwell within your heart and soul and mind. Is it not written that We make Our Home in you when you have said 'yes' to Us? And so, that is why We speak today of individuals being other Christs. You are the temple of the Living God, and your light is shining. This annoys Our mutual enemy, who attempts to attack to no avail, for he is rendered harmless by Me, the Living God. Do not be afraid, I am with you, I am always with you. You are My beloved one, you are never alone! Thank you Lord Jesus. As I was planning a song of praise, Omen received a Charismatic song "His Name is wonderful, Jesus our Lord," silently ,and said we should sing a song of praise. I had been singing in my heart, "Christ Jesus Victor, Christ Jesus Ruler, Christ Jesus Lord and Redeemer."

As I arrived home from these prayers, I saw in a cloud near my home about five to seven angels moving rapidly back and forth within the cloud, becoming very bright when they came to the fore; but they never came right out of the cloud. I watched for 10 to fifteen minutes in awe, but they showed no sign of leaving and it was very cold so I had to go in. The next morning I saw the grey serpent back again though not as clearly, in my right peripheral vision. At Adoration fortunately I was alone, and I screamed asking our Lord to help me. Immediately, Our Lady of Guadalupe stood exactly where the serpent had reared himself to the right of the Tabernacle. She did not even look at him but he seemed to know immediately his place and he shrank down and wriggled under Her foot. From then on every time he tried to appear I saw Our Lady of Guadalupe again and he went under Her foot, till over the course of that day he gave up.

I saw Genesis 3:15(He will strike your head with his heal.) enacted by The Woman clothed with the Sun (Rev12: Our Lady of Guadalupe. Thank You Jesus and Mother. Amazing!

<u>St Michael speaks.</u> *St Michael attends upon you. Little children, be at Peace. Fierce is the warfare about the earth today. Know well that all the beloved Holy Father is doing is the Will of the Father. Know well that the enemy writhes in torment because of these words and deeds, and thus the enemy most assuredly is making haste to make war on the children of the Woman Clothed with the Sun,(Rv12:17) scattered about the globe, in a desert of Faith. Oh little children, the Lord is with you, the armies of God, the cohort of angels, are as a vast shield, encompassing the Body of Christ(1Co12:27),, the Church of God securely; therefore be at Peace!*

<u>Prayer to St Michael.</u> *St Michael the Archangel, defend us in this day of battle; be our safeguard against the wickedness and snares of the devil. May God rebuke him we humbly pray, and do thou oh Prince of the Heavenly Host, by the Power of God, cast into hell satan, and all the other evil spirits who prowl about the world seeking the ruin of souls. Amen.*

CHAPTER TEN
SORROW AND WOE

MARK OF CAIN Gn 4:15
JESUS:

In suffering and sorrow they come unto Me. (Rm 5d)Oh My little one, sorrow, grief and wrath are in the Heart of your God for what Humanity is now doing. Oh woe! Little sister, hold My hand, it is your Jesus who speaks; and hold Mother's hand. Let Us walk together with Our beloved Joseph, in Faith and Hope and Trust and Love and patient perseverance. My gifts to mankind are always contingent upon the Laws of your God; and thus, mankind, to your sorrow, they fall under a curse, rather than a blessing. What will you do when you run out of body parts? It will become expedient simply to kill another for the body parts. You are already aware that this can and does occur in various nations. Walls of flame surround those who are behaving in this manner. The mark of Cain is upon many on earth. They are Mine yet they elect to kill their brothers, for their own motives.

A haunting sorrow is in the Heart of the Lord your God, because of the tragedies of mankind's pride in the works of their hands, not consecrated to Me, but to power and to greed. Oh, My little one, there is sorrow in the Heart of your God at what is happening in the field of medicine and all the sciences; both sorrow and grief. The walls which surround the hearts of the many prevent them from knowing Merciful Love, Agape Love, Compassionate Love. In a sterile, loveless way they work their works of iniquity upon My Creation, Humanity. My little one, you know each person you speak to has their individual free will, and many of them who are professing Christianity, hold in contempt the Word of God. They neither live in My Commandments nor teach My Way. Oh sorrow and woe, that so many souls of My gifted children are so tarnished. Oh sorrow and woe, that so many minds are so full of conceit and deceit and pride and arrogance. Oh sorrow and woe, that they heed not the example of Myself and My Mother and Saint Joseph and the many faithful.

The crusade is about the world to stop legalized abortions. The people of God know the sorrow of this malady of death but of Me do not hear, they cannot comprehend the Words of Merciful Love! Oh Woe, suffer oh earth, for your deliverance is at hand, but not without a great battle, a great route of the foe. It holds the many with great impact about the world and those who think they have great impact, in the embrace of eternal death. I give you Love, in the ravishing beauty of the Woman Clothed With the Sun (Rv 12:1), the Mother of God, but you choose not to heed Her call to Love, choose not this Gateway to return to the Lord Your God. You choose rather error, sin, death and destruction. Oh woe, oh My people, oh My people, what have I done to you? How have I offended you? Answer Me. (Mi 6:3)

My wounded one, thy wounds are indelibly marked upon thy soul, yet through these wounds radiate My Healing Light upon the many. Persevere in the Mission -My Mission- Our Mission; for it is in embracing thy cross, for Love of Me, that the healing miracles of Our Love occur. Smallest instrument, I bless thee. We confess that you are appealing most profoundly for their mercy, but yet there remains such a black cross over the medical field. *Lord what more can I do?* You are doing that which I have requested of you. Be at Peace in this matter (1 Th 5:14). We bless many with Enlightenment now. It is just to let you know little one, the great Mission to which you are assigned. The power of darkness is immense. There is grief in

Heaven for the behaviours of many doctors, research scientists and many more; and yet as My Church walks the *Via Dolorosa*, you must know, as I did, and as Our Mother did, *that it had to be*! Little children, it is so for the Body of Christ.

Little children, be not distraught, come now into the Peace of My Presence. My little ones, when you come to Me as the Holy Infant of Prague, as the Holy Infant in Bethlehem, it is pleasing to Me. When you come to Me at the foot of the Cross, it is pleasing to Me. My little ones, Mother's in tears of joy at your faith, your persevering faith despite all the obstacles. There are many about you who speak well but do not know Me. Oh sorrow; enmeshed in the world they cannot seem to find Me, and yet I am knocking at the doors of their heart (Rv 3:20). My Own as you know are tested like gold in the fire (1 Pt 1:7), that all the impurities be removed, for it is only in the perfection of the soul that the individual comes to the sanctity I desire before he can be an instrument, a true instrument of My Peace. Many there are, who believe they are working in My Name. Oh sorrowful lot; they barely know Me.

Bread of Life, Bread of Life I give to you (Jn 6:35). The angel of death is defeated today! Little children, as Mother loved Luke, so she loves Her physician children. Mother weeps copious tears of sorrow at some of the events that are happening in the medical field, and yet glorious tears of joy at the many beautiful successes in healing Love, for the use of the God given intellect and capabilities on behalf of the suffering brother or sister is so pleasing to God. Many, many physicians are precious and blest of the Lord God, yet the grave error of this humanist wave of atrocious medical actions is grievous to both Our God and to the Mother of God. Indeed send him a letter and a copy of the scroll for it is our desire that none of those in key positions can say, "I did not know". Those who are open to My Words, should be motivated to say to you, "tell me more, what is this about" and when they do that their learning is enhanced, because you have at your disposal much, much more to give to them. Soon this will be happening with specific individuals. Little one, do not be distressed at the slow response. There is an immense store of knowledge in the Information you have been given by your God, which takes man a little time to absorb, and to ponder upon and decide upon. Patience dearest children; patience.

Little children you are My Own, and you will be buffeted about even as I have been, and even as I am to this very day! Little children, it is part of being part of My Family. My little ones, you are privileged to be as it were, key witnesses to the sorrowing concerns of the Heart of Jesus. Persevere (Heb 10:36), I am with you (Mt 28:20), I go before you (Is 45:2); I Am your Strength (Ps 18:1). Trial by fire; Go! Even as the three men in the fiery furnace (Dn 3:20), go proclaiming Glory to God through it all. Sorrow and pain are the lot of those who do not believe you little children. It is the Lord Your God Who speaks! Little children, you live in a time of great of peril for all mankind. Dear children you, each one of you is aware of this; but few on earth are aware of the imminent danger which is upon them. Their understanding is darkened in these times, for insidious inroads by the evil one have occurred in their minds and hearts. Yes Mother weeps for all the sorrows upon the earth today, and yet amidst the sorrowing tears are tears of Joy at the stamina in battle which you have shown today little children. You are blest and blest again.

Little children, the harsh words hurled at you throughout your lifetime will fall on your Jesus like so many whiplashes (Rm 15:3); they too are no more. Little children, I ask you; do not look back on the sorrows of yesterday, for I have erased them. When you dwell on the sorrows of yesterday you become immobilized spiritually, or mentally or emotionally; in some ways you become limited. This is not of Me. I ask you to live each God-given moment united with Me, living in My Life, My Light, My Peace, loving those whom I set about you in Christ-Love. Time is a gift of your God, a healing Gift. Use it well My precious ones. Little children, you are as lighted candles in the darkness of the world today. Prevail little ones, for the darkness is so dark that My people walk in confusion, unknowing which way to turn, for the hireling shepherds have not only abandoned My flock, but they have debased My Church, and harmed My flock! Do not concern yourselves about these matters; just know that My faithful remnant, is like unto the small faithful remnant in the Old Testament. [like the army leader Gideon that chose his men when they went to drink water-Jg 7:5] . This remnant I strengthen, I protect, I train them in the way of spiritual warfare, and I hold them strongly united to Me; and under the great mantle of Love, in the power of the Holy Spirit, it is so. Little children, you are included in this army.

You have now entered a time of world diplomacy, which will wreak further havoc on humanity. Therefore persevere little children (Ps 18:1). Peace; We bid you rest. In all things give thanks little one (1 Th 5:18). I am here, I reiterate. You are surrounded in a fierce spiritual warfare, the likes of which has not been seen on the earth up till now. This is now the time of the Chastisement. In My Mercy, I shorten it and make it less severe, for Heaven hears the prayers of the faithful. Your Faith, your prayers are pleasing to the Lord. Living waters flow upon you. I am attendant in such a manner that the prevaricator cannot assail you!Dearest children of a merciful and loving God, I remind you that you are My Own by virtue of your Baptisms. You are in the world, but not of the world (Jn 17:16) for you belong to Me, you are My Own. Therefore do not concern yourselves unduly with all that is happening in the world, at this time of Chastisement it has to be; but since you are My Own, you are safe in Me. Little children I remind you that My Own are safe in Me, whether they are yet in the battle on earth, or in their purifications in purgatory, or have attained the Glory of Heaven; they are My Own and I take care of My Own, I am the Good Shepherd (Jn 10:11).

Therefore little children, take and hold the Hand of your Jesus in Spirit and Truth, and take and hold the Hand of Our Beloved Mother as We walk beside Saint Joseph, Guardian of the Holy Family of God, through all the hills and valleys of this life's journey, through all the trials, walking always in Faith and Hope and Trust and Love, in patient perseverance, enduring all things little children, this is the only way. This is My Way; indeed I am the Way, the Truth, the Life (Jn 14:6) and I light your Way, for you are My Own little brothers and sisters and precious to My Heart. Therefore know that each of those faithful priests are precious to Me, the Lord God. They shall live on this earth in their mortal bodies as long as I Desire and at a moments notice they are taken Home to Glory where great crowns and a place of Perfection awaits each and every one of My faithful little ones. You both are numbered in this. Be prepared to fight for your Faith little children, for the time of peril is imminent! Heaven hears your plea; continue to pray for all the patients being sent to you and be at Peace (1 Th 5:14).

A Living Flame of Love is the Spirit of the Living God. I bid all of My Own to invoke the Living God, praying unceasingly in these difficult times. Hosts of angels and a goodly number of saints I set about you, to assist in all that is occurring. I tell you, people of God, at this time every soul is experiencing testing and trials, and all are called to persevere, patiently enduring all that is occurring, and the more they are yielded to Me, the more they trust in My Love, all-holy Love; the more they are strengthened, and the more rapidly their problems are resolved. In these times you are noticing an increase in physical illnesses especially cancer; you already have AIDS now for some time in the world. You notice an increase in the numbers of depressed ones and an increase in the numbers of marriages breaking up, and break-ups of various groups, various relationships; all these are signs of the times, and yet I am with My people. You are living in a world where the Christians, for a generation or two, seemingly have forgotten about their God, the God they are given over to, consecrated to in Baptism and Confirmation; thus you find yourselves in a pagan world, for they have failed to baptize their children, failed to teach their children in the way they should grow, failed in all that they could have done, should have done, and might have done for their children, and now it is unto another generation and this lapse, this opening of their armor of God, for themselves and for their offspring, the enemy has found many areas to send his fiery darts of deceit and lying assailing My beloved Humanity. Therefore I bid you, be not surprised what you hear, what you see, what you experience, what you suffer; these things have to be at this time. I ask My Own to stay prayerfully united.

Little children, know that I the Lord Your God am attendant upon you and each and every one of your hearts concerns little children, for nothing is hidden from Me. My little children I ask you to just trust in the Lord in all things (Pr 3:5); you know well that you are living in stormy times, in unsettled times, in this world, and the Body of Christ is sorely tested by those who know Me not! Little children there are people who read Holy Scripture as one would read a history book. They do not Invoke My Spirit and do not receive the anointing to Understand the Love of the Lord God for every human being. Little children, continue invoking the Holy Spirit of the Living God in all your works in all your readings in all prayers. This Way Enlightenment comes to you to understand what is hidden from those who know Me not. *He's showing Omen it's like when He spoke in parables and the disciples went to Him and understood when others did not (Mt 13:10-16).* So it is with My Spirit. Little children, I ask you to rely on the Holy Spirit. My Delight is in your invocation to the Holy Spirit to come through the Immaculate Heart of Our Mother. This Way Blessings and Graces come upon you. Be assured that the Lord God is attendant upon every soul who has said "yes" to the Will of the Father. Therefore rejoice in this Our Love's Union. Rest often in the Peace of My Embrace of Love.

I am attendant upon you little children; Mother is attendant upon you. Graces flow upon each one of you, for the true children of God are profoundly anointed in blessings and graces, in this time of trial, for it is you little ones, whose soul is filled to the fullest, in the River of Life and Light and Love, to be poured forth upon the needy ones whom you meet on your daily journeys. This is the Mission of the true Christian, to pour My Love and My Mercy upon everyone in your pathway of Life. The irritable ones, the unfriendly ones; these ones I ask you to just simply say a little prayer for them as they pass through your life, and persevere (Ps 18:1). Oftentimes it is the only prayer these unhappy souls get. It is because no one is praying for them, that is why I call you to pray, and the Virgin Mother of God, visits the earth pleading the cause of Humanity and calling them to pray and pray and pray again. Little ones, do it joyfully; give Me the joy of your morning offering, and I, with the Mother of God, visit those whom I would contact. Many know it not, and yet My Love is falling upon them too. That is why I call you My faithful ones, precious precision instruments in My Hands, to see yourselves always as just that!

I am attendant upon thee. I ask you to persevere in going there My little one. Your eyes see, your ears hear, you know what is happening in the world about you, both in the material world and in the spiritual world; you perceive the insane direction in which the medical professions, the alleged scientists are going. This is a far cry from caring for an afflicted patient as you know. I desire that you attend to make mental note of the various ways in which the human mind, the finite mind is plunging into darkness, despite the prayers of the faithful, despite My Call to holiness! I would desire to have these individuals working in Unity with Me, for the well being of each individual, yet they go off at a tangent which is alien to Me and not good for the patient. I simply wish you at this time to attend upon the meeting making observances of the noticeable trends in the health movement for future reference. The concept of free enterprise versus socialism is at the root of these circumstances, and always little children you see, in this type of battle the egos and the self centeredness of the individuals involved. Therefore the only solution for the true believers is again prayer.

As you have noticed the desolation is in the places in the world which should be the most holy. It is but the beginning. My little ones, continue to pray for the conversion of the many. Mother magnifies your prayers, presenting them to the Father, and more and more My people come back to Me. You are witness to the great need of conversion in the cities of Europe; in Jerusalem. I call these people. My people, I call to them; My people, My people; what is it that fascinates you in the world to the forgetfulness of your Creator? A Day of Reckoning comes upon the earth as is written in Holy Scripture; and indeed a Day of Reckoning comes for each individual soul when it comes before Me at that crucial moment; therefore little children, persevere in all prayerfulness.

I Myself attend upon the many, and again, in the Will of your God, you must be instruments in the healing of your brothers and sisters, all you who know Me and have unity of Love with Me. I call you to be healers in My Name, for the suffering ones. You know that some, in My Will, I take home to Myself; some I heal that they may remain longer in the world in Me, even though they are My Own, for My Own reasons. Little children, love Me and trust Me. He shows us all the technical apparatus that man is using for healing today in the scientific world and saying…I ask you if it is necessary? Some of it works for good, some of it works for harm. If they would ask a blessing from Me upon their undertakings, much, much more good would come upon their works, but they prevail in finite reasoning to do what they do. Little children, you are as it were, strategic instruments in My Cause, which is Healing Love! At this time of darkness upon Mankind, Mother weeps copious tears of Sorrow for the children of God, for there can be no turning back from the fate that awaits those who have allowed themselves in free will, to be ensnared in this culture of death. Those who promote it are already in bondage to satan. Rest assured your God is aggrieved over each and every soul who in free will, elects to serve Our enemy. An end of this evil reign is in sight!

I Myself, it is the Lord Who speaks, make haste to help you now. Counted on earth, is every soul which is yielded unto Me, and those who are yet to come unto Me. I have called again and again to Mankind; come back to Me with all your hearts. A goodly number have, but there are those who do not, and are fast running out of time, the necessary time, the Great Hour of Mercy which is yet upon the earth briefly. It is assuredly that time of darkness covering the earth, and the thick clouds, the people. The Light of Christ prevails in the Faithful Church, and in the souls of the true Faithful.

I tell you again, I am your Jesus, All Powerful God, Wonder Counselor, Great Physician, and I desire to hold every precious little one to My Heart of Love, even as Mother does, for the Healing of soul and body. My precious little ones, the times in which you are living, have brought distress and unpleasant disorders and diseases to humanity. Oh My people, I am calling all to come back to Me like the prodigal son (Lk 15:11-32). There is only suffering and sorrow and hardship where they choose to wonder, and they find it so difficult, for the return journey back to Me, and yet I await them with open arms of Love. How I long to clothe each one with Salvation. Tell Me their names in prayer at the Adoration Chapel and leave them there with Me. I am your Jesus of Mercy, your Jesus of Love. Upon whom I will, I have Mercy (Ro 9:15). At this time I have Mercy upon all of mankind. I await their response to My Call. For the sake of His Sorrowful Passion" you pray, and Heaven hears and answers. Oh dear little ones, I am He who Lives and Loves eternally. I am your God; I address you as the Triune God. Holy Angels of Light surround you in this place which I have claimed as a Sanctuary, a sacred place, yet the enemy taunts you hither and yon in all your endeavours. Yes you find it frustrating. Don't wonder where I am; I am with you (Mt 28:20). In this the time of times it has to be. The fight is great, yet My Victory is before My Eyes; and in My Victory is your own victory. Little ones, believe!

Little children, the Call to Christianity is far greater than many Baptized Christians recognize in these times, and it is essential then, that they might know Salvation and wellness, increased testings and trials to bring them to the needed Faith, the needed Fortitude, before the purification of soul can be established in them. Little children, when they seek the false idols, they make their journey more complicated. Pray for them, but stand by your word and your Faith. I am Jesus; remember children, I am the one Who Loves each one of you most tenderly, most totally and eternally. I tell you that again and again! Little children, you are My beloved; and the patients in the hospitals are My beloved also. Many of them are suffering prayerfully. Some even though they are deathly ill, know Me not! Yes, dear little children, pray for every person I set in your pathway of Life; I do not say do an immense, long, formal prayer, but simply a little "God Bless you", or "Jesus heal this one," or "Jesus Mercy. Mary help," any such little words of Mercy and Love upon these other ones.

I give you the needed resilience to work where you are placed, for I am with you always and remember little children, I do indeed carry the brunt of the Cross, but I let you feel it. It is for your formation little children, therefore persevere a little longer. I have plans for you for your good; I bless you in your adherence to Truth; I Bless you for your patient perseverance in enduring all that you are enduring in My Name. Bless Me! We adore Thee oh Christ and we bless Thee, because by Thy Holy Cross Thou hast redeemed the world! Little beloved ones, My Peace is upon you; a great Blessing is upon you. Little children, love Me as I have Loved you; this is the pathway of holiness, the narrow Way. Little children, many there are who seek Me but they do not follow in the narrow Way. Little children, in the world today there is so great a temptation to follow the ways of the world, to seek the material gains, not realizing in so doing, you are being caught up in the snares of the foe, in idolatry and the like. But little children of Faith, be not unduly concerned, for I seek your loved ones out. I am the Good Shepherd, I bring them back to Truth in due course. Even so, in Our Father's great Design, the prayers and the penances of the faithful, play an integral role in causing those who are in free will, yet in the world, to have a conversion of heart. You don't realize at what moment, after so much prayer, one soul will come back to Me, in all repentance, and be embraced in Love once again.

That is why Mother is one earth, frequenting the earth, calling the children who can see, who can hear, who know, to pray and pray and pray again, for the conversion of sinners, the Salvation of souls. Hosts of angels assist in the works of My Church upon earth. Hosts of angels assist each one of you now in these unusual times. My little ones, pray much and trust Me, the Living God, the Giver of all life. No matter what is happening on this earth, your prayers do indeed resound in Heaven in unity with the saints, and much good is brought forth. Also always remember that in your faithfulness in prayer, in word and deed, you are storing treasure in Heaven, to be known to you only on a glorious day of the Lord. In the interim, walk in My Light and My Love and My Life, persevering.

The visionary has done well in enlightening many, but many remain in darkness. Faithful Missionary is assigned to enlighten the peoples of great intellect; Omen is assigned to the peoples of the first nations, many of whom have great intellect but lack true spirituality, and to assist the street people as you call them, for they too are My Own, and many intellectuals find themselves there in the streets at rock bottom, despite their wisdom and knowledge and understanding ; for they have taken a wrong turn, and need to come back to Me with all their hearts. Indeed I seek them out, I am the Good Shepherd.(Jn 10) I seek them out in you and through you, and all those who work in similar manner on My behalf. Thou hast worked well; thou art well advised from Glory. Things are going according to Heaven's Design. Be at Peace. The virtue of Love is such that I am present to you. A severe testing, a severe attack is upon your works little children; prevail, We are with you. Believe, We are with You. Be at Peace therefore!

A sorrow is that the many will not to heed. But there is rejoicing for those who do indeed heed, discern, begin to believe in the true sanctity of each God-given life. Your work is immense, greater than you can comprehend little children, therefore be not dismayed at any obstructions; the enemy is wrath. Through this Portal of Light, the Heart of your Beloved Mother, the Mercy Gate, blessings flow upon each of My Own among whom you are numbered little children. As to the meetings of the Catholic physicians in unity with the priest, it is a tragedy, a sorrow, that they do not choose to believe, but seek a burden of scientific truth before they would believe. Though you present this to them very clearly, they are reluctant in their great intellect to accede to these Truths. Be not dismayed; it has been ever thus. Thou hast asked that We rebuke in the Name of Jesus, it is the Lord Who speaks, the spirit of pride which assails many intellectuals. This has been an ongoing war throughout the course of the centuries, and continues to now; yet some will yield. A certain yieldedness-in-Faith to the Living God is essential, before the thoughts of this people, the minds and thoughts, are opened to Truth. I the Lord God AM Truth.

What sorrow this is to the Hearts of your God and of your Loving Mother, who pleads unceasingly on their behalf, and to them, that they may know Salvation. In this manner you see the immense battle which is occurring in this time; and why each little effort, each little prayer, each little penance which you perform dear children, is so precious, is so important to the Lord your God. That is why I the Lord God ask you so often, to Love Me for those who do not The Lord your God sorrows at the rejection of these precious Gifts of My Love for mankind; Gifts of new Life, planned to give a unity between a mother and father in each case. Their very existence is denied by those who parented them. Do you see the Sorrow of their Creator, your Creator in this matter? Those who do not come back to Me, were never Mine, to their sorrow and ruin, and to My Sorrow. I ask you little children, to abide with Me as you do, in My Presence in the Mass, in the shrine, and as you go about your days, for truly I am with you.

Be at Peace; it is well known by you, little children, that it is in suffering and sorrow that the many come back to Me with all their hearts, for it is only then, that so many little ones fall on their knees seeking assistance from God, and I Your God, do not refuse. I attend upon them most profoundly in their hours of need and it is thus that they become safe in My Love, safe in My Embrace. It is happening to multitudes upon the earth even as We speak, and it continues to happen. It is a Sorrow of these times. It is at best, a symptom of the Great Apostasy which is upon the earth, that Mankind has gone so far away from their God; that Mankind disregards the Laws of God; that Mankind has brought itself to this state of ill-health that causes them to believe that body parts are warranted. I the Lord am completely shut out, and the field is totally black—-a great Sorrow to Our Mother and your God. It is as you say, in suffering and sorrow they come back to Me; I would they would come by other means, in Joy, and yet I ask you to persevere; I assist you profoundly; I cast out the foe at every instance in his attack on My Own. Remember, you are profoundly assisted by your God in all that you are doing. Giving me His reactions to some patients as they speak, so intensely that I can hardly speak to them. Lord I need Your Guidance; what do You wish me to do when this is happening?

The Virtue of Love is that I am Feeling in Your Heart, the intense Sorrow and Pain to Me, by the offenses of these persons, who seek healing not knowing that I Am the Healer! My little one, as you have become aware of these circumstances, I take consolation in your heart, and I ask you to simply pray for the troubled ones' conversion of heart, for the softening of hearts. Indeed, the pardon prayer is a good instrument for it is rapidly prayed and most effective, but any prayer you choose, to speak a word or phrase, asking that their hearts be softened, that their minds be opened unto Me. They remain resistant to My Call to Love, and in this very resistance, they find themselves ensnared in these afflictions! There is much Sorrow, that they are, at once wilfully doing what they do, and yet seemingly they are ignorant of what they are doing. Therefore one must continue to treat them with all compassion until enlightenment comes. You may not see it in every instance, yet simply pray for them; I will move your heart with inspirations of prayers on their behalf. *Our*

Lord showed Omen Pharoah, and each time He gave him a plague He would say, "then he will know that I am God! (Ex 14:18)" Sometimes little children, it takes much affliction, much suffering, before a human yields to their God, for I am God of all! .(cf Ex 14:18) Persevere dear little one, persevere. My precious little ones, you are sprinkled as salt about the earth,(Mt 5:13-16) in the midst of multitudes of people who have either their minds or their hearts closed to Truth. I am Truth.(Jn14:6) My Spirit, the Spirit of Truth,(Jn16:13) comes upon many now, and they begin to seek detailed Enlightenment on what is actually occurring in the deaths of these people , these patients who have been labeled "brain dead." Poor, poor, poor souls who know Me not; how I grieve for them. He is feeling His Sorrow, in and through our hearts. These people are like the ones that the wall fell on in the Gospel; its not their sins *per se*. (Lk13:1-5)Dolours, dolours are all around little children in this time of sorrow.

Militant angels surround you; militant angels under the leadership of St Michael, protect My Church, the Body of Christ. (1Co12:27), My Own faithful ones are safe in Me, but you gaze out from the security of My Presence and you see suffering and sorrow, which because as I have told you, the weeds also mingle with the precious wheat,(Mt 13:24-30) My Own also suffer and die through no fault of their own. The times in which you are living should be clear evidence to all, that they are signs of impending Judgment.(Rv20:11-15) Little children, you will linger a little longer, pleading for the conversion of sinners, the Salvation of souls. Continue to pray that none of those experience a sudden, unexpected death. Be ready to come before Me, to come to the Embrace of Eternal Love. With regard to the woman who is My Own and was deceived by the world and suffered in the world; as you know little children, a humbled contrite heart your God cannot refuse. (cf Ps51:17) In the confessional I absolve each one of My Own from past transgressions, the errors of judgment, all such; and I remind you, the sorrows of yesterday are no more! Live therefore in each God given moment in My Life, My Light, My Love. I Love you most tenderly, most totally and most eternally. Keep your eyes fixed on your Jesus. Little one, you and your spouse, speak to your God in all loving prayerfulness and ask always for the Gifts of the Holy Spirit. Seek to live the virtuous life; cling to your Jesus, invoke the Mother of God prayerfully and choose some favoured saints and invoke their assistance. Nothing is impossible to the Lord your God.(Lk1:38) You live in a time of trial little children and I ask you, remain faithfully in My Church founded on the Rock of St Peter(Mt16:18), present even today in the person of John Paul II. I assure you that My blessings are profoundly upon you. I am the God Who Loves you most tenderly, most profoundly and most eternally. You will recognize the blessings that have come upon you as the days and weeks go by. Rejoice in this Our Love's union and be at Peace. (Jesus told us she may even become pregnant without the surgical reversal.)

Little children, I am Jesus! You know, you are living in a great hour of Mercy, and yet it is punctuated by great sorrow and great tragedy round about the earth, because of man in free will responding not to the Living God, but to the eternal enemy. Thus there is much suffering and much grief. Dear little children, these things have to be as you know, before the fulfillment of Scripture! There is a great spiritual warfare all over the earth as you know; many are dying in wars and famines-all man made- and this is a great sorrow to Your God; and those who are dying in a coldly calculated manner, at the hands of the alleged physicians; this abomination is more grievous to Me, than what cruel dictators are doing to My little helpless ones who are My Own. Little children, it is a grave affront to Your God, for an individual to choose when one shall be born and when one shall die bodily death, and I address this warning in My Epistle of Love to the scientific world, and I address this warning increasingly so, through the beloved John Paul. All those who are attending the conference become most clearly enlightened, for many pray on this issue of bodily death, of clinical death. Much suffering has occurred for many families in their time of need, their time of crisis, in the illness of a loved one, when these body parts are transposed to another human being and the beating of a human heart, which belongs to Me, is stopped! You will hear further on this matter when the beloved John Paul speaks, imminently now. Be at Peace.

Little one, sorrowful as We are with regard to that doctor, you may believe that I Myself shield her from that which is unclean, for thou hast prayed much for her. Continue to pray for the conversion of the doctors in this world today that are in the darkest degradation of soul. Continue to pray for him and such as him. I give all that opportunity to repent and to come back to Me, for example, Dr Nathanson's conversion. Little children, you recognize the epidemic that cancer has been upon the face of the earth. At this time these diseases have to be! It is a great sorrow to the Lord Your God. Little children, simply pray for those who are stricken, by this disease and many other such serious diseases and trust in the Lord. Little children, at times the disease goes into remission, and others are taken home. Dear little children, simply pray for those stricken and trust in the Lord. Sorrow, sorrow has been a lot of this woman's life. Little children, in your anointing of the gifts of healing, believe that even she can be healed. Therefore know that healing anointing comes on this woman in due course. It is not yet for she is not fully receptive yet. She seeks solace, she seeks comfort, but not of Me, the Living God. Nevertheless, I will fetch her back to Truth and heal her brokenness. Persevere in all prayerfulness attending this woman.

The poor woman will come to you seeking solace for sorrow, and will find it. You will be empowered by the Holy Spirit, to do so without jeopardizing your practice, because of your profound Faith. I Myself will give you the Words. When something so tragic happens in a life as you know often, there is an obsession which lodges itself, in the individual and becomes as it were, unshakable, and in all gentle Healing Love, you and I and Mother, will work a Healing Miracle on this poor soul, for it is only in her healing, that the members of her family, also come around. It is sufficient for today. She is already medicated; it will be suffice until she sees you. It is not in My Trust, and yet, as you well know, she cannot cope without it. The sorrow which encompasses M is known to Me, therefore I bid thee M, son of Peace, to be at Peace. I fill thee with My Peace and My Love. Your actions were actions of Charity and Love; Enlightenment. There is so much misinterpretation of Truth, that those whose loved ones are wounded to the point of death in accidents, are indeed often persuaded, even manipulated to commit to the organs being stripped from their beloved ones. This remains a haunting memory to them which is not easily healed. Therefore We ask each one of you to pray for this mother, for her healing to continue. I bless you little children, for your prayers for this woman.

More and more of the scandalous behaviour of the physicians throughout the world today is a great sorrow to your God; that these gifted individuals use their capabilities for the destruction of God-given life. A time fast approaches when those who are My Own will recall the words in Holy Scripture, "James: is there any sick among you? Let them be brought to the elders, let hands be laid upon them. (James 5:14-15) In My Name they are healed. You will see this happening more and more among the believers in My Name. Our Lord is showing the physicians about the world and saying, "I place before you a blessing or a curse(Dt28 etc); choose Life therefore! **Our Lord causes us to share His** *Pain* Little children, to be near death and to be dead, are separate conditions are they not? I am in Sorrow that this bodily death is dealt with so lightly, so casually even! There are grave consequences to such an attitude of modern doctors, which many may not be aware of until they are Enlightened, before they come before Me in Judgment. That is why you are called to much prayer for them. The beloved John Paul II speaks of a "Culture of Death," and this is what is evidenced throughout this book, and evidenced throughout all the medical fields at this time. I, the Giver of Life, the Giver of free will to mankind, am aggrieved about all that is occurring today. I am with you always. I pour out My Spirit upon My loved ones most profoundly. I pour it out on many who shield themselves from My Spirit, to their sorrow and My Sorrow.

In suffering and sorrow they come back to Me. Again I remind you as I have spoken in the past, when I call them gently, they do not heed Me. And so they wait a time when they need Me and they cry out to Me, and I attend upon them. For some, the way of the prodigal is the only way. Pray much for those who are lost and confused little children; they are yet My Own! A Solemn Oath I have given to you for every Word I utter is Truth; it shall occur. We release to him vital information as to the hypocrisy of what has been going on and been covered up as Charity and Love. A Great Sorrow is upon your God and indeed upon Our Mother over man's betrayal of his fellow man and the many underhanded activities which are rampant about the world, within the medical profession, and within the general population as you have noticed the insurance companies; they are not the only ones, for none abide by My Commandments, none but a few faithful ones, for greed besots their minds, power besots their minds. That is why My faithful ones endure much, and in so doing are blest!

The errors and sorrows of the world today are grievous to your God. You will recognize the major false idol of money, of greed, and you know well that the love of money is the root of all evil(1 Timothy 6:10) and you see these evils being perpetrated against My suffering little ones day in and day out! I am God..(cf Ex 14:18) and I am not oblivious to what is occurring here. You pray, "come Lord and do not delay." You ask My intercession for the many causes and I am attendant upon each and every precious little one, and those who in free will have chosen to follow the father of lies in an earthly quest for material things and greed and power, they do not go unpunished. Though they think they have deceived all, they have not deceived Me! Beloved little ones, graces and blessings in the Power of the Holy Spirit flow freely upon you and upon those whom you carry in your heart. Ask Me for every needed thing, for even the smallest cause and I assist you, for you are My Own, My beloved ones. I am a God of Justice! Have I not spoken "Vengeance is Mine says the Lord?"(Dt 32:35) Do not doubt little children, that those who are behaving so cruelly, so unjustly to those without voice or power, go unpunished. Except they repent in true sorrow, woe unto them! Little children, I have filled your hearts with My Merciful Love; you shall persevere, (Rm 5:1-5) and I am attendant upon My Own. The Body of Christ(1Co12:27), is secure in the Power of the Spirit of the Living God. Little children, manifold are the blessings and graces coming upon you and the true faithful all over the earth.

It is a time of trial and you are aware of it, and in each testing you are strengthened to the necessary courage, the Fortitude, the perseverance(cf1Cor13), the all -powerful Faith to resist the deceits and the snares, for I am with you always. I AM YOUR STRENGTH!(Ps. 144)I Love each one of My Own as I have spoken, most tenderly, most totally and eternally. I am aggrieved by those who choose to know Me not; especially those who do not recognize Me in the suffering brother or sister on earth. The Lord's planted grain, and the enemy's planted weeds intermixing.(Mt 13:24-30). Little children that is how it is today. Oh sorrow! Little children it is with Sorrow I gaze upon multitudes of the depressed. Some, even many are Baptized unto Me, but they know Me not! You pray to Me as Almighty God, Great Physician, Wonder Counselor, (Is9:6) but so few know Me in this Way. Yes little children, you know well that I have already won the Victory over satan, sin and death. In My Name, Jesus, is each souls Victory. Do not worry about the signs of Death, the 666 and other such signs of that which must be, before My Return. I protect My Own, I shield My Own. Yes you will see sorrow, and yet you will see Victory. Be not afraid, I am with you always. Hosts of angels surround the children of God all over the earth now. Remember that twice as many angels were loyal to Me. Therefore cling to your Jesus, cling to the Heavenly Host prayerfully and be at

Peace.

I ask you to pray for all factions in this war, for this war brings no good to anyone on this earth. My little ones, as I gaze at the Middle East, I am heavy burdened with a Great Sorrow. Woe and again, Woe! Now is truly a time for all believers on earth to, as it were, don sackcloth and repent not only for self, but for all of humanity, that your God, in His Merciful Love, bring release from this dark bondage. In this sorrowful matter, I the Lord God address you. Little children, as you see, numerous such cases of loved ones, as it were disappearing from their homes and families. Do not think that I am unmoved; untouched! I respond to the prayers. All that occurs in the lives of humans as you know, is related to free will given to every individual, and as you well know some use the free will, not as the gift that I give them, but inappropriately. They use it to the detriment, the harm of others, and of their own souls. This is grievous to the Lord your God. I would also give you to know that these too, are the signs of the times which you have been called to watch for, even as fellow humans abscond with other people's loved ones, so the enemy absconds with My loved ones, and I am aggrieved about this also.

Little children, there is a connection between Faith and lack of Faith, and the disastrous events which are occurring upon the earth now. The enemy has much of humanity bound up in fear. Faith, Faith-in-action, defeats fear; therefore children, pray much! In this way your Faith is strengthened according to the needs of these times in which you live. Trust Me; I attend upon this heart-wrenching request which you have just read! On whom I will, I have Mercy; I am the Lord your God (Ex34:6-8) Who speaks. I have Mercy on My beloved Humanity, and yet the multitudes as it were, shun Me and go their own way, or worse still, heed the enemy who brings death to the world, death to the souls of those who follow in that direction, and so this is a time of sorrow on the earth.

Know that in Our Mercy as We have assigned the Queen of Heaven, the Queen of Angels and All Saints to intercede for the beloved humanity, in a special way in these times, She is attendant upon this suffering humanity now, as Mother of Mercy and Mother of Sorrows, and yet Mother of Perpetual Help. Little children, you have given Our Mother many titles because of her Merciful Intercession before Me, the Living God, and She attends upon you in those titles, calling the children of God, toward Light and Love and Peace; rousing them to turn towards Truth, towards Salvation. How long oh Lord,"(cfRv6:10)many cry in prayer, before an end of this suffering, and yet it is a time of decision which is upon the world, decisions for Light and Love and Peace, or decisions for the opposing factors. I give time for the multitudes to choose Life, to choose Love, to choose Peace, that they may know the eternal Victory, and in this interim of time, there is rampant suffering about the earth. That is why true believers, all of you are called to pray; pray for Mercy from your God.

It is indeed true; the Lord your God is wrath about the transgressions of His Laws which are great, occurring rampantly on the face of the earth. A measured beat of time is upon the earth, and at the end of it, then comes the sequence of events which are forecast in Holy Scripture and hold fear for the many. Be undaunted by these fearful messages. Those who are Mine, are ever Mine. There are those who were never Mine. Do not concern yourselves about this matter. I Will you to know that I am God and nothing is impossible to Me. And yet there is a Sorrow in the Heart of Your God, when the ashes of a human are scattered far and wide, or just sat there in a corner somewhere, neither honored nor recognized, for all Creation is sacred to the Lord. There is no exception to the rule! At this time, as I gaze upon the so-called civilized nations, I see great lack of Faith. They are calling themselves a Christian nation, but they do not live holiness; they do not honor the Birth of the True God-man on earth, but rather they persevere in pagan idolatries even in the Holy Season. This is an abomination to the Lord your God, and so it is a time of sorrow.

Little children, always remember, it is only Death of the soul which is a grave problem for the soul, and a grave sorrow to the Living God, when such an event occurs! At this time, clinical death is occurring among My Own and those whom I Love, in a matter not acceptable to Me, for I am the Giver of Life and I chose a time to be born and a time to die, (Qo3:2) for each soul! Thus I have Commissioned you to work on the Epistle of Love Mission to the Scientific World. My Soul is sorrowful even unto death."(cfMt26:38) I am Jesus, Eternal Victor. Even at this time I call you to trust Me.(Jn14:1) Hope in Me when there seems no reason to hope at all! Hope in Me; do you not know that your God brings good out of all this wickedness, that I am ever Victor in the battle for souls! Little children, love Me as I have Loved you; this is the pathway of holiness, the narrow Way. Little children, many there are who seek Me but they do not follow in the narrow Way. Little children, in the world today there is so great a temptation to follow the ways of the world, to seek the material gains, not realizing in so doing, you are being caught up in the snares of the foe, in idolatry and the like. The little ones need not suffer, were there any measure of justice and fairness on this earth. Our Lord goes quiet and gazes at all the killing and suffering, and He Sorrows. He is looking at the world and weeping. We get Scripture, [He gazed at Jerusalem and said, Jerusalem, Jerusalem...Mt 23:37-39]

(Romans 3:10-18; Isaiah 59:7-8)

There is not a good man left, no, not one! There is not one who understands; not one who looks for God. All have turned aside, tainted all alike; there is not one good man left, not a single one. Their throats are yawning graves; their tongues are full of deceit. Viper's venom is on their lips, bitter curses fill their mouths. Their feet are swift when blood is to be shed, wherever they go there is havoc and ruin. They know nothing of the way of peace, there is no fear of God before their eyes.

CHAPTER ELEVEN
HIS BLOOD. The Covenant: The Blessing and the Curse

MARK OF CAIN Gn 4:15

Pilate was vexed and said impatiently, "what I have written, I have written!" Annas and Caiaphas thus left off disputing in vain with Pilate, because he wrote the inscription, "Jesus of Nazareth, King of the Jews." They went away in haste, fearing they would be late for the Pascal sacrifice which was but a symbol, unknowingly leaving the true Pascal Lamb, Who was being led to the Altar of the Cross. They were most careful not to contract exterior defilement, while their souls were completely defiled by anger, hatred and envy. They had said, "His Blood be on us and on our children,"[Matthew 27:26] In the name of all sinners they solemnly accepted the curse! Thus were the two paths formed-the one leading to the altar belonging to the Jewish law, the other leading to the Altar of Grace. But it is excruciatingly painful if, with the recognition must come the claiming of a part in the Crucifixion of that Messiah, as all of us must, for we are all sinners. Besides Mary, all humans from the beginning to the end of time, have contributed by sin, to that load which the Sinless One bore, for the Salvation of all humanity. Yet, in His great Mercy, He assures us of forgiveness, whatever we may have to repent, and then Salvation for all eternity! That is a two thousand year-guarantee, repeated again in these His Words.

Over one hundred years ago, on 28th May 1898, the Shroud revealed, in an unforeseen and unpredictable way, the secret of its Image. During the exposition organized for the wedding of the future King Victor Emmanuel III, an enthusiastic amateur photographer, Secondo Pia, a lawyer by profession, attempted to photograph the Shroud with two exposures of 14 and 20 minutes each. "Closed up in the dark room, I felt an intense emotion when, during the development, I saw for the first time appear, as a *positive* on my photographic *negative*, that Holy Face, with such a clarity that I remained frozen on the spot said Secondo Pia. Thus began a century of scientific study, still ongoing. Science reveals that the image is not a painting; it is caused by some form of radiation, and seems to be "illuminated from within;" the image of an executed man, who had been scourged, capped with thorns, crucified with nails, pierced in the side, who had abrasions on the left knee due to a fall, wounds, swelling and bruises to the face and the bridge of His nose was broken; inexplicably imprinted as a three dimensional *negative,* whereas the blood stains are positive. Science can never *prove* the Man of the Shroud is Jesus Christ because there is no archival evidence that might confirm it. But, "if it be a hoax, we will have to rewrite the whole history of technology, because for it to have been created as it is, more than a thousand years ago, they would have had to be aware of techniques unknown to us today", says Luigi Gonella, scientific consultant to Cardinal A Ballestrero. There are at least seven "coincidences" between the Gospel accounts and the image on the Shroud, notably by St John who the Gospel tells us was an eyewitness.

On September14th,1578, Duke Emmanuel Philbert transferred the Shroud of Turin to the Turin Cathedral, where it was permanently installed in its own chapel in the Cathedral of St John the Baptist, on June1st,1694. In 1983, King Umberto, last King of Italy, bequeathed the Shroud to Pope John Paul 2 before he died The Shroud of Turin is unique. There is no other burial linen in existence which bears the image of a crucified man. As with the image of Our Lady of Guadalupe of Mexico on the tilma of Juan Diego, the image on the Shroud is indelible and as vivid today as it was over the centuries. The imprints on the Shroud of Turin are those of a human corpse in a pronounced state of *rigor mortis,...* just under six feet tall and of good physique. The Image is of a man, and determinations suggest he was laid on his back on the lower half of the cloth, and the upper half drawn over the face and front of the body. There is no evidence of decomposition of the body, suggesting that He was in the Shroud less than 48 hours, in keeping with the Gospel account. Of course to Christian believers, the absence of decomposition of the body presents no mystery whatsoever, because death was part of the Divine plan, decomposition was not.

The Image bears the marks of lacerations from a severe scourging and a badly bruised and swollen, but none the less dignified, face. The chest cavity is expanded, as of someone agonizing for hours to inhale air into his lungs. As for the crown of thorns, it was not a wreath-like circlet as is commonly depicted. Instead, it was a crude cap covering the entire skull, and its thorns dug into the scalp vessels which are well known to bleed profusely. There are thirteen blood flows which can be traced to puncture wounds on the head. The knees of the man on the Shroud also revealed extensive damage such as would be incurred through heavy falls. There were also two oval areas of excoriation in the region of the left and right shoulders, caused by the carrying of the patibulum, or the cross beam of the Cross. There is also clear evidence that nails were driven into the wrists, not the palms of the hands...A nail was also driven between the second and third metatarsal bones, with the left foot on top of the right, with a gaping hole between the fifth and sixth ribs on the right side, and upon close examination, clear serous fluid is seen mixed with the blood which flowed from the incision.

The Shroud also testifies that all across the back, shoulders, buttocks and legs, there were severe welts and shredding of the skin from flagellations of the Roman flagellum. Many other scientific details are discussed such as the carbon dating controversy, the photographic enigma, molds and pollens, the discovery of the coin on the left eye.... but there are several aspects to the Shroud which loudly attest that it is indeed the Cloth of Christ, e.g. the wounds caused by the thorn-cap. This is truly exceptional because there are no other documents reporting any such head cap either among the Romans or any other peoples. Moreover, after death the man of the Shroud was wrapped in a sheet...very uncommon in antiquity, as in most cases the crucified men were left on the cross to be eaten by wild animals, or at best buried in a paupers grave... "In fact I do suspect science will acknowledge that the Shroud of Turin is indeed the Shroud of Christ. It will certainly be all part of God's plan and timing As Dr Pierre Barbet, the Author of *A Doctor at Calvary* said: "Science can do no more than keep silence, for the phenomenon is outside of its domain. But for the man of learning, at least there is proof of resurrection. And so, the physical body, with its thorns and punctured flesh, has left a lingering testimony to scientists and faithful alike. It was a horrible mutilation. But will it help us to show more gratitude to the man on the Shroud for the suffering He endured for us?

Dr Barbet and several other physicians over several years performed a number of experiments on cadavers, their students and themselves to determine the cause of death of Jesus. One example dealt with the argument over the Gospel of St John [19:34.35.]*But one of the soldiers with a spear opened His side, and immediately there flowed out Blood and water.....*Critics ridiculed the historical veracity of this. But performing a number of autopsies, Dr Barbet verified that by carefully inserting a syringe, he drew out serum first, "hydropericardium" before entering the ventricle and drawing blood, and further making the point that in the case of the exceptionally painful death-agony of Jesus, this serum would be superabundant. Hence an eyewitness as was St John would indeed be able to see the "Blood and Water" flow out. The Holy Shroud then, is a magnificent confirmation [in many ways] of the historicity of the Gospels, especially St John's Gospel. Dr Barbet continues; *"the bloodstained pictures were clearly not drawn by the hand of man...no artist would have been able to imagine for himself the minute detail of what we now know about the coagulation of blood, but which in the 14the century was unknown. The fact is that not one of us would be able to produce such pictures without falling into some blunder. It was this homogenous group of verifications without one single weak link among them, which decided me, relying on the balance of probabilities, to declare the authenticity of the Shroud, from the point of view of anatomy and physiology, is a scientific fact."* Dr Barbet published several preliminary studies be fore his definitive summary, A Doctor at Calvary," one of which was *"Les Cinq Plaies"*[The Five Wounds].

(St. Paul's Letter to the Hebrews 9: 24-28): It is not as though Christ had entered a man-made sanctuary which was only modeled on the real one; but it was Heaven itself, so that He could appear in the actual Presence of God on our behalf. And He does not have to offer Himself again and again, like the high priest going into the sanctuary year after year with the blood that is not his own, or else He would have had to suffer over and over again since the world began. Instead of that, He has made His appearance once and for all, now at the end of the last age, to do away with sin by sacrificing Himself, since men only die once, and after that comes judgment; so Christ, too, offers Himself only once, to take the faults of many on Himself, and when He appears a second time, it will not be to deal with sin, but to reward with Salvation those who are waiting for Him.

JESUS: The Rock of Ages bids thee Peace! Precious children of a Loving Father, speak your heart's requests. *Lord You know what is in my heart; I would not mention it except if it is Your Will.* You may well speak it.

On Christmas Eve a benefactor unknown to us sent 2000 beautiful roses from Mexico to our parish in celebration of Jesus' 2000th birthday. On New Year's Eve, I went to the evening Mass, then cleared out the roses that were dead. But at the foot of the altar I saw that I had been pricked by a thorn in my right ring finger, and a large drop of blood had fallen on the lowest step; which I initially just swept away without a second thought, but Our Lord said to me in Adoration this morning:

We have a covenant written in blood now! *Lord, I know that You have bled and died for me, and that I receive Your Body, Blood, Soul and Divinity every day at Mass, but what is the significance of a drop of my blood?*

My beloved, My beloved, My beloved, are we not one? My little children, every sacrifice, every suffering, every penance, united with your prayers, rises up as pleasing incense before Me, the Living God, for we are one![*Our Lord shows us again the Gospel of St. John 17*: "Father, may they be one in Us..."]Little children, each one of you has become one in Me(Jn17:21), and so our hearts are one, our sufferings are one, our relations are one, our Joy is one. Little children, believe that the miracle of roses is not yet over. Many, many, will come in Adoration in this Church, for I have selected it in honor of My Mother, who is reverenced in that parish beyond that of many parishes. Militant angels of God are watching over the Documents; the obstructions are prevented, a free flow of printing occurs. Heaven assists profoundly. And is it not First Friday? *The Sacred Heart; thank You, Lord.*

I will pour out My Spirit on all mankind and they will live! Our Lady of the Miraculous Medal wills to help you in all of these undertakings, and so it shall be. [I am] Lover of souls. The vortex of the storm is hanging over the Holy Land now. Do not be distraught at anything you hear now. Even the media may not be carrying truth, as you understand Truth. Little children, We keep that area of the world and the people

142 — Medicine of God

We draw there in your prayers. I have a Plan and I have a Design, as you know. It is the Lord Who speaks! Yet this people on both sides, these people are not yielded to Me. And those who proclaim to the world that they are working to a peaceful solution are often just meddling, for their own cause, their own agendas, as you know. The political expediencies, as you know, are often brought into play. Dear little children, at this time I ask the faithful to simply continue to pray that your God's Will be done and that Peace comes without a horrendous cost to mankind. *We prayed an Our Father, Hail Mary, Glory Be...*

Therefore remain at Peace, little children. As ever, I am with My Own always. My Name is before you and on your lips.

Little children, in these Missions of Love which I have entrusted to you, as it were, although I am profoundly united with you in all that you are doing, great blessings come upon you. Indeed, each one of you shall persevere in all that you are under-taking. Do not be dismayed at anything that occurs in the world today, for you live in most unusual times, turbulent times. My precious little one, itemize and ask of Me what you will, on each subject of your heart's concern. *Lord Your command, "If you love Me, keep My Commandments [John 14]," is the reason for this Mission to the scientific world especially, and to the people of this time. And Lord, the vision You gave me last year on the eve of 11th February, is almost exactly the words You spoke to the Samaritan woman [symbol of a woman missionary] in John 4: "The water that I shall give will turn into a spring inside him, welling up to eternal Life."*

Little children, you have been told through the many visionaries and locutionists of Our Mother, that these are the turbulent times, these are the trying times, and yet, My Love, that River of Light and Love is pouring forth upon My precious Faith-filled little ones, even as now, and you *shall* persevere. Again, I tell you, each one of you, I am your Strength, your Dignity. My Power, it comes upon you helpless little ones, to persevere in all that I call you to, and I carry your cross, My beloved ones. I let you feel it upon occasion, and yet I do indeed carry the brunt of the cross for each of My Own. My beloved one, rejoice in Our Love's union. In this way, when you are united with Me, as you often are in prayer *[the times in the Adoration chapel]*, I am with you profoundly and I fill you with all that you need to carry you, moment by moment, step by step, day by day, through-out your Faith Journey. Beloved, you know well that I have chosen you for this most specific Mission, and yet it is essential that you continue the work of your hands that you are doing in the Healing Ministry. You recognize that the little ones are in darkness and affliction, sorely afflicted, most particularly those who know Me not. Even so, I bless you to be My Heart, My Voice, My Hands in the ongoing healing. Do not be frustrated with the troubled and troublesome ones. Give them the specified measure of time and leave all the rest to Me. Give them over to Me often during prayer, especially at the Church, at the chapel. Just give them to Me; leave them with Me. Attend upon them for the allotted time and leave all else to Me, for I am with you in a remarkable unity of My Love. Your Love for Me and Mother and My Love and Mother's Love for you – is it not a beautiful trinity? Therefore, be at Peace.

Blood Transfusions

JESUS: The only blood needed is the blood of the Lamb!(cf Rv5:9-10.) See, I set before you now a blessing and a curse(Dt 28); Look what you have chosen! If you had before you a blessing and a curse, I ask you this: Would they stop because of My Word or your word? Even so, speak your Words! I, the Lord your God who lives and loves eternally(Rv 4:9-10), bless you. Scripturally, it is written: 'thou shalt not eat blood.' There are many ways in which this is comprehended by My people. I believe you know well now, that there are ways of substituting and even ways of using each patient's own blood or blood products. Yet in dire emergencies, blood transfusions are indeed used. My little children, this whole catastrophe of medical science is because man does not follow God's Law, the Will of God as taught even unto Moses and even unto this day. The principle of blood transfusion has been accepted by the medical profession and yet it is not without hazard, as you well know.

They must be aware of what they are doing. There is no blessing upon this generation of mankind, which snatches the infants from their mothers' wombs, destroying them in a bloodbath of death. It is written: 'the firstborn belongs to God.'(Ex13:11-16;Lk2c;Rv1:5) Where are the firstborn? They *are* not! A cry greater than Rachel's is upon the earth now!(Jr31:15) The timing of this document which you are writing is important to Me. I will leave to you how to write about the blood transfusions which have been in existence now these many years, but you will be inspired by Heaven. A haunting sorrow is in the Heart of the Lord your God, because of the tragedies of mankind's pride in the works of their hands, not consecrated to Me, but to power and to greed. My little sister, I am anointing you and blessing you profoundly. Be at Peace in all these things. My Voice needs to be heard. These people need to at least revise what they are doing, because it is true that a day comes when they stand before their Judge;(Rv20:11-15) and since thou art the one I choose to forewarn a multitude, thou art profoundly blest.

Remember, you are not alone. There are others of like heart and mind amidst your people and Heaven is with you. *The Blood and Water, Living Water I give you from My own Heart.* (Jn19:34-35)To all the faithful: a great blessing, a great anointing, at this time, this period of the year in which you are living, is assisting the faithful most profoundly in all that they do. A Great Ingathering is occurring now. Little children, love one another and be at Peace! *Blessed be God in His angels and in His saints. Blessed be the great Mother of God, Mary Most Holy. Blessed be God forever! Dear Lord, I would like to have further enlightenment on the subject of blood transfusions.*

I make it known to you that there is no need of blood transfusions, were mankind using their free will for the love of God and the love of neighbor (Mt22:35-40). Alas, it is not so and, thus, is blood transfusion deemed necessary now for sustaining life. What would you have Me do? Because I have given you free will, humanity, you use it to maim and to injure and to wound; and then you use it to attempt to repair that which you have mutilated. This blessing of the great Pentecost is upon the faithful all over the earth, those where Love yet reigns in their hearts and controls thus their rational thoughts and minds. You believe you have great rational powers, but you do it without My merciful Love. I bid you know that you use your brothers' and sisters' blood and you have reaped a harvest of AIDS and Hepatitis and more. Blood given from an unknown donor to another conveys with it, as you well know, many, many, dangers – until recently, not fully comprehended by the scientists. The resulting ailments do not aid the poor victims but, rather, harm them.

I set before you a blessing and a curse mankind; look what you have chosen. Even so, in My Great Mercy, I hold My wrath in abeyance. I bless and I heal, for I hear the prayers of the faithful, little children, with hearts of love pleading with God to spare this life, to spare that life, here, there, everywhere all over the earth. I hear and I heal. In spite of the errors the scientists make, I heal as I Will. On whom I will, I have Mercy! It is thus with the one you have met in My Presence." *[Jesus is referring to one who has had a liver transplant, kneeling in Adoration of the Blessed Sacrament.]* My precious little one, daughter of faithfulness, prevail. The stonewalling is temporary. You shall succeed in your Mission, for I am with you. Mother is with you. You are profoundly assisted. Continue to pray and address this matter. 'By what authority?' they ask! By the Authority of the Name of Jesus. By the Blood of the Lamb. This is your Authority! (Rv 5:9-10)

Cling to Me;(Ps91:14) your weakness is My Strength. United with Me, you shall not fail. You may be scorned in the eyes of the world. This is nothing new. This has happened with My sainted holy ones and yet they prevailed. You are anointed in so profound a way that you cannot separate yourself from Me and My Will any longer. Yet in your abandonment to Love, the Lord your God has accepted your surrender, and thus these great and powerful graces pour forth upon you and Heaven is at hand to you. This is a testing of your very soul at those moments(1P:3-11); and yet I am with you, and together We do it. And Mother, in all delight, is also with you. United in the two Hearts of Love, thou shalt not fail! Be at Peace. Look at the prophets, at the warriors in the Name of the Lord in the Old Testament and the New. Follow them.

MARY: *Continue, little children, for there are not enough yet that are so enlightened. My little one, I am your Mother; I am the Mother of all.(Jn19:26-27) The graces given to Me at the time of the Annunciation(Lk1:35) flow through Me still. For it is the Will of the Father, Son and Holy Spirit that it be through* this *Vessel that the graces flow. I come to earth here, there and everywhere. All over the earth, beckoning them, calling them to come back to the Lord their God, that the disasters on earth, the afflictions, the miseries, be at least ameliorated. Some are, and some are defeated all together. But the people of mankind need to read the Scriptures, the journey of the chosen people. As soon as the Good Shepherd got them on safe ground, they wandered off again to false idols. This is not new, except that there are many more false idols and many more temptations that are happening on the earth. And, tragically, there are many, many more people affected by this falsehood, which is taking shape in many forms all over the earth. Thus, My little ones are called and armed to be brave warriors of their Christ. Know that God is with you, even as He said in Holy Scripture. He is ever with you, even unto the end of time.*

Peace! A great anointing of Love, Peace, Joy and all the accompanying graces and virtues are attendant upon you as you continue your work of Love in the Name of Jesus. I am donning sackcloth like Esther and going before the Great King to gain the release of multitudes of children from the bondages of sin and death. Night and day, the river of Light flows to dispel the darkness, for now is a time of great Redemption upon the earth.Rv14:3-5) Believe and be at Peace. You may take your ease now, My precious little ones." Blessed be the great Mother of God, Mary Most Holy! *[Angels are singing: "Faith of Our Fathers, Holy Faith. We will be true to Thee till death; we will be true to Thee till death!" We sing the verses.]*

What I am telling you is that were man to return to the Covenant of Love written in My Blood,(Jn14:21-24) there would not be this additional spilling of blood, this continuous spilling of blood, this continuous need for blood transfusions and the like, for I by Myself am the Healer of all. Little children, I heal many in spite of the use of human blood; and I heal many who the doctors would say require blood and yet do not receive it. I heal them Myself, restoring them to fullness of health. Peace! I am the Lord your God and I am with you. I bless you, little children, profoundly this day which is Holy to the Lord. A great anointing of My Love is felt by you now, is it not? We release now an obstruction that had been hurled against this Mission. Thou art the ones chosen for this work of Merciful Love and enlightenment to My people, to the intellectuals, to the scientific mind. These people do indeed recognize the beauty of Creation and specialize in certain aspects of My created beings. Often times, as they limit themselves to one area, one specialty, they see only, as it were, blood cells or heart valves or specific tissues. And they intensely devote their studies and works and healing arts to that small area to the point where they cease to see the entire being or the entire complexity of Humanity and of Creation. Yet I bless them. I bless them with the necessary skills and intellect to do research, to do healing works on behalf of My suffering humanity. The blessing is there. The fact that it is not freely flowing on each individual physician is because of certain barriers they themselves, in free will, have placed between us. I believe you are familiar with these sorts of barriers. My little children, now is a moment of sweet surrender to Love in the Peace of My Presence, which is upon you. Ask of Me what you will.

MARY: *A sorrow is that the many will not to heed. But there is rejoicing for those who do indeed heed, discern, begin to believe in the true sanctity of each God-given life. Your work is immense, greater than you can comprehend, little children. There- fore, be not dismayed at any obstructions. The enemy is wrath. Through this Portal of Light, the Heart of your Beloved Mother, the Mercy Gate, blessings flow upon each of My Own, among whom you are numbered, little children. As to the meetings of the Catholic physicians, in unity with the priest, it is a tragedy, a sorrow, that they do not choose to believe, but seek a burden of scientific truth before they would believe. Though you present this to them very clearly, they are reluctant in their great intellect to accede to these Truths. Be not dismayed; it has been ever thus.*

JESUS: Thou hast asked that We rebuke in the Name of Jesus – it is the Lord Who speaks – the spirit of pride which assails many intellectuals. This has been an ongoing war throughout the course of the centuries, and continues to now. Yet some will yield. A certain yieldedness-in-Faith to the Living God is essential, before the thoughts of this people, the minds and thoughts, are opened to Truth. I, the Lord God, *am* Truth. Another Gateway of Truth is opened elsewhere in the Americas, in agreement with what you are given, converging as it were with what you are given, and this assists you. Little children, those who serve the Lord do not work alone. Much help is given you.

MARY: *My daughter, it is your Heavenly Mother who speaks, in conjunction with the Holy Spirit, which is indeed so at every time I speak. My little one, when the Holy Spirit came upon your Virgin Mother of God, all Graces flowed upon Me, and My mantle is essentially the mantle of the power of the Holy Spirit of the Living God.* (Lk1:35) *You see, Jesus' Body and Blood were formed in Me. I gave Him My Love. I gave Jesus to mankind.*(Lk1:32-33) *But Jesus in turn, gave Me to mankind at the foot of the Cross of Calvary*(Jn19:26-27). *The only blood needed is the Blood of the Lamb. My little one, you know well that My life, as Joseph's, the beloved saint, are, as it were, hidden in Scripture. But We are present in both Scripture and Tradition most profoundly. My little children, you are My children. If you read the book of Revelation, you are My other children*(Rv12:17), *for you keep Me and you keep the Name of Jesus ever on your lips. It is these, My other children, in unity with Me, the Woman Clothed in the Sun*(Rv12), *who defeat the dragon, in the economy of our Father's Design, since He has called you to be little brothers and sisters of Jesus. Therefore, you work in unity with Jesus to defeat the enemy.*

In your own prayers and sacrifices, which are pleasing to God, you cause multitudes to convert. Little one, you wonder why you are tested and tried. It is because you are working works of merciful love, which is angering the dragon, and so you have these testings, these trials as you claim the Name of Jesus, as you claim the Presence of Jesus, yet on earth these 2,000 years in the power of the Eucharist. (Jn6:32-63)*The gift given to My priesthood was to consecrate the Bread and Wine*(Lk22:19-20). *This was the work Jesus promised that He would cause His Apostles to do greater than He Himself. They bring Jesus to all who yield to the Faith of the Apostles. My little one, you may feel at times little; a very small light, a dim candle in the darkness. It is not so. The Spirit of the Living God has anointed all followers of Christ as apostles and disciples with a flame of Love. Once He has claimed His Own by Baptism, Confirmation and the anointing by Faith in the Holy Spirit in the Word of God, you are His great flames, lighting up the darkness as so many candles all over the earth.*(cf Jn 6:64-66)

[*Jesus is saying: "My Love...My Love...My Love...My Love..." as His Blood is dripping. "My Love...My Love...My Love ...My Love..." Mother Mary, help humanity to understand His Love.*] I died that you might have Life to the fullest. Scientific facts to the contrary, there is *one* body attached to *one* soul. This is the Design of your Father, your Creator. This is the way it is; this is the way it should be!Mankind's hands are now stained with the blood of the innocents (Proverbs 6:16,17;Genesis 9:6:Ecclesiastes 12:7; Job

1:21).). and cannot be washed off no matter what they do – except they kneel in penitence and humbly ask forgiveness of their God. The Blood of the Lamb alone washes the sin of murder from a soul.*(1 John 3:12-15)* Oh My people, oh My people, oh that you would choose Love. I give you Love, in the ravishing beauty of the Woman Clothed With the Sun(Rv12), the Mother of God, but you choose not to heed Her call to Love, choose not this Gateway to return to the Lord Your God. You choose rather error, sin, death and destruction. Oh woe, oh My people, oh My people, what have I done to you? (cf Matthew 27:21-26) Continue to work in Faith as thou art taught. In the tape I have inspired your friend to show you, there is a wonder-working power in the Blood of the Lamb. Claim the Precious Blood of your Jesus to heal the individuals spiritually, mentally, emotionally and in every aspect of their being as you pray, and it is done. And your patients will be healed most rapidly. Do you believe?

MARY: *Every time you attend upon the Lord in His Body and Blood, you are anointed. It is the Will of the Lord your God.*

[Jesus asks us to do a symbolic act of Faith. Put your finger on My Heart. We touch His Heart on the Crucifix. Take the drop of Blood and place it on yourself, and the healings proceed! You do not know what is happening here, little children. You are being drawn closer to the Sacred Heart of Love. Encased in My Love, you will go forth as apostles of these times in great Works of Mercy. The anointing is complete and profound. Give glory! *Glory be to the Father...* Mercy is extended to the multitudes on this evening, which is holy to the Lord! By Faith are the victories won!"(Hb11) In obscurity was Our Lord born. In obscurity did He grow up. Now Saint Joseph, ever holy, obscure and humble, remains so to most of the world. Yet He is of the highest order of saints. These are the Keys: humility and obedience. Especially at the time of Consecration, ask what you will of Our Lord, for this is the moment of Divine Mercy! Little children, understand that by the Faith demonstrated here this evening, Heaven is profoundly united with you, and the Church triumphant is in union with this My faithful remnant, among whom you, little children, are numbered. Herein lies the Victory for each believer. My little children, it is known that some are called home to Heaven promptly, rapidly. Some remain in suffering for a time, for the good of their own souls or the good of those whom they carry in their heart or for My Own reasons. Yet I am ever a God of Mercy and Love. None of My Own will be lost to the Glory of My Presence. Therefore, teach the little ones with afflictions to persevere in prayer.(Hb10:36) Teach them that I Love them, that the Mother of God loves them. Teach them that in the Name of Jesus is their Victory. Remind them that I have already defeated satan, sin and death(Rv20:10; 21:4) and that it is only a matter of defeating self. And that with the assistance of your Jesus, and of Our Mother, and a myriad of the angels and saints in the power of the Holy Spirit, they defeat all that comes against them. And in this battle, defeating the foe and self, they give glory to the Father. All the children of God will be clothed in the Sun, like unto the transfigured Christ, like unto the Woman Clothed with the Sun. On that Glorious Day of the Lord, for each and every one of My Faithful, it is so! (Rv22:3-5)Thus are saints able to attend upon those who pray asking that saint to plead their cause. And I, in My delight, allow the many miracles to happen.

With every affliction, firstly We heal spiritually then – as the Lord your God Wills – mentally, emotionally, physically, socially, sexually, in every aspect of their beings. I am the Creator of each one of them. I know their weaknesses, I know their strengths, their vulnerabilities, their utter helplessness when they have been entrapped and ensnared by the enemy. I am the Good Shepherd. I work My healing Love upon them as I Will. You know well that Faith is imperative and that, in their frailty, I send my beloved ones of great Faith, like unto the Faith of the Apostles, to release them from their fears, their anxieties and then their afflictions. Prevail, little ones, prevail.

The Krever Commission. *Commission of Inquiry on the Blood System in Canada: Final Report (Krever Commission)(Published by Canadian Government Publishing, 1997)The three-volume final report of the Commission of Inquiry on the Blood System in Canada, by the Honourable Commissioner Judge Horace Krever, is a detailed overview of the events surrounding the tainted blood scandal of the 1980s, as well as an account of his findings from the testimonies of over 400 witnesses who appeared before the Commission. In his report, Justice Krever provides a series of fifty recommendations formed after hearing evidence from various provincial and national authorities and health officials, as well as from individuals who had been infected, or whose lives had been affected, by the contamination of the blood system......*

In June 1996, a federal judge ruled that the Red Cross Society and those who ran it in the early 1980s could be named by the Commission if Krever found they were to blame. The federal government, provincial health ministries, pharmaceutical companies and people who guided the blood system when the tainted transfusions occurred could also be named if they were deemed responsible. Douglas Lindores, the Secretary General of the Red Cross, complained that Krever had been given the green light to assign misconduct against the Red Cross and more than a dozen of its officials, but other players in the blood system——such as the provinces that funded the Red Cross blood program, and the federal government that regulated it——were essentially left untouched.

The Krever Inquiry ended its public hearings after three years of investigation on December 1996. In July 1997, with the Krever Report still not released, Minister of Health Allan Rock declared there would be no meaningful role for the Red Cross in a new Canadian blood agency. The Red Cross, which had been running the country's blood system for more than half a century, was to be reduced to recruiting blood donors under a new agency that would operate at arm's length from the government. On November 26, 1997, and after a long arduous process, Rock released the Krever Report, the final report of the Royal Commission of Inquiry on the Blood System in Canada. Also worth noting is the particular attention given to a cross-comparison of the Canadian blood system with other international blood systems. France and Japan are two countries that underwent blood scandals similar to Canada's. In France, "l'affaire du sang contamine," as the scandal came to be known, resulted in the transmission of HIV to almost 3,000 people, including 45 per cent of French hemophiliacs.

In 1992, three senior public health officials were sentenced to four years imprisonment each for using up stocks of unsafe blood and blood products before using heat-treated blood—the Krever commission heard similar testimony concerning the Canadian Red Cross. In addition, the three were ordered to pay $1.8 million US in restitution. In response to court challenges against government ministers, the French National Assembly took the unusual step of making current and former ministers more legally accountable, amending the constitution to that effect in July 1993—three months before the Canadian government had even started the Krever Commission. The French government even expressly set up a court to try its ministers. ...In addition, the European Court of Human Rights has ruled three times against France, saying the rights of HIV/AIDS patients had been violated by government delays in compensating them for their infections.

In Japan, about 2,000 hemophiliacs were infected with HIV through tainted blood. In a series of lawsuits, the three directors of Japan's only HIV/AIDS-policy organization in the 1980s were accused of using non-heat-treated blood products when they knew they were unsafe and refusing to import foreign-made products. A criminal investigation of the three was begun last year and trials that began this year and are still ongoing. In addition, three former presidents of a company accused of knowingly selling tainted blood products pleaded guilty to professional negligence in March. The Japanese government did not wait until the issue came to court to apologize. In October 1995, Health Minister Churyu More offered his government's regrets in a formal ceremony before the families of dead hemophiliacs and said, "We cannot deny that delayed government measures led to the tragic increase of victims."

The Canadian government, instead of displaying such candor, took its own Krever Commission to court three times and only apologized within minutes of the report's release, after it was clear that no individuals were directly accused of crimes. The Krever report was, after over a year of delays due to court battles, released five days before World Aids Day, Dec. 1. In it, Justice Krever states that "The compassion of a society can be judged by the measures it takes to reduce the impact of tragedy on its members" and that "A system that knows that these consequences will occur... has, at the very least, a moral obligation to give some thought to the question of appropriate relief for those affected by the inevitable events." Krever's 50 recommendations all have to do with "impact" and "relief"—and make no mention of blame. The major recommendation is no-fault compensation for those infected with HIV and/or hepatitis C, since he calls lawsuits too costly and time-consuming. But beyond compensation—no amount of money will give these victims their health and their lives back—is this little matter of justice, which is supposed to be a fundamental precept of our society. If you do something wrong, or if you fail to do something right when it is your responsibility, you go to jail—that's what all Canadian kids and immigrants are taught. Everyone is, of course, presumed innocent until proven guilty, but the Krever report does not even suggest any criminal investigations—let alone trials—to determine guilt in a scandal that has robbed tens of thousands of Canadians of their health...

.

I ask mankind to come back to Me with all your hearts. Hear Me. I bless, I heal, I cure, I regenerate. For those with deep Faith, united in prayers with their brothers and sisters of deep Faith. Even so, little child of God who is injured and gravely ill from whatever cause, I again bless even the unbelieving doctors and scientists to heal My little one. Much of what is happening in the various fields of medicine is not according to My Will. Yet My sheep are there(Jn10). Because of them, the blessings flow in spite of the great errors being made! The ultimate goal is enlightenment to physicians and associated scientific minds throughout the world. It shall occur! I call each of My Own to assist and I call them while yet leaving them in free will and in their own discernment. Unique events occur in M's life and in the lives of those about him also. And so he has a time of, as it were, bathing in My Love, immersing himself in My Love. And subsequently, he is open to understand My Words to you, which have come to him through you. I come in Love and Mercy in the power of the Holy Spirit. Through those who believe, I am able to heal whatever affliction befalls persons of Faith, should they approach prayerfully – two or more gathered in My Name – in the Faith which you call the Faith of the Apostles, in total Faith. I want to heal that person. I repeat, when they come to Me, as it were, as dead men – unbaptized, unconsecrated to God, unknowing of God, living outside the Law and the Commandments – do you not see that help is not forthcoming from the Lord your God in these circumstances? Come closer to the Hearts of Jesus and Mary.

MARY: *"Mother Mary is praying: God Our Heavenly Father, through Your Son Jesus, Our Victim High Priest, True Prophet and Sovereign King, pour forth the power of your Holy Spirit upon us and open our Hearts. In Your Great Mercy, through the Motherly mediation of the Blessed Virgin Mary our Queen, forgive our sinfulness, heal our brokenness, and renew our hearts, in the Faith and Peace and Love and Joy of your Kingdom, that we may be one in You.*

I bless all that pray for him. We work a miracle of Love. You are a formidable pair. You have stolen My Heart. Remember always that I heal first spiritually, and then as I Will. I Myself comfort the afflicted in a profound manner. I bring the Peace of Christ into your workplace. I bring the Good News to your patients. I bless you in a great anointing of My Love. You are called to be My Hands, My Heart, My Voice. Simply claiming the Blood of your Jesus is suffice. You may ask that it be instilled in the heart; you may ask that the individual see himself at the foot of the Cross and in the Blood of the Lamb, bathing away the affliction. By Faith are the miracles wrought, and this month [July], consecrated to the Divine Mercy of My healing Blood and Water pouring forth, it is a good time to instigate this type of prayer hither and yon about the earth to all those who will listen! I am He Who lives and Loves eternally. I, too, seek the spiritual healing of My People. I bless them with additional healing as I Will.

Simply give all My Words over. Indeed, the Jehovah Witness cult which you mention took the Word of Holy Scripture, but to use it as a bone of contention, and not as it should be, from a truly spiritual position. They are, as is every cult, unstable even in this issue, which shall be clear to My faithful, for it is already recognized in the media and in the Jehovah Witness cult, that this ruling varies from country to country and from nation to nation, and is not a tenet of True Faith as they are using it. Little children, prevail in all prayerfulness, for those who do not know Truth. I the Lord God am Truth. Many do not see Me in the Holy Sacrifice of the Mass. They do not see Me in the Blessed Sacrament, the Thanksgiving which you give to the Father, in Me and through Me. A time comes when all on earth will recognize this Truth. Little children, since it is not yet, prevail, pray for the conversion of sinners, the salvation of souls, prevail and trust in My Mercy. What I am telling you is that were man to return to the Covenant of Love written in My Blood, there would not be this additional spilling of blood, this continuous spilling of blood, this continuous need for blood transfusions and the like. For I, by Myself, am the Healer of all. Little children, I heal many in spite of the use of human blood; and I heal many who the doctors would say require blood and yet do not receive it. I heal them Myself, restoring them to fullness of health. The Sacred Blood of Jesus, attendant upon thee, is truly profound. There is a profound anointing occurring now, the Grace and Enlightenment to assist you further for you have noticed the spiritual warfare is increasing in leaps and bounds. Rest assured, even though demons abound around the Earth, angels and saints and the grace of your God abound even more. My Own remain safe in Me. When you have such attacks as you have experienced, little children, you realize your unity with Me is all that is necessary for the defeat of the foe, for the banishment of the foe, in his attacks against you. Would that all mankind recognized the spiritual warfare. Alas, it is not yet!

Additional Meditations

1. On the Precious Blood of Jesus By Gerard Manley Hopkins. S.J.

2. St. Michael and the Angels. Copyright 1983; Tan Books and Publishers Inc.

{previously titled *The Precious Blood and the Angels*. Copyright 1977; Marian Publications, South Bend, Indiana. ISBN: 0-89555-196-9 LCCC no.: 82-62040

CHAPTER TWELVE
THE TEN COMMANDMENTS

MARK OF CAIN Gn 4:15

JESUS: The Lord your God gives you a great and glorious anointing. Now is Love come upon the Earth in the Power of the Holy Spirit. All those who belong to Me on this earth will experience an anointing of the Holy Spirit - the Spirit of Love; the Sanctifier; the Comforter. The Spirit of the Living God anoints each and every one of His Own, and as the Mother of God continues to beckon and call, it will be through the Faith of such as you, which will cause others to come back to the Lord their God with all their hearts, that they too may know Salvation. It is indeed true; the Lord your God is wrath about the transgressions of His Laws which are great, occurring rampantly on the face of the Earth. A measured beat of time is upon the Earth, and at the end of it, then comes the sequence of events which are forecast in Holy Scripture and hold fear for the many. Be undaunted by these fearful messages. Those who are Mine, are ever Mine. There are those who were never Mine. Do not concern yourselves about this matter.

Scientific minds are, as it were, small reflections of the mind of the Creator of all that is. But you must remain in obeisance before the Lord God. Is it not written that those to whom much is given, much is expected?(Lk12:48). It behooves men therefore to remain within the walls of the Commandments of God. The vaunted halls of scientific learning have come to an aberration where they no longer respect God-given Love. Respect life, My faithful little ones proclaim, but few heed. This is true in many aspects of science now today. The virtue of Love is such that I wish you to address these intellectuals, these scientists in these matters. They proclaim the Gospel contrary to the Will of God. Yet they proclaim it so loudly, so profoundly that now it is seemingly drowning out the Word of God given forth by Me, that of My faithful little ones. Even so, repeating and repeating it loudly does not make something Truth. My little ones, I call all back to the Faith as profound as that of the great prophets, the great patriarchs; and indeed as profound as that of My Apostles. Because of the inroads in certain scientific minds, in certain as you call it 'new age' beliefs and attitudes and pronouncements, it is a much more complex time than that of My Apostles. Even so, Truth remains Truth.

In My great Merciful Love, when one shares out of love (He shows the kidney transplant of a loved one to a loved one), the living donor risks his life to give that loved one a portion of himself. In My great Mercy I accept this as an act of love. Little children, the quandary is that it should not become necessary, were mankind all living within the walls of the Ten Commandments. These afflictions which are prevailing in the bodies of My people would not be; and in the Name of Jesus, the healing would occur without taking such dire measures to prolong life. Then, in all Charity of Love, I bless with certain healings some of these procedures. When it is love in action I forgive, as it were, the invasion of the human body to remove the part so that a loved one might live. It is a time of great action and yet great sorrow, where mankind elects not to live in the Design of our Father; elects not to be protected by the Ten Commandments of Love. They are not Commandments for the Lord God; they are Commandments for the people of God. Those who live within the walls of the Commandments, rarely have the afflictions which are occurring upon the Earth now, which the scientific members of your community try to correct in many and varying manners, not always successful, and not always pleasing to the Father.

I come in Love and Mercy in the power of the Holy Spirit; through those who believe, I am able to heal whatever affliction befalls persons of Faith, should they approach prayerfully - two or more gathered in My Name,(Mt18:20) in the Faith which you call the Faith of the Apostles; in total Faith - I want to heal that person. I repeat, when they come to Me, as it were, as dead men - unbaptized, unconsecrated to God, unknowing of God, living outside the Law and the Commandments, do you not see that help is not forthcoming from the Lord your God in these circumstances? Thus, they decide in dismay and confusion, to study science and become gods themselves. Little children, it does not work that way. They put their own souls in peril. Even so, I am a God of Mercy and Love, and I cause Enlightenment to be presented to each and every one. I cause little miracles to happen round and about each one, that they will know I am God. Yet in their blindness, they know Me not! I send many little faithful souls to tell them of My Mercy and Love. When will they heed? How long should I the Lord, hold back My wrath? The Lord quotes Scripture; "I played them a song, but they did not dance; I played them a dirge, but they did not mourn."(Mt11:17). They heed rather the din of the world, the cacophony of lies they swallow readily ![Ezekiel 13vs19]

*On this day I show My wrath in certain areas of the world. You will hear of it. Be not alarmed; it has to be ![later, on the news We heard of the earthquake in Turkey, and the floods in New York State. Two days later there were the horrible fires in Florida, and the Church burnings in Ireland.]*As to your Mission; prevail. You shall attend the conference clothed in a great dignity -the dignity of Truth! I reiterate. Those who will come back to Me with all their hearts, are welcomed with open arms of Love! Those who do not, were never Mine! I have taught you many things which are clear and coherent and Scripturally sound; and not at variance to Love and Charity. Little children, go forth boldly in My Name, for indeed I am your Strength and Security and Providence and you are blest! Let Us gather in this manner of prayer perhaps weekly, that you be strengthened little children, ever in the Peace of My Presence. We shall speak therefore at the next meeting; a meeting of Love. You will sing Faith of our Fathers...Now the Lord shows us how, like little children we keep coming back for Our Fathers' blessing.

I am the Living God, I address thee little children each one as the Triune God. Yes I am a doting Father to those who love Me and keep My Commandments. I address thee each one as thy Saviour, a Victim of Love. Have I not told you, you have stolen My Heart ? I address you as the Spirit of the Living God, My Great Life Force, which is as essential to your wellbeing as the oxygen you breathe, it is so essential to you, both body and soul. Therefore be at Peace. You dwell now and always, in this, Love's Union. Mother attends upon My beloved little Faithful Missionary, small sister of Jesus, small sister of St Luke of whom you inquire. Medical healing is good, can be good. There are many acceptable practices in the healing ministry of physicians, and this is pleasing to the Lord God, the Giver of all the gifts, and all the intelligences, and all the arts. These are gifts of the Living God to His sons and daughters, among whom you are numbered. Used within the walls of the Commandments, in obedience to Holy Scripture, most especially in loving ones neighbour as oneself, there is no harm. It is when one ceases to see an individual as a unique Gift of God, and treats them, one might say, like so much merchandise, that the harm comes into effect. At times, from My view, it is that My people are processed like so much livestock. How can this be pleasing to your God!

But certain of mankind is ever proclaiming themselves gods in grave error and transgression of My Laws. They control, and even terminate, the lives of their fellow men. This is known to Me. This is not pleasing to Me. This is bringing upon the Earth, all mankind, My Wrath! 'Are you not afraid to play God,' I call to them, but they shun Me in their greatness. They do not serve Me. They believe only in their own free will - not knowing it is My gift to them, My gift that they might choose Me, choose Love - but they kill Love. My gifts to mankind are always contingent upon the Eternal Laws of your God; and thus, mankind, to your sorrow, they fall under a curse, rather than reaching joy under My Blessing. What will you do when you run out of body parts? It will become expedient simply to kill another for the body parts. You are already aware that this can and does occur in various nations. Walls of flame surround those who are behaving in this manner. The mark of Cain is upon many on Earth. They are Mine yet they elect to kill their brothers, for their own motives.

They appear to be drowned out by the action and sound of the worldly; but it is not so. My Peace is spreading all over the earth now. "It is a time of great action and yet great sorrow, where mankind elects not to live in the Design of Our Father; elects not to be protected by the Ten Commandments of Love. They are not Commandments for the Lord God; they are Commandments for the people of God! (cf Jn 14:20-21) Those who live within the walls of the Commandments, rarely have the afflictions which are occurring upon the earth now, which the scientific members of your community try to correct in many and varying manners, not always successful, and not always pleasing to the Father. Ask of Me what you will, My little one, that I may answer specifically I remind you, little children, that your bodily health itself is a gift from your God. Many of the afflictions upon mankind today are manmade, and many are caused by the sins, the dissipations of the various individuals. Little children, I repeat: I am a God not of chaos, but of order. I set the stars on their courses, and the planets and the moons. I set life on the earth in its cycles. Each child I create has a pathway of holiness to walk; even as a star has a pathway in the Heavens. My little children, when you break the Laws of God you are not on that pathway any more, and the fallout is sin and suffering.

My Cause is Love. Thus I have given the Great Commandment of Love, that My little ones truly love one another, even as I Love each one. Verse and phrase of your Words are in Scripture! I the Lord God, heed and answer. I have come to Earth to give freedom and Salvation to all mankind You are My own the works of My Hands. The beloved Holy Father, the Bishop of Rome is aware of the Epistle of Love and has many working on a paper, a thesis, regarding the grave matters at hand. You know well that he prays and discerns intently, and is thus able to make the great documents of Truth which he does, for he is in Unity with Me.[the Lord shows a great big horn that he is speaking through loudly to the world]and it shall be thus! You see, he is a Pope of profound discernments. In this time frame that you delivered the Message to him, he must verify each and every concern, and validate each and every concern, and remain ever in My Truth, while dealing with ever so many complexities. In due course, this changes. In the interim, know that your God is working powerfully with many, many individuals involved in these very concerns. They are instruments of My Peace and Healing Love, and together a frame- work of Truth in this field of Medicine is set up. A bulwark of Faith is set up and My Will is done, and all those who are My Own heed! Be at Peace therefore!

This(ESCR) is a hideous crime, and not pleasing to the Lord who is Wrath, for the wages of sin is Death.(Rm 6:23). Death of the soul is the Death to be dreaded! There can be no exchange with evil; there can be no compromise with evil. This political leader attempts compromise with evil to no avail; it cannot be! It is either Truth or deception! There is no middle ground, even for the most politically astute. It is an impossibility to try to appease both sides, destroys trust and character and much, much more. I am not oblivious to all of this! " His Eye is on the sparrow, His Eye is on us. *Lord convergence of Your Mercy and Your Justice, which the Holy Father discusses so well in Dives in Misericordia.*

My Mercy remains upon My beloved humanity in a prolonged hour of My Love. In the context of My Will, in the matter of Life and Death, it is the Lord Who speaks; you see the scientists usurp the role of God. They have been Enlightened scientifically but not spiritually.

You cry out, Lord where will it end, when will it end? Those who belong to Me I will hold secure through all these perils, for the time of Holy Freedom on Earth is not quite yet. If it were, there would be no cause for this book. But it is yet a little longer, and in this time frame, science attempts that which is undesirable for humanity as a whole, and displeasing to your God. I have My Eye on each one of them; <u>My Will IS done!</u> In due course, they become aware of this. Trust Me! Continue to walk, hand in hand as it were, with your God, and I bring you to the understanding I desire for you! When others read the book, they will obtain an understanding, each one for himself, because My Words, though not in Scripture, are yet from Me, and they bring Light for those in darkness, and are fully compatible to those in Scripture! Let the book remain under the convenorship of the Mother of God and all falls in place. Little children, recognize that She does indeed attend upon the Living God, in all that you pray about, and you know well the response you receive. The ones with the space will have the big pictures. Those towers and the Pentagon are symbols of death and I do not really want them in a book of Life; yet there will be instances of Victories in My Name which you may in due course, include. This will come to you in due course. You get the Picture. I am with you; call on the Names of your Jesus and Our Mother and We assist you profoundly. It is always thus. It was that way for the saints who have gone before you little children. Cling to your Jesus; cling to Our Mother and We guide you, moment by moment, in all that We wish you to accomplish.

Therefore I must first warn My beloved mankind, for I do not cease to love them! Even when they walk in error, I love them. Little children, think about the Words you are placing on your typewritten pages, as each one being as an arrow of My Love, to reach the heart of someone somewhere on the earth , and do not cease pouring forth these Words which are the Way, the Truth, the Life, the Light for My poor confused Humanity. I speak in a manner to cause man to contemplate on these issues himself , each individual , and make each of these decisions in the Godgiven free will which they possess. Sacrifices of human beings to pagan gods were often by means of hurling that individual into the fire. Ask those who cremate what god are they honouring! It is suffice for this conversation! Oh My people, I am calling all to come back to Me like the prodigal son. There is only suffering and sorrow and hardship where they choose to wonder, and they find it so difficult, for the return journey back to Me, and yet I await them with open arms of Love. How I long to clothe each one with Salvation. Tell Me their names in prayer at the Adoration Chapel and leave them there with Me. I am your Jesus of Mercy, your Jesus of Love. Upon whom I will, I have Mercy. At this time I have Mercy upon all of mankind. I await their response to My Call.

Indeed! The Presence of the Lord is profoundly upon you little children. I am He Who Lives and Loves eternally. Each one of you is blest in a profound anointing of My Love and My Peace and My Joy. Little children, I remind you that I have long told you, in the battle in which you are front line warriors at My Desire, you would be wounded, battle-scarred, weary, but ever victorious in My Name; Jesus! **Those who read the documents you have presented, must from then on answer to Me! It is incumbent upon each one who reads the documents to come before Me prayerfully, and choose whether they wish to live under a blessing or a curse[Dt 30:19] The physicians of the world themselves, are precipitating the wrath of God, in unison with certain other malefactors.** I am the Living God, I address thee little children each one as the Triune God. Yes I am a doting Father to those who love Me and keep My Commandments. (Jn14:23-24) I address thee each one as thy Saviour, a Victim of Love. Have I not told you, you have stolen My Heart ? I address you as the Spirit of the Living God, My Great Life Force,(cfJn14:26) which is as essential to your wellbeing as the oxygen you breathe, it is so essential to you, both body and soul. Therefore be at Peace. You dwell now and always, in this, Love's Union.

I am your Jesus of Merciful Love. Little children, you serve a God of All-Merciful Love, and on the purified earth little children, there will be a Body of Christ(1Co12:27), which encompasses this Law of Merciful Love and none other . On that day, all mankind, each and every one on this earth, will live the Great Commandments of Love. To this end We work, to this end We prevail in the face of a militant foe, a foe who uses insidious and underhanded methods in this great battle for Truth. To whom I Will, I have Mercy! Each one of you has touched My Heart little children praying for this people in My Name, you live the Great Commandments of Love, and the Blessings flow! Tell Me you believe for those who do not! My God, I believe, I adore, I trust and I love Thee; I beg pardon for those who do not believe, do not adore, do not trust and do not love Thee! Those who are truly faithful in their abandonment to the Living God as you are; pledged to Love as you love, are solace to the Two Hearts of Love. Little children persevere; there are so few who live the great Commandments of Love today and there is so much need upon the earth.

My little ones, I know that each one of you has a heart of love for your God and for your fellowman. This is living the Great Commandments of My Love, and it is bearing much fruit. See, I have interlocked you with the true faithful round about the globe, in what I have described to you as a great tapestry, a seamless Garment of Love. This is the Mystical Body of Christ(1Co12:27), many and varied are the Missions of each one in this great tapestry; put together, all is accomplished in My Name. It is a period of turmoil for a little longer. The groundswell of Faith is occurring, and Faith is always accompanied, since a Gift from Me, with Love and Peace and Joy. Now people will begin to understand the meaning of Great Commandments of Love. You worry because there are many factions; the atheists, and shall We say religions which are rather alien to Christianity, in their beliefs, as well as presence of paganism and New Age. You will see this happening more and more among the believers in My Name. Our Lord is showing the physicians about the world and saying, "I place before you a blessing or a curse(Dt 30 etc); choose Life therefore! Heed the Commandments of Love, be true to Your God, be true to your oath, be true to yourselves, love your neighbour as yourselves." (Lk10:27)

Beloved, I am attendant upon all the victims of the disasters everywhere, those living and those who have come before Me. At this time little children, pray for both the living and the dead; and little children, I bless all those who assist in any way the victims who are now without food, without shelter, without drink,(Our Lord shows us Beatitudes, Mt 25:34-46). Those who are able are attendant upon them, those who have gifts to give are doing so, those who are not able to do either are called to pray much on behalf of the suffering little ones on earth, and for the deceased. Therefore be at Peace little children, when each human is doing all they can prayerfully or in material ways, physical ways to aid, they are living My Great Commandments. Peace; I attend upon the matter. Little children simply continue to love as you do loving your God and loving your neigbhour as you do. I tell you again, you are thus living the Great Commandments of Love. These Two Commandments encompass the entire Ten Commandments(Mt22:36-40); thus you are living the Way your God Desires you to live. Little children, I simply on this evening, bless you in an anointing of My Healing Love that you may pour it forth upon all those whom you meet, those who permit you to bless them and pray for them.

It is indeed true; the Lord your God is wrath about the transgressions of His Laws which are great, occurring rampantly on the face of the earth. A measured beat of time is upon the earth, and at the end of it, then comes the sequence of events which are forecast in Holy Scripture and hold fear for the many. Be undaunted by these fearful messages. Those who are Mine, are ever Mine. There are those who were never Mine. Do not concern yourselves about this matter. My little ones, it is a time where much prophecy is upon the earth through various places; some are Truth, some are not, but I just ask you My little ones, to live the Great Commandments of Love,(Mk12:28-34) and remain in joyful anticipation for all that is coming forward to you. Remember, I live within you and about you and you are safe in Me. I lead you in the pathway of holiness.

I am the Lord, your God; I am attendant upon you, little children and upon your heart's intentions. Little children, it is still to simply live the Great Commandments of Love, (Mk12:28-31)loving Me, your God, and Loving your neighbours, whomsoever I set about you at any given time, as you love yourself. Love them with My Holy Love; strive, strive to pray unceasingly.(I Th 5:17) Your good morning offerings strengthen you for the entire day little children, and the enemy has great difficulty in taunting the little ones who are faithful to their morning and evening prayers. Hear Oh Israel, the Lord your God, is One God! You must love the Lord your God, with all your heart, with all your soul and with all your mind. This is the greatest and first commandment. The second resembles it: you must love your neighbour as yourself. On these two Commandments hang the whole Law and the prophets also! (Dt 6:4-5 and Mt22:34-40).The opportune moment arrives rapidly now, for the Vatican has been apprized of what is happening in the many so-called civilized nations. The culture of death has insinuated itself into every stage of the human life of individuals now, and the cloning and other activities occurring which are abominations to Me, cause My Wrath to fall as I will on this earth, where My Commandments are ignored, where I the Lord God am shunned, I the Giver of Life!

Even as the great nation of America, and other nations self-destruct as it were, for lack of obedience to My Will, lack of obedience to My Ten Commandments of Love, lack of obedience to Truth, so will these scientists suffer in strange and varied ways. Surprising events occur because they reject the Shield of Protection of the Holy Spirit! (Ep6:10-20)Little children, I ask you each one to live the Great Commandments of Love to the utmost of your being and to trust the Lord your God. There are great areas of darkness, upon the earth now. At times the Church seems to have but a dim light of Faith shining in all of this darkness, and I am calling each child of Faith to be a lighted lamp, bringing My Love and My Peace, My consolation, to all people. You know well, it is a world starved for holy Love.

Ezekiel 36: "I shall put My Spirit within you, says the Lord; you will obey My Laws and keep My Decrees!"

Matthew 5:17-19 Jesus said to the disciples: Do not think that I have come to abolish the Law or the prophets; I have come not to abolish but to fulfill. For truly I tell you, until Heaven and earth pass away, not one letter, not one stroke of a letter will pass from the Law until all is accomplished. Therefore, whoever breaks one of the least of these Commandments, and teaches others to do the same, will be called least in the Kingdom of Heaven; but whoever does them and teaches them, will be called great in the Kingdom of Heaven.

The Ten Commandments. Exodus 20:2-17; Dt 5:6-21; CCC 2052. see also Mk 10:17-22.
1. I am the Lord your God. You shall have no strange Gods before Me.
2. You shall not take the Name of the Lord your God in vain.
3. Remember to keep holy the Lord's Day.
4. Honour your father and your mother.
5. You shall not kill.
6. You shall not commit adultery.
7. You shall not steal.

8. You shall not bear false witness against your neighbour.
9. You shall not covet your neighbour's wife.
10. You shall not covet your neighbour's goods.

Dt 30:15-19.

15 Here then, I have today set before you life and prosperity, death and doom.

16 If you obey the commandments of the LORD, your God, which I enjoin on you today, loving him, and walking in his ways, and keeping his commandments, statutes and decrees, you will live and grow numerous, and the LORD, your God, will bless you in the land you are entering to occupy.

17 If, however, you turn away your hearts and will not listen, but are led astray and adore and serve other gods,

18 I tell you now that you will certainly perish; you will not have a long life on the land which you are crossing the Jordan to enter and occupy.

19 I call heaven and earth today to witness against you: I have set before you life and death, the blessing and the curse. Choose life, then, that you and your descendants may live.

CHAPTER THIRTEEN
CONVERSION

You know well there are some who will accept; others will reject. Do not worry about that. You will have done what I have called you to do in sending out those Words .Be at Peace, all is in the Hands of your Saviour Who desires the conversion of the physicians, a profound conversion like unto a U-turn in their thinking. You know well this is not readily acceded to by the many. It is a slow process, an ongoing process; it is in the time-frame which I the Lord God desire. Be at Peace. Little children, you are indeed apostles of these difficult times and you are bound to meet with opposition here and there. Do not let it discourage you. I have blest you with so great a fortitude, that you shall indeed prevail in spite of all that is coming against you. The winds of change are now. Those who did not believe yesterday, believe today, and this is an ongoing miracle of Our Love. My little ones, I call all back to the Faith as profound as that of the great Prophets, the great Patriarchs; and indeed as profound as that of My Apostles. Because of the inroads in certain scientific minds, in certain as you call it 'new age' beliefs and attitudes and pronouncements, it is a much more complex time than that of My Apostles. Even so, Truth remains Truth.

The virtue of Love is such that I, the Lord God, adjust the ways of mankind very profoundly, very soon now. In the interim, I yet would address the scientific minds to know that I bless them with many abilities for healing and curing. There are certain things that go beyond My Will in the realm of science and this is not pleasing to the Lord your God. My people have forgotten that Eternal Life is in Heaven. There is no fountain of youth upon earth. It is but a temporary journey. You are called in Holy Scripture to keep your eyes turned towards Heaven your True and Native Land. Therefore, the perfection of soul is always the priority. Choosing, in your eyes, that which is the lesser of evils, does not make anything right in the Eyes of the Father. Those I desire to hear shall indeed hear, because of you. I choose you; and in you and through you, and those believing priests to whom I direct you. A goodly number will heed, who have not considered the many aspects clearly. Do not worry about numbers. I tell you that if even one has a change of heart, it is a worthy effort, a worthy project and I bid you know that more than one will change, more than one will consider, more than one will come closer to Jesus and the Truth.

The Message I give to mankind is for *all mankind*, all Christians to receive. National borders do not count in this My Work. Send them out to be read by the eyes of those whom I choose to read. Do not worry about the others. Simply send it out - it is at the least, thought-provoking. Address those to whom it is possible, fairly soon. Carry with you these Words to the conference. There are means readily available for translation into various languages. Be at Peace in this regard. Be at Peace in My Love. Know that I have tested you and trained you these many years for this time and this Mission which is singularly yours. Be at Peace therefore - I am with you always. I cause rivers of Light and Enlightenment on those in the profession whom I am calling by name now; and in September, My Enlightened ones will be in every nation! As We gaze upon those whom you carry in your hearts little children, and see their trials and agonies, in Our Great Mercy, We lift their suffering, We take away pain, We bless them with the Peace of our Presence. Some return Home quickly now; others remain yet with their loved ones and healing occurs. All are before My Eyes; each one is My beloved. Some know Me, some know Me not. I Myself attend upon them; those who know Me not, again and again. The prayers of the faithful break down the barriers of discord. Therefore it behooves you little children, to first persevere in prayer proclaiming the Name of Jesus to those in suffering relationships, that they have yet an opportunity to come to Me. Leave everything else up to your God. The Lord loves each one of His Creations, most tenderly, most totally and most eternally.

Be at Peace ; all works out for good to those who love the Lord, among whom thou art numbered. You know very well the burden that humanity is saddled with at present; the legalization of abortion. You know well the so-called scientific experimentation and usages of My small Creations, is grievously wounding the Heart of your God; and My beloved Mother. Remember, I the Lord God elected to be born in a stable, a cave, a place of lowliness; and yet in these humble beginnings , the Church was built in My Name. You do not realize that small efforts you make, though they may seem large to you as you are doing them, are being expanded and multiplied by the Lord your God. You are not alone in these beliefs. There are many with you. It is a matter of opening eyes and ears and hearts and intellect. Trust Me, I know what I am about ! Enlightenment comes forthwith from you, in slightly varied and different ways than others who know Me and love Me and elect to serve Me, that they may be My friends forever. Be at Peace. You are not alone. Generous loving hearts I set about you to assist you. Little child, the overflowing Love of the Father, the Son, and the Holy Spirit is pouring forth on Humanity, who may accept or refuse. Little child, you are now blest in My Love. You are blest by God! A profound anointing is upon you. You are called to be My Heart, My Hands, My Voice, in the Enlightenment of your fellow man!

Remember, I am building up the Family of God on earth! Remember, the earth is the Lord's, and the fullness thereof! (Ps24:1)Know that I am the guardian of the rights of My Own, among whom you are numbered; little one, you are protected. Be at Peace, therefore! There are many gifts of healing graces given to doctors who operate ethically and with love and compassion for their patients. The medical profession is in need of this essential component in the world. My blessings are upon those who in all conscience prevail in a holy belief in the wellbeing of their patients. My blessings are profoundly upon them. The Work which I have assigned to you, is to explain My Stance - which is opposed to the stance of certain doctors and scientists. Don't worry about those who do not heed or believe. Enlighten your fellow physicians, that they have this God-given opportunity to remain spiritually, morally and ethically pure in their works; that their works be truly that of the healer in every sense of the word. I, Jesus, bless you and assist you in all that you are doing."

Discernment on March 25, 1998, Feast of the Annunciation: GOD THE FATHER: "Fall on your knees to the Father, Who deigns to attend!"*(we pray prone)* Mighty is the Lord your God; all-powerful indeed! Whosoever falls on their knees in all surrender to the Father knows Salvation; for it is at this time in the Power of the Holy Spirit, that the Works of conversion and healing occur. Mother and I busy ourselves in these Works of teaching those who come unto the Lord God, the Ways of holiness. It is written; I would that none of My Own be lost.(Mt 18:14). The Father, in total agreement, attends upon each of My Own, among whom you are numbered, little one. Do not be afraid, do not be dismayed; this Mission of Love is given to thee for Our Own reasons. It shall be completed in and through thee, when those whom the Lord God wills to hear, to read, to heed these Words, do so! Do not worry about others who will not pray or ponder on these Words. Ask of Me what you will, My little one,(Lk 11:9) that I may answer specifically.*[I prayed for unity of the physicians, in doing God's Will]*.The many will unite with you. We ask your associates to continue to pray for your intentions supporting you in this work. For those who do not heed, do not worry; I call them back in due course. As you know, each one is at a different spiritual level. This is, you might say, a rather profound and intense separating of the wheat from the chaff. A profound discernment is called for *now*. The Tree of Life is being shaken *now;* the bad fruits fall and they are devoured by the birds of prey and by the insects. The good fruits remain securely attached to the Tree of Life.(Jn 15) Some day, little children, you will understand all that Holy Scripture teaches you; and that which is being preserved in the Tradition of My Church. Triumphant angels are in attendance now, My little one. The Will of the Father is done in and through such as thee. Therefore, be at Peace!"

The Lord is giving the Words - a book called Materia Medica, a doctors' book. The knowledge of science prevails yet in the mind of that physician. (Our Lord named him.) Do not be distressed by this. When one has been trained in a specific discipline, in a specific manner for a long time, it is hard to uproot that which has been instilled in the mind of man. My little people, many have trouble in the area of trusting the Lord God in all things. Each one of you has been trained well by your God and by your Heavenly Mother, and this trust is present in you. Little children, it comes at various times to each one. Had it occurred to you that the movement of the Holy Spirit occurs in and through the Words of the Lord your God, which are in and of themselves a blessing? It is given to each and every one of them. Have I not told you that My Word shall emanate from this point of Light throughout the world? Many believe, many do not believe; many are confused feeling a pull of the world and of human intellect. They reason it cannot be, that the Lord is speaking to some unknown on so profound a subject.

Even so the tug of My Words being Truth, shall We say haunt them, causing them to linger in attendance upon these Words, making an opening in the door of their heart, that the Spirit of the living God may enter. Rejoice; it happens to the many. Do not worry about any hard hearted individuals. Leave them over to the Lord your God. Love conquers all. Continue, no matter what happens, as you are; for your prayers, your love, your obedience, your humility, your patient perseverance are the hallmarks of sanctity, and are pleasing to God. Believe little children, We are not giving you Words which might inflate your ego. We are simply blessing you with Our Words. Persevere in Faith and Hope and Trust and Love and patient perseverance relying on your Jesus. Remember, in your weakness is My Strength, and that I am with you always.

Many rejected Me, many will reject you, yet I have strengthened you to persevere, and that you shall do! Little children, those who heed the Words know a Great Victory of Love, and begin themselves to evangelize, and to propagate the Faith of the Apostles, which is in sore disarray upon the earth at this time. Persevere little children of Faith, persevere. My little one, do not wait; do it now. My little one, the enemy propagandizes in the name of world peace. Dastardly deeds are done in the Name of Charity, by the medical profession.

Cling to Me; your weakness is My Strength. United with Me you shall not fail. You may be scorned in the eyes of the world. This is nothing new. This has happened with My sainted holy ones and yet they prevailed. You are anointed in so profound a way, that you cannot separate yourself from Me, and My Will any longer. Yet in your abandonment to Love, the Lord your God has accepted your surrender, and thus these great and powerful graces pour forth upon you, and Heaven is at hand to you. *Help me to remain joyful when I feel bruised in my ego at these times.* This is a testing of your very soul at those moments; and yet I am with you, and together We do it; and Mother in all delight is also with you; united in the two Hearts of Love thou shalt not fail. *I have the Authority of my beloved Lord; but I do not have the approval of any bishop or priests; is it sufficient for me to leave it there Lord?* Be at Peace; look at the prophets; at the warriors in the Name of the Lord in the old Testament and the new. Follow them. In unity with Mary, greater graces occur in regard in particular to conversions and the salvation of souls. I have already won the Victory; the triumph of the two Hearts is at hand. Yet the enemy works furiously, attempting to capture and deceive the many. I Myself bless the words of the book you have at hand, and We ask you to pray for Cuba, asking, Mother of the Americas, to hold My people of Cuba under Her mantle at all times.

The physicians of the world themselves, are precipitating the wrath of God, in unison with certain other malefactors. And yet your merciful God, causes a turn-around in this affair. Little children, the dark days and all the trials *have to be*; before the dawn of Light is upon the world. It is rapidly approaching, yet you have time to save the souls of those who by their atheist beliefs, their humanist beliefs, are hurling their very souls into eternal darkness. This is your Mission. I would that they be spared such a fate*!*

Shunned by the many, do not be distraught. In your humble obedience, you are doing what I ask of you. My little one, you know each person you speak to has there individual free will, and many of them who are professing Christianity, hold in contempt the Word of God. They neither live in My Commandments nor teach My Way. Oh sorrow and woe, that so many souls of My gifted children are so tarnished. They put their own souls in peril. Even so, I am a God of Mercy and Love, and I cause Enlightenment to be presented to each and every one. I cause little miracles to happen round and about each one, that they will know I am God. Yet in their blindness, they know me not! I send many little faithful souls to tell them of My Mercy and Love. When will they heed? As to your Mission; prevail. You shall attend the conference clothed in a great dignity- the dignity of Truth! I reiterate. Those who will come back to Me with all their hearts, are welcomed with open arms of Love! Those who do not, were never Mine!

My little children, it behooves you therefore to seek aid from your God Who is Love, and indeed is the Author of Love. Those who proclaim themselves atheists or agnostics, seek to win the victory in a purely scientific mode by reasoning and logic alone, and they are entangling themselves in a quagmire of confusion. How can they extricate themselves? A Raelian priest(doctor), promoting cloning (in Medical Post) says they do not believe in God or souls, but science is their God. Here you come face to face with those form of so-called scientists, who know Me not, nor do they desire to know Me! This kind have chosen in all free will, to be not of Me. It is their decision. Will they change because of prayer? Many atheists have changed because of the power of prayer, the power of Love! You see little children, before this type of scientist does too much damage, <u>I the Lord God must act and act I shall indeed!</u>

I have given the world many messengers in these times, for example Mother Theresa, who spoke My Truth, the only Truth. My people, how many ways can I tell you that I love you, that I am Love, that I am Truth , that I want that which is good for you; and I am forced to stand by and watch you follow the liar, the master of illusion, the darkness. Yet in My Merciful Love, I go forth and draw you out of the darkness and back into My Light. I send many more of My instruments to be My Heart, My Hands, My Voice now. Faithful Missionary is but one, and I have given her this singular Mission. Heed My Voice in her. Recognize the sanctity of each God given Life. I place My wholesome Life in you; do not deny it to another human. Seeds of destruction of human life are rampant about the earth , yet in the midst of this remains My Light, My Life, My Love. Now is a moment of Enlightenment. Open your hearts, your minds, and together with your God, you will readily work great miracles of healing. The vaults of Heaven pour forth the needed Enlightenment now. I repeat; *now* is the opportune time. I am your God of Merciful Love. Be not surprised at what is happening. Each one of you who has truly said yes to your God, like unto the Blessed Virgin Mary, their soul becomes like unto a mirror; reflecting My Love, My Truth, upon mankind.

My precious little one, your assignments are manifold. Therefore, make the prayer card as you have described and been inspired to do and be at Peace. You will also be inspired as to who you should give it to, even as you have been inspired in the past as to whom you should speak My Name to - it shall be so! You will just know because I am working in you and through you. You are My Heart, My Hands, My Voice; believe, little one, and be at Peace. We call all unto Ourselves in this time, which is short now, and We have positioned you that you have access to those who have need of the Name of Jesus; and as I send them unto you, you will proclaim My Name and great blessings will fall upon you. Believe, little one. You know always that the blessings bring you joy; and yet often they bring more work for your hands. We bless you with busy hands and busy voice. We are with you. I pray that any Jehovah Witnesses may read Your Words and be converted Lord. Little children, prevail in all prayerfulness, for those who do not know Truth. I the Lord God am Truth. Many do not see Me in the Holy Sacrifice of the Mass. They do not see Me in the Blessed Sacrament, the Thanksgiving which you give to the Father, in Me and through Me. A time comes when all on earth will recognize this Truth. Little children since it is not yet, prevail, pray for the conversion of sinners, the Salvation of souls, prevail and trust in My Mercy.

Even as We speak, all these things which we have discussed are occurring all over the earth. My people are being denied their Godgiven rights all over the earth and the hearts of so many remain unmoved. Be like a little child , be like a little child I'm calling to all My Own, because then your heart is not cinctured by the cares of the world. Little children, in each of you here, I have removed any obstruction in your hearts and minds. Yet the enemy attempts to put obstruction in your thoughts. This is ongoing; as he pours forth his arrows of hate, We in Unity of Love pour forth Our Arrows of Love. I am victorious. Hearts as cold as ice melt in the warmth of Our Love. You shall see many changes in many people. You will realize that the process appears slow to you and the conversions, but I ask you to prevail. I Myself will fill your heart with love for My priesthood, My suffering priesthood, as you write to Father Francis and give him Words held in My blessing for him , for He too is My instrument in the unique way I have chosen for him. Understanding comes. The need for money for every activity on earth is quite abhorrent to the Lord your God. The great need for so much money in these times. It is a sign of the times. It is forewarned to you in Holy Scripture and it is so. The year 1999 fast approaches . Little children, proclaim the Good News now while you have the opportunity for it is not always with you. My Delight is in all those whom you have touched. In any of these expressions the enemy is attempting to stop you totally, to shut you down. I shall not permit this to happen, yet the foe persists.

I hear the hymn 'hear I am Lord, 'and the Lord said, See, you have hearts of Love, you little ones, but many, while they are partially of Love, they are still partially of the world; and some are yet stony cold hearts, in the world. Little children they are Mine. You are My instruments in all that you have done in connection with your fellow physicians and with the priests, it is launching My Arrows of Love at their hearts, to change them from stony cold hearts, or from fearful hearts or from disinterested hearts. I wish to take all this away from them. I wish them to know that indeed I am God, supreme among the nations; that My Laws are immutable! Were all the stars in Heaven to disobey, as My beloved mankind has, all the constellations, what would happen to creation! Man is in a chaotic state on earth; like so many shooting stars out of control. I must act must I not?

The Mercy Gate of the Immaculate Heart is wide open. All these little ones who appear to be tormenting you and instruments of the foe, will indeed be given an opportunity in the very near future, to examine their souls in My Light, and choose Me. Yet again this opportunity is given to every person living on the earth. My little one, rest as you do often in the Peace of My Presence, giving over all your hearts concerns to Me, for it is in this total abandonment to Love; I the Lord God Am Love; that you begin to work the many miracles of Love, the conversions of hearts , souls and minds, that I desire you to work. Stay as you are; never disappointed, never discouraged, but ever going forward; plodding on, in Faith and hope and trust and Love and patient perseverance. This is the very story of the saints is it not? It is your story too little one. Living Waters; Light, prevails all about you, surrounding you in the Light of Christ Jesus your Lord at all times. The Lord your God has gifted you long ago, for these works of Love to be performed at this time. I assure you, they shall succeed. I take away all the roadblocks now. You will succeed. Let us go forward in Faith and Hope and trust and love in all patient perseverance My little sister; for you and each one with you are part of My great Family of Peace. Enlightenment must come, that many hearts are changed and true conversion occurs in Our Great Design.

The energy , and the cumbersome weight of the world is obstructive to the Will of God. As it is flowing through the little faithful ones, you'll realize , let us say, the intellect of a doctor is at times obstructive to the free flow of the Holy Spirit. Thus there are delays! Even so, pray for each and every person who will be there. Place them on the altar at My feet, and believe. I work My Own miracles of conversion in the hearts of the many. All that happens is, as it were step by step, expanding exponentially. Little children, prevail in all prayerfulness, for those who do not know Truth. I the Lord God am Truth. Many do not see Me in the Holy Sacrifice of the Mass. They do not see Me in the Blessed Sacrament, the Thanksgiving which you give to the Father, in Me and through Me. A time comes when all on Earth will recognize this Truth. Little children since it is not yet, prevail, pray for the conversion of sinners, the salvation of souls, prevail and trust in My Mercy. You are instruments of My Peace, instruments for conversion; and yet I bid you always remember that you carry within yourselves the Secret of God, the Great Secret of Love. You are [it might seem far-fetched to the logical mind], as small secret agents of the Loving God. Ever be open should any of My faithful choose to contact you.

You children, as it were , you seem to be defying *the establishment* as it is called, rather shockingly, rather blatantly in the eyes of certain individuals. Yet you have chosen to say '*yes Lord*," in obedience under the example of Our Beloved Mother and Our Beloved Joseph. This is so pleasing to the Lord your God that many blessings accrue and flow freely upon you. Despite all these trials you have remained doggedly faithful to the Lord. Believe it or not, such holy obedience is rare on this Earth, for there are billions on the Earth and so few respond to My Call of Love, My Call of conversion. Let us therefore pray together with the whole Heavenly Court, and in unity with those yet in their purifications, the miraculous prayer, the *Memorare*, that Mother begin to work on these two , Her children as well as Mine, and the miracles begin; the miracles of conversion and Enlightenment. We pray for many at this time.[Christmas]They give Me lip-service at this time of year; they claim the Light is for all time, and the Love is for all men, but they do not go further than that. What would you have Me do? Peace; all who are to come unto Me, come unto Me. Pray as you do, it is pleasing to your God. Omen sees someone holding a bell calling all for the ingathering. *The spiritual song," Mary and Martha just come along to ring those golden bells; They're crying, free grace undying Love; free grace undying Love Oh hear the Word of the Lord."* We pray a special blessing upon the Moslem People. May Your Holy Will be done.

You live in a time of trial little children and I ask you, remain faithfully in My Church founded on the Rock of St Peter, present even today in the person of John Paul II. I assure you that My Blessings are profoundly upon you. I am the God Who Loves you most tenderly, most profoundly and most eternally. You will recognize the Blessings that have come upon you as the days and weeks go by. Rejoice in this Our Love's union and be at Peace. I am the Lord Your God. I hear your pleading, I hear your love, I hear your compassion. I have permitted you to discern the division in My Church which is not pleasing to Me. My Church is attacked on every possible front in these times, but there is one staunch shepherd in My Name, John Paul, who as you know is yielded to Our Mother, the Woman Clothed with the Sun(Rv12:1); the One Who crushes the enemy's head(Gn3:15); and I ask you to stay, like him, united with him, in all surrender, to the Love of God, and in all tender loving abandonment, to the Love of Our Mother. This is My Way; let it be your Way as well. Little children, do not worry about those who have permitted themselves to go astray. Those who are My Own come back to Me wholeheartedly. Those who do not come back to Me, were never Mine, to their sorrow and ruin, and to My Sorrow. I ask you little children, to abide with Me as you do, in

My Presence in the Mass, in the shrine, and as you go about your days, for truly I am with you. As you know, the Lord your God indwells the hearts of those who are truly abandoned unto their God, such as you. Therefore, do not be dismayed at all that is occurring; simply persevere; continue in all-patient perseverance, enduring all things in My Name. Much Heavenly assistance is given to you and the true Body of Christ upon Earth.

The works of iniquity prevail yet a little longer. I strengthen you, My Power comes profoundly upon each and every one who is truly My Own. You will readily know, you will instantly recognize the wolves in sheep's clothing, for I gift you to recognize them, that you are not wary of everyone that you meet. Lord, how will we recognize them? Your very soul, and your guardian angel will allow you to know. You may call it Divine Inspiration, or intuition, or some such thing, but it is the Lord God permitting you to know, that your armor remain always intact; and I teach My little ones, when you come upon such a one who is seemingly one of you, but causes distress and obstruction and destruction, these fruits are not of Me, pray for that one, but do not become overly emotional about it; simply claim your place in Our Hearts. "I am someone Jesus Loves, I am someone Mary Loves; I am safe in the Arms of Jesus, I am safe in the arms of Mary, " and be at Peace. It is the Peace during these moments that is powerful in the conversion of the many. Little one, sorrowful as We are with regard to that doctor, you may believe that I Myself shield her from that which is unclean, for thou hast prayed much for her. Continue to pray for the conversion of the doctors in this world today that are in the darkest degradation of soul. Continue to pray for him and such as him. I give all that opportunity to repent and to come back to Me, for example, Dr Nathanson's conversion. Continue to give a little prayer for each one before their attendance upon you, as you do, little children. You have no idea about the power of one "Our Father," and then My little sweetheart, I will assist you in discerning what medication to place each of these individuals on temporarily, until My Healing Love encompasses them for it surely shall.

They have come to know a way of life which is alien to Peace and Truth. Little children, it takes much prayer for this type to begin to respond to the Call of Almighty God to come back wholeheartedly. I Myself assist you with the dealings with the one, and this will spread to the family rather like a contagion; therefore be at Peace. We bless the works of your hands with the healing Love of the Living God. Little children, persevere in your works and prayers as you do, for I am with you always. Little children, each one of you in anointed profoundly this day; additional charisms are given to you to assist you and those whom I will set in your pathway, for the bringing of My Healing Love upon them who are in sore need of My Love. You will recognize this as you go forward day by day, one might say, in this anointing. In the power of the Holy Spirit it is so. Welcome the little stragglers back into My Presence in My Name. There is a feast day quickly approaching which will bring blessings upon the many; I believe it is the feast day of St Therese[October 1st.] It will bring blessings upon the many. Little children, recognize each holy day in the calendar and pray in unity with the Communion of Saints. Little children, Heaven is powerfully attendant upon the Church Militant on the earth at this time. You will see more miracles occurring for I am bringing rapidly back into the Sheepfold, many stragglers and even many who have never known Me, I cause to know Me at this time.

CHAPTER FOURTEEN
INSTRUMENTS in the INGATHERING

JESUS: I choose those who will be My instruments very carefully; I choose them in a unique manner; you do not know the lengths your God has gone to, to choose each one of you for what you are doing, and for all those who serve Me in Spirit and in Truth, in every aspect of their Faith journey. Each one, I have handpicked for these times, and for these Missions. Your hearts and souls and yes indeed your minds, as it were, interlocking one with another, to make the Great Victory invincible, like people become an invincible army. Little children, do not wonder why you are chosen for these various Missions. Just remain surrendered to your God as you are and let My Merciful Love and My Words flow through you. They truly will fall upon the ears or eyes of those who need to know them. It is always not necessarily so, that those who read or hear them will respond in the desired fashion, for they too remain in free will; and yet many shall; and the others may well move their positions at a later date. And those who in all stone-heartedness reject My Words, are in essence rejecting Me; they are themselves to blame for the consequences of their acts and of their attitudes. Leave them over unto your God. Little children, always remember that I am a God of Merciful Love; I change hearts.

The battle is fierce. Those who interfere, those who interlope into these Missions I Myself readily remove. All shall indeed go according to Heaven's Design. You have a demonstration for example last Tuesday, of how your God works in and through His beloved instruments of Peace and Love. In My Hand, you do what I call you to do; it is the same for G and the many others. Little children, continue to cling to your Jesus and Our Mother, in this time of change which is upon the earth. My little children bless Me! We adore Thee, oh Christ and we bless Thee, because by Thy Holy Cross Thou hast redeemed the world. We are in a time of Redemption of the little ones. I am counting them through the Sheep Gate little children and I ask you to continue to evangelize in My Name. My little children, I ask you to continue to be My Heart, My Hands, My Voice, in the Ingathering. There are many who are seeking Truth and few there are who are teaching Truth.

1 His Holiness, Pope John Paul II

The Holy Father, though you have already quoted him in many places. You may lead with him. God the Father recognizes the Jubilee year that Pope John Paul has asked for and He reminds us of what Jesus said to St Peter, the first Pope," what you hold bound on earth, is bound in Heaven, what you release on earth, is released in Heaven."(Mt 16:18-20) So it will be with what the Holy Father asks for the jubilee. Little children be at Peace; it is a time of great Mercy on earth yet; and the Holy Father, the beloved one of God, is fully aware of the documentations. He has many loyal followers in the Vatican, and he has as it were, an ear to the pulse of the world, on all that is happening. He has been handpicked to be the Pope of these times. His task is not easy and We ask you to continue always praying for his well being and his intentions. Thou art blest in this man, and discussions will be occurring ongoing. Continue to pray therefore, that there is no interference by the foe in all the infiltration of all the Causes of God. As it is written that many were healed by simply being in the shadow of the beloved Peter, this man who holds the Chair of Peter, is singularly blest in a similar way. His presence, his voice are instruments of My Healing Love, thus the enemy strives to silence him, but is at once fearful, for I have already defeated the foe who has no power over Me and no power over the beloved John Paul. Still, it perseveres in all wickedness. Children, be at Peace but continue to pray for the beloved one.

The fruits of his most recent trip are already showing. Reported in L'Osservatore Romano, was an unusual letter of conversion, a week after the Holy Father had returned from Kazakhstan. Svetta Barbassova, a 22year old woman who had worked as an interpreter during the papal visit, wrote that after being personally touched by the Pope's message, she had decided to join the Catholic Church and become baptized. She said she had followed almost all the papal events and "was amazed at the Pope's personality; so weak physically but so strong in spirit." "In those few moments I stood near him I immediately experienced a sense of wonder and peace. The clarity and strength of his spirit is incredible." "No one has ever spoken to me like that before, and the Pope spoke to me in the Name of Jesus." "When the Pope told young people that the Lord loves each of them personally, he struck a chord with many," she said.

A great Blessing comes upon him. A holy priest will speak of the wellbeing of the beloved Pope. Trust Me, We carry him in Our Embrace, every step of his journey. Astounding blessings flow from this holy man of God, upon all Mankind. He rests in Our Embrace; Mother is ever lovingly attendant upon the beloved Pope John Paul. Blessings upon you both for your love of this holy man of God. Wretched, wretched, are the ones who assail the beloved John Paul. I am the Lord Your God! The walls of flame lick about the boots of those who assail the beloved John Paul, all those who obstruct My Intent yes, even in Israel as well! Little children, you are at the time long foretold. You begin to see now, the fierce warfare which is epidemic all over the earth. It is intensified for most assuredly, the enemy's time on earth is extremely limited. Mother and I attend upon you little children. The Rock of St Peter is being, if it were possible, shaken by the attacks of the foe on earth today. At every aspect of life these attacks are coming upon Truth. I am Truth, there is no other! That is why I have called you little children, to persevere in bringing this Enlightenment to those who will heed. Fear not, and concern yourselves not with those who turn a blind eye, a deaf ear to Truth.

That which must be done in this My Cause, is indeed being done in the Vatican at this time, and that which you are called to do at this time little one, you have done most pleasingly to the Lord, your God. Those whom I Call will heed; those whom I Enlighten will heed, and there will be sufficient numbers of them to effect changes, for nothing is impossible to the Lord your God! My darling, the Holy Father John Paul, has won a great victory-over-self many years ago, and thus he has remained a constant instrument of My Peace and My Love, and his has been a Joy filled journey. He is assailed cruelly, but this is how the prophets were treated, and worse; and I Myself. He is blest above all men on earth today, for he is unyielding, unswervingly faithful to the Law of Almighty God, and thus great Blessings and Graces are upon this man who is holy to the Lord.

His name, long written in the Book of Life, will be remembered before God in Heaven for all time and all eternity. Little children, there are many great saints unrecognized throughout the generations. This one, John Paul, I choose to have recognized on earth by all believers, and those who denigrate, who deny, who defy, do so at their own peril, for he is My victor. He represents Me, as a calm, clear voice of wisdom, of reason, to a world gone awry, a world confused and deceived. Many believing they are enlightened in one way or another, are but victims of deception who do not even understand what they are proclaiming against Me and My Church. These times have to be, little children. My Peace remains upon My Own, for the Mission of Love is yet ongoing. Persevere little children, your prayers are pleasing to the Lord Your God.

Little children, be at Peace. Great things happen when God mixes with Man; you sing this to your God.

Believe; it is true. I am with you. Many and varied miracles are happening not only in the realm of healing but of Enlightenment of many. Dear little children, the Bishop is cognizant of what happens in St Paul's on Cordova Street and what happens among the First Nations Peoples. He is aware of the Epistle of Love most fully, and is aware of the Truths enclosed in this My Letter to the doctors. I ask you to just be patient a little longer; endure a little longer in all prayerfulness and trust Me, for most assuredly, good news comes to you in the many aspects of the works that are emanating from each of you because of your 'yes' to the Living God, through the Immaculate Heart of the Beloved Queen of Angels and All Saints. Dear little children, trust a little longer.

Traitors and Betrayers. All shall account to Me! Dear little ones, rest assured your prayers accomplish much! Little children, at this time I ask you to just Trust. All is falling into place according to Your God's Design. Little children, at this time I remind you, you are front line soldiers; foot-soldiers like infantrymen, and your major Call is obedience without question. This is where you find yourselves in these very grave issues at this time; these grave issues in which you are playing active parts according to My Design. My little children, persevere. You are instruments in the Hand of Your God Who loves you so; and in you and through you, ongoing Blessings flow upon My needy Humanity. Triumphant angels surround the Pope, the Holy Father; triumphant angels surround all those who are fighting for Life. Little children, you are both surrounded by triumphant angels. Little children, persevere! When John Paul speaks, it is like in Scripture, Gabriel's Horn.

It is known to the Holy Father at this time, for many of these like stories come to him from about the world and he realizes, he recognizes the evil intent of certain physicians who are atheistic in their view of Life and Death. I Cause him to speak soon now; I am in unity with him profoundly. Little children, your God is not unaware of these practices which are abhorrent to the Lord God and yet the timing of the Holy Father's words must be at the moment I Desire [He shows Omen a vision of interlocking clockwork] for the good of the majority. Walk in Faith and Trust and continue in Faith to do all that you are doing in My Cause. The beloved Holy Father, the Bishop of Rome is aware of the Epistle of Love and has many working on a paper, a thesis, regarding the grave matters at hand. You know well that he prays and discerns intently, and is thus able to make the great documents of Truth which he does, for he is in Unity with Me.[the Lord shows a great big horn that he is speaking through loudly to the world]and it shall be thus! You see, he is a Pope of profound discernments. In this time frame that you delivered the Message to him, he must verify each and every concern, and validate each and every concern, and remain ever in My Truth, while dealing with ever so many complexities. In due course, this changes. In the interim, know that your God is working powerfully with many, many individuals involved in these very concerns. They are instruments of My Peace and Healing Love, and together a framework of Truth in this field of Medicine is set up. A bulwark of Faith is set up and My Will is done, and all those who are My Own heed! Be at Peace therefore!

2 Saint Francis of Assisi

The Prince of Peace desires that the saint of Peace be next to the Pope of Peace who leads the group of My instruments.

St Francis of Assisi, born in 1181or 82, was inspired as a young man to embrace a life of poverty by the grace of God. After coming from quite an affluent home, with lots of friends, he began to spend more and more time in prayer. One day while praying before the Crucifix in the then dilapidated Church of San Damiano, he heard these words, "Francis, go and repair My Church which you see is falling into ruin." He first thought a physical or material ruin was meant, and later realized the spiritual restoration was more *necessary. He gave up all his material possessions to live as poor as Christ, relying on the Providence of God. He followed radically the Gospel :"take no gold, nor silver, nor copper in your belts, no bag for your journey, nor two tunics nor sandals nor a staff...in writing the Franciscan Rule, which he and his followers observed with the approval of the Pope. From there in 1211 he and his followers set forth on their apostolic missions, preaching the Gospel and urging the faithful to repentance and prayer; healing and helping the poor. St Clare who was his contemporary and follower, started the Poor Clares, a contemplative order of women also following the Franciscan Rule. His order was enormously successful attracting thousands of friars. From 1221 he became more and more contemplative in his life and two years before he died Francis received the sacred stigmata of Christ, on September 14th [other places say September 17th], during a time of intense prayer in union with Christ.*

On the 31st October, a Muslim theologian, and biblical scholar said that the "Spirit of Assisi" is more necessary than ever. Shahrzad Houshmand Zadeh was referring to the interreligious prayer meeting convoked by John Paul 11. This week the city of San Fransisco, California held several commemorative meetings attended by Muslim, Buddhist, Hindu and Christian representatives. She told Vatican radio that, "following the meeting convoked by the Pope in Assisi, we have seen that interreligious meetings, for reciprocal information, have intensified." This new era of contacts is known as the "Spirit of Assisi," which is especially necessary following the September 11 attacks on the United States, the Muslim stated. ....

"The meeting of religions is to bring peace on earth among men." Jesus says this to Christians, but his word is valid for all peoples of the world: "love one another as I have loved you"Haddad Zadeh, who publishes books on Islam and Christianity in Italy. "He Himself came to make us understand that we are brothers and that we must love one another." The Koran says this when it states, "In truth all believers are brothers. Therefore take peace among your brothers, "and "peace is always better. Believers in religions, even if they are of different religions, must have total peace and fraternity between them, to be able to be true believers of the message of peace in the world."

A Eucharistic meditation of St Francis:

let everyone be struck with fear, the whole world tremble, and the heavens exult when Christ, the Son of the Living God, is present on the Altar in the hands of a priest! Oh wonderful loftiness and stupendous dignity! O sublime humility! O humble sublimity! The Lord of the universe, God and the Son of God, so humbles Himself that He hides Himself for our salvation under an ordinary piece of bread! See the humility of God brothers, and pour out your hearts before him.{Ps62:8 V61:9]}Humble yourselves that you might be exalted by him cf1Pet.5:6;

Jas4:10

3   Saint Padre Pio.

At 4.25am, this morning [8th October 2001], I was woken by the sounds of sobbing and opened my eyes to see a vision of Blessed(now saint) Padre Pio who I saw close to me but not looking at me. I saw just the top half of his body; he was first crying and then speaking earnestly and continuously, but I could not hear his words, even when I was fully awake and listening intently. I was puzzling over what this meant, when I saw him again, still talking earnestly, but I could not hear anything. The vision lasted about a minute or so each time. Later on in the day I saw him again for a few seconds exactly as before. Dear Lord, I thank You but what does this mean?

You have prayed much for the beloved John Paul to address the issue of the unity of the human body and soul. Who better knows of that unity than the beloved Padre Pio? Assistance is given you and knowledge is given to the beloved John Paul which is distressing for him, to learn about what science- calling themselves physicians -is doing to many persons, and he, at last, shall speak! He is Our Pope of Peace, in a time of war! He has journeyed to Israel, to Palestine, to the many nations of Islam, as well as to the Christian world and the pagan world, to bring about the message of Love and Peace. Like yourselves he prays his utmost for the power of Almighty God to prevail upon humanity. Like yourselves he loves the Lord God and has a loving allegiance to the Mother of God and loves all his brothers and sisters on this earth.[Omen is given a vision of the Pope going to the prison to forgive Ali Agca who had shot him].My dear little children, the Lord does not give you this Mission idly, but asks you to persevere despite the signs of the times about you. The priest Padre Pio has an Assignment of Mercy from the Living God to assist you in all your works and in the Healing Ministry. Doubt not but believe! Beloved, let the people know that I am God, supreme among the nations; that I am the Great Physician, the Healer; that I am Wonder Counselor; I am much, much more, but this is a beginning! Let them know of My Healing Love! I work My Healing Love through those who have been chosen as My Instruments, such as the beloved Padre Pio, the beloved Teresa Neumann [stigmatist ;see below.]The Lord your God attends upon each of these individuals in tender and merciful Love. Mother also attends. A great healing saint attends; Padre Pio. Little children, remain walking in Faith. Do not ask in advance, simply believe. By Faith are the miracles wrought, by Faith is the Victory won! Little children, with your Faith, your love, your compassion, it is as it were, compensation for certain individuals themselves, and certain ones round about them, and since you unite your prayers always with those who have attained the Victory in Heaven, the healings flow. Be at Peace. Sweetheart, the confessional is the best thing for the multitudes who need healing.

Pope John Paul II recently visited the historic monastery where Padre Pio lived and died. This was the third time he had come to the remote village in southern Italy, San Giovanni Rotondo. On his first visit many years ago, His Holiness was just a simple priest and it was then that Padre Pio told him he would, one day, become Pope and that he would be covered in his own blood. Both prophecies have come to pass! On his second visit, John Paul II was Cardinal of Krakov, in his native Poland. But on his third visit he came as Christ's Vicar on earth to celebrate The Holy Mass. It was 25 May 1987, the 100th anniversary of Padre Pio's birth.

One of the greatest stories ever told. As recently as 1968 Padre Pio died in a Franciscan Monastery in Southern Italy. For 50 years he bore the wounds of Christ's Passion. Thousands visited him every year when he was alive to be cured of their bodily and spiritual ills. Even more visit his tomb today. Why? This video includes personal testimonies of healing, bilocation, powers of conversion, prophecy etc., and Pope John Paul II's visit to San Giovanni Rotondo. A CELEBRATION OF PADRE PIO was directed by award-winning English filmmaker, J. Paddy Nolan with the spoken word by Sir Michael Hordern. (As seen on EWTN).http://www.marianland.com/Padre02.html

I, your Mother, Queen of Angels and All Saints, assure you that the sainted Padre Pio, will assist you more profoundly! *They're showing Omen that our Pope was a lay Franciscan in his early life and the charism remains with him.*

4 Theresa Neumann

A stigmatist who I had been reading about this weekend, who lived 31years on the Holy Eucharist alone, receiving the stigmata from mid-Lent of 1926 accompanied by visions of our Lord's Passion, and co-

pious bleeding from the wounds, at times liturgically connected with the events of Our Lord's Passion; her life of suffering started the same year that Padre Pio received his stigmata. Padre Pio is the only priest with the Stigmata of Jesus in the history of the Church. She was born 8th April 1898, and died September 18th, 1962. Padre Pio was born May 25th 1887, died 23rd September 1968, and was beatified on May 2nd 1999.

Jesus Speaks of His Blessing to Theresa Neumann

My dear Child, I wish to teach you to receive My Blessing with fervor. Realize that something vast takes place when you receive the Blessing of My priest. The Blessing is an "outpouring" of My Divine Holiness. Open your soul and let it become holy through the Blessing. The Blessing is a heavenly dew for the soul, through which all that is done can be made fruitful. Through the power to bless, I have given the priest the power to open the treasury of My Heart and to pour out from It the 'rain' of graces on souls. When the priest blesses, I bless. Then a vast stream of graces from My Sacred Heart flows into a soul to its fullest capacity. By recollection, keep your heart open, in order not to lose the benefit of the Blessing. Through My Blessing, you receive the grace to love, strength to endure suffering, and assistance for body and soul.

5   Mother Theresa. Of Calcutta

JESUS: Mother Theresa never could be put in a time slot , because she would say she never could say how long the Holy Spirit would want to speak. For the Spirit of the Living God is beyond time. Even so I will keep order in the conference. Place it all in the hands of Our Mother, Mediatrix of all Graces. The blessings flow. Things fall into place. Walk in Faith little children, ever in Faith. [He gives me Hebrews 11 and 12.] and there are more evidences of Faith in Holy Scripture as you well know. The one who is Mother Theresa is secure in the Lord; secure in Glory. She was called a living saint while on earth; yes indeed you may quote her, you may use the words given to you in Spirit. The beloved Mother Theresa of Calcutta; little ones she worked healing and medical care and feeding and sheltering the poor; is she not one of the saints of the Beatitudes?[Mt5:3-10]You may mention her again with a short quote of some of her inspirational quotes like 'do everything with love or it doesn't count at all.I have given the world many messengers in these times, for example Mother Theresa, who spoke My Truth, the only Truth. My people, how many ways can I tell you that I love you, that I am Love, that I am Truth , that I want that which is good for you; and I am forced to stand by and watch you follow the liar, (Jn 8:44) the master of illusion, the darkness.

MARY: *Do not let these inroads take away from your peace. We give you Mother Theresa, We give you John Paul, and We give you your own Father P as examples. Peace prevails within such hearts no matter what is occurring around them. You are called little children to love and trust Our Lord Jesus no matter what is happening. I reiterate, though the earth quake beneath your feet, keep your eyes upon Jesus. Thus, thus is your victory won; and I bring your sacrifices of love to the Father , that Love may emanate upon the needy upon earth. Little children, in the power of the Holy Spirit thou art blest in the Name of the Father, and of the Son, and of the Holy Spirit.*

Jesus tells us Mother Theresa of Calcutta wishes to speak to us.

Little ones, your works of merciful love, are powerfully assisted by the Communion of Saints; for the saints of Heaven are powerfully united in all the spiritual warfare that is going on on the earth at this time. I myself attend upon many on earth, including you my small ones, my small sisters. I unite with you in your pleas for the many, as do the myriad of saints. Heaven is in all delight when little ones on earth comprehend this way of humble holiness before the Lord and develop an attitude of prayer which is pleasing to the Living God. Mother is ever rejoicing in her precious faithful children on earth. You are counted among them. You have no idea what you are accomplishing small sisters of Jesus, small children of the most wondrous Mother in all Creation. Continue as you are doing. Holy angels of Light also profoundly assist. The one who is called WD is attended upon now by healing angels and saints in the accompaniment of the Mother of God. Let the healing begin. C is profoundly attended upon likewise. Be not surprised what you hear next. Little children, rest assured that it is good to repeat the Words of Our Saviour," by Faith are the miracles wrought, by Faith is the Victory won." In every instance it is so!

More of her quotes.

"Yesterday is gone. Tomorrow has not yet come. We have only today. Let us begin."

"Like Jesus we belong to the world living not for ourselves but for others. The Joy of the Lord is our strength."

"There is only one God and He is God to all; therefore it is important that everyone is seen as equal before God. I've always said we should help a Hindu become a better Hindu, a Muslim become a better Muslim, a Catholic become a better Catholic. We believe our work should be our example to people. We have among us 475 souls - 30 families are Catholics and the rest are all Hindus, Muslims, Sikhs—all different religions. But they all come to our prayers."

"There are so many religions and each one has its different ways of following God. I follow Christ: Jesus is my God, Jesus is my Spouse, Jesus is my Life, Jesus is my only Love, Jesus is my All in All; Jesus is my Everything."

Jesus is God, therefore His Love, His Thirst, is infinite. He the Creator of the universe, asked for the love of His creatures. He thirsts for our love...these words, "I thirst,"-do they echo in our souls?

You may use any other of the officially recognized words of the beloved saints. It is good to pray to such saints for their intercession, that greater understanding comes upon you in these circumstances. Beloved, use the words of any saints, as you will. Be at Peace.

7. St Theresa Of Jesus

[Theresa of Avila,[1515-1582], founder of the Discalced Carmelites, Doctor of the Church. From her autobiography:

O *Wealth of the poor, how admirably You know how to sustain souls!. And without their seeing such great wealth, You show it to them little by little. When I behold majesty as extraordinary as this concealed in something as small as the host, it happens afterward that I marvel at wisdom so wonderful, and I fail to know how the Lord gives me the courage or strength to approach Him. As soon I asked about her our Lord quoted her*

JESUS Quotes her: Love Love and live to Love again! :

(When I prayed)Lord please never let us say or write any word that will harm Your Missions in any way, or Your priests, in pride or in ignorance.

A great saint, Theresa of Avila, ensures that this is so! Do not worry about what others think about you, even those priests, even unto bishops because I am with you and I remind you of the works of the great saints, [Teresa of Avila and Catherine of Sienna,]who corrected the Pope when she felt he needed it.

MARY: ***St Teresa of Avila; let nothing disturb you, all things are passing; God alone is constant!***

8 ST THERESE` OF THE CHILD JESUS AND THE HOLY FACE.

The patron of Missions, on whose birthday the Words of this Mission was given me. (Jan 2ⁿᵈ 1998)

You may include her there. A great blessing is upon you, Faithful Missionary, for this work.*" Jesus says* 'there is a great Doctor of the Church who assists you.' It is Therese'(Don't be surprised little one, you are Our delight. Forthwith be at Peace. I, the Lord your God, have anointed you in this Assignment. I repeat your own words: with God, nothing is impossible.(Luke 1:38) It shall be done. *Jesus shows us my beloved Therese' again and He is saying,* "How appropriate is she not, the Patroness of Missionaries; and is this not a house with a great Mission; and are not your' Words', as a missionary of " the Epistle of Love to the scientific world." *Our Lord showed us how-*St Paul converted the Greeks in the great' Logic ' of their minds; they too surrendered to Truth and Love. (ICo 1: 17-31; Ac 17:17-34)Little ones, prevail fearlessly for I am with you, and I am with Father Francis, and I am with a myriad of people who will come to your assistance.

<u>Her Prayer.</u> *'Everything is a grace, everything is the direct effect of our Father's Love-difficulties, contradictions, humiliations, all the souls miseries, her burdens, her needs, -every- thing, because through them, she learns humility, realizes her weakness- everything is a grace because everything is God's gift. Whatever be the character of life or its unexpected events-to the heart that loves, all is well.'*   Spirituality of St Therese`.

<u>Prayer of St Therese`of Jesus to The Holy Face of Jesus;</u>

Oh Jesus, Who in Thy bitter Passion didst become , 'the most abject of men, a man of sorrows,' I venerate Thy Sacred Face, whereon there once did shine the beauty and sweetness of the Godhead; but now it has become for me as if it were the face of a leper! Nevertheless, under those disfigured features, I recognize Thy infinite Love and I am consumed with the desire to love Thee and make thee loved by all men. The tears which well up abundantly in Thy Sacred Eyes, appear to me as so many precious pearls that I love to gather up, in order to purchase the souls of poor sinners by means of their infinite value. O Jesus, Whoes adorable Face ravishes my heart, I implore Thee to fix deep within me Thy Divine Image and to set me i=on fire with Thy Love, that I may be found worthy to come to the contemplation of Thy Glorious Face in Heaven. Amen.

9.St Juan Diego

For about three weeks I have felt something is changing for me spiritually; I have been seeing something that was just a wavy horizontal line almost continuously; I told LT two weeks ago that I could not speak of this because I did not know what it was or how to describe it. But I have been experiencing the indwelling of the Holy Spirit each time I see this "seeing" this off and on but knowing it is not externally visible. Now in the last two days it has become wider and I see that it is many feet; they have sandals, they are covered with desert type sand, and they are walking in every direction back and forth. Yesterday suddenly I saw a door frame and the feet are going in and out through the door frame, but there is no door. The word EVANGELIZATION is appearing on and off in my "minds eye;" but there is no sound. Then suddenly today I see a man, short and stocky, swarthy in complexion; with curly black hair, about three or four inches long, with cropped black moustache and beard. He seams between thirty and forty years old. He is just standing in the door frame and smiling. He is wearing a kind of cloak made of a coarse thick weave, which is striped longitudinally. The broad stripes are cream and orange, the thinner stripes are brown, green and maybe reddish. I thought the cloak may have a hood, but I'm not sure. I see him very brightly but I have no idea who he is. It seems like   Old Testament times and I first thought he was Joseph with the coat of many colours. I phoned my prayer partner to pray together, but as soon as I put the phone down I had a strong intuition that he is Juan Diego. When we were praying Our Lord said;

It is of Me. It pleases Me to give you this vision in progressive steps for My Own Purposes. It is My Will to use you as a precursor of things that are to come, that are to be The Holy Spirit, the Holy Flame of Love is upon you. You will be experiencing an exciting time.

At Adoration this morning,[Friday] Our Lord says that St John the Baptist and Bl Juan Diego had similar roles in their times in the history of mankind, and also that they looked similar.Our Lord also told me that I would be contacting the Monsignor who contacted me from Mexico City last year, telling me of the movie being made of Juan Diego; The Prince of Eden.[April 26th, 2000] I have received the letter regarding Juan Diego from the Canon of the Basilica of Our Lady of Guadalupe; Msgr Rosada; I have no idea if or how you wish me to respond Lord, or even if it is of You. After a period of silence our Lord says, There are many facets to what is occurring now. Continue to obtain the information that is obtainable on the internet, and yet I bid you wait on the Lord a little longer. *After a few months the information about the movie disappeared off the internet.*

10 Marshall MacLuwan

Dear Jesus, You are the One who reads all the hearts and minds of the many who are calling from the media; You know that I would not respond at all; yet You have called me to come to ask who, which and how to respond, according to Your Will.

The Voice of your God pours forth through your lips at this time on behalf of My beloved Mankind. I say do not hesitate to proclaim the Good News and all the variations of the warfare which is now ongoing against the ruthless foe; yet one must use discretion for certain interviewers indeed are not of Me. They would present a very biased Message; distorted. *Lord, how am I to know which ones would be one of Yours?* The Virtue of Love is such that I attend upon you. You may, at a convenient time to Yourself, attend upon each call; and yet you will question them as to why they wish to interview you and whether they would present an unbiased and objective report. You will immediately discern those who are working for the foe; you will immediately say it is not a convenient time to take part in what they are doing. One or two you will recognize as valid and objective reporters. Marshall MacLuwan will assist. *I do not know who that is Lord.* I am the Lord your God! I set about you someone who has wisdom; a saint who has wisdom about matters of media, and you will be powerfully assisted. A great Canadian saint, yet unrecognized, is this man of letters. You do not realise how powerfully you are assisted little children, for these Enlightenments, I AM THE LIGHT OF THE WORLD; which I have assigned to you dear little children, are so important to Me that great Heavenly assistance is attendant upon you in these times when your Words come to the fore. The Illuminator, the great St Clare also assists you. Little children, many saints assist besides My Own powerful angels who surround you. Do you believe now little children, that this is a Work assigned to you by the Lord your God? *Yes Lord we believe; we just sometimes feel too little as instruments entering into deep and unfamiliar territory ; I could not survive without You.* Continue to pray this prayer; without You Lord, I can do nothing at all; without You Lord, I am nothing at all. *After this discernment I read that Marshall McLuwan was a University Professor who became Catholic and understood the forces of spiritual warfare and he is the originator of the famous slogan ; "the medium is the message" and nobody could understand but now we see that he who controls the media or the medium ; his message gets through. He[MM] saw it all his life.*

With Marshall McLuwan and St Clare there is no battle.

11   JUDY BROWN OF AMERICAN LIFE LEAGUE.

Lord what about Judy Brown of ALL [American Life League]. You may include Judy Brown.

The ALL philosophy, as stated in its Web section on euthanasia, maintains:" A human person has value, no matter how old. Or how sick." "Every preborn child, from fertilization on, is a human being who is entitled to both social and legal protection." Even a "single cell zygotic child" is "not a potential human being; she is a complete human being."

12   Mary Wagner.

Lord may I quote Mary Wagner who has been in prison repeatedly for speaking out against abortion, especially the speech she gave the judge at her trial. It would be good to show her firstly what you choose to do. It is a time now when many are in great trepidation and fear in speaking out on behalf of the pro-life movement, and yet she is not afraid, even as thou art not afraid to stand up and be counted in the battle for Truth. Therefore I bless you and I bless Mary Wagner and I bless the works of your hands, for it is, in each instance, bearing much fruit for the Kingdom of God. (MARY WAGNER ADDRESS TO THE JUSTICE. Where she told the Justice that he too, was an embryo once as we all were.)

And there are many others as specified by Jesus in this Scripture;

Scripture: John 15:14-16a

You are my friends if you do the things I command you. No longer do I call you servants, because the servant does not know what his master does. But I have called you friends, because all things that I have heard from My Father I have made known to you. You have not chosen Me, it is I Who have chosen you.

Comment

'You, your Honour, were created at the moment of conception'

Mary Wagner and Glenn Reed were sentenced July 19 for sitting in front of Vancouver's Everywoman's abortion clinic. Reed was given 2 years probation while Wagner received a jail sentence of 3 months and a day in addition to the 24 days she had already served.

The following is Wagner's statement of defence.

Your Honour,

My friend and co-accused, I myself, and many others are deeply troubled. We are troubled by the hard truth, that in our country and throughout our world, child after child is being killed before she has left her mother's womb.

What is most shameful is that we, who are grown, continue to allow our tiniest sisters and brothers to be destroyed. We do little to protect the vulnerable child who is at risk of being aborted. We allow her mother to make the grave mistake of aborting, instead of welcoming her child.

We are guilty of both the avoidable deaths of countless children, and of the unimaginable damage to their mothers. Were we on trial today for the neglect of prenatal children causing death, and harm to women, we would surely be convicted.

Instead, we are on trial for attempting to protect some of our young sisters and brothers, who were scheduled to be killed on June 25, 2001.

We have no legal defence for peacefully intervening where children are routinely killed. We have no legal defence, because those of us who had the power to do so, have passed laws which say that you, Your Honour, were not a person from the moment you were conceived, until the moment you totally emerged from your mother's body.

In other words, our law says that personhood begins when a "non-person" comes forth from the womb of the "non-person's" mother. The first nine months of your life, as you grew and were nourished in the warmth and security of your mother's womb, were, in law, irrelevant. You existed, but not legally were you acknowledged.

Your Honour, most of the laws of this country are based on reason, though this is not always so, nor has it always been the case. As recently as last century, women and First Nations people were not considered people in Canadian law. With the clarity of hindsight, we can see how unreasonable and unjust this was.

Must we live as blindly as those of past generations, defying reason and justice to preserve the legal status quo? How can we, when the legal status quo permits the killing of over 100,000 Canadians each year?

Henry David Thoreau, in his essay On the Duty of Civil Disobedience, remarks, "Must the citizen ever for a moment, or in the least degree, resign his conscience to the legislator? ... It is not desirable to cultivate a respect for the law, so much as for the right." Thoreau was an American citizen who was writing in opposition to slavery, which at that time, 1849, had the endorsement of his government.

Thoreau made an important observation. "It is not desirable to cultivate a respect for the law, so much as for the right," simply because the law can be wrong, the law can be unjust.

Your Honour, many have proposed that one may voice opposition to abortion by means other than by breaking the law. We agree with this point. However, opposing abortion was not our sole intention. We must do more than that.

We believe that we are to live in such a way that we serve our Creator, and we do so by serving His creatures, our brothers and sisters. We believe that you, Your Honour, were created at the moment of conception, and that you are a unique being of infinite worth. We believe the tiniest of human beings has been made in the image of our Creator, is more precious than any thing, and must be respected.

This belief must be lived. In our hearts, it has become clear that we will go, by God's grace, to the places where our brothers and sisters are at risk of being killed, intervening for them by whatever peaceful means we can.

By such direct intervention, some might think that we are being disrespectful, or behaving unjustly towards mothers, fathers, abortionists, or associates who are present. However, someone once made the astute remark that, "An injustice anywhere is an injustice anywhere." When there is injustice towards a tiny child not yet born, there is injustice towards her mother, father, and ultimately, towards each one of us.

Treating a tiny child justly does not deny justice for others. Justice, by its nature, is incapable of breeding injustice.

Thank you, Your Honour.

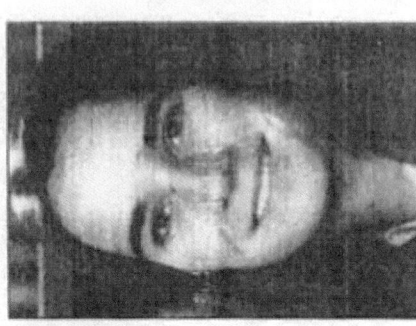

Mary Wagner

CHAPTER FIFTEEN
HEALINGS, BLESSINGS, ANOINTINGS

JESUS:

Expound upon mankind little children, that I am God! There is no other; none other! Those who will believe are known to Me already. Those who will not believe at this time are known to Me already. Those who will never believe are known to Me already. They reject the Blessings of My Messages. But for those who believe now, and who shall believe, proceed little children without doubt, knowing that this is the Desire, the Will of your God <u>It shall come to pass!</u> Little children, when you pray with Omen and she captures the Words of Love flowing freely upon you in the Light of Christ, in the power of the Holy Spirit, through the Love of the Blessed Virgin Mary, these Words do not stop when Omen leaves you or you leave her; they are ongoing ; flowing upon you, and thus you absorb then as Divine Inspirations and are just having thoughts to do the Will of the Father. In your surrender to the Will of the Living God it is so. Your 'yes' is accepted like unto the Mother of God's yes; like unto Joseph's holy and humble yes, and the blessings flow, the graces flow.

Little children, do not be fearful of poverty. Many of the great saints willingly chose poverty over riches that they might be closer to the Living God. Fear not poverty; embrace any and all that is given to you by your God. Little ones you know well that My Heart is with My poor little ones. The rich maintain themselves in a pampered array of riches not sharing with the needy and yet as you pray giving Glory to God, I bless you little ones with anointings, blessings, providences which carry you moment by moment throughout your Faith journey. In this abandonment to Love, I the Lord God Am Love, the blessings flow. This is the Faith walk each one of you is called to. Little children live joyfully and peacefully, all that comes upon you each moment of each day. Little children, in your rejoicing in Our Love despite the needed sacrifices, great blessings and healings and graces, come upon My people, the people of God. Little children, do you love Me?

The Holy Spirit is speaking in tongues; *Pray for us, pray for us you cry. Heaven hears and responds. The song of Love comes into the heart and soul and mind of J at an anointing, a receiving, a claiming of Faith is given to her; hosts of angels attend upon her and indeed a few saints. Darling tell her there's a reason for everything , and that the Lord God knows the reason; and to leave behind all the past; and to live in the immediate moment in the Light and Love of the Lord, and blessings flow. We are given Revelation and" Hear Oh Lord the sound of my cry, hear oh Lord and have Mercy."*

Little children, your prayers are pleasing to your God, and therefore, in conjunction with J's own prayers We attend upon her. A resolution is at hand even as We speak. We are consoling her in an anointing of Our Peace. Both I your Jesus and Our Mother, are attendant upon her. Turbulent is the world in which you are living little children, yet I take care of My Own. It is so for J. Be comforted, I am with you always. Little children, even when things look very dark or bleak I am with you, and a sudden enlightenment is yours and release is yours. Little children continue in all Faith. By Faith is the Victory won, by Faith are the miracles wrought .Guardian Angel's name. The name is Holy Key. All the children of God will be clothed in the Sun, like unto the transfigured Christ; like unto the Woman clothed with the Sun; on that glorious day of the Lord, for each and every one of My Faithful , it is so.

Thus are saints able to attend upon those who pray asking that saint to plead their cause; and I in My delight, allow the many miracles to happen. I reiterate! Love conquers all. Little children, you who know love, who embrace each other in love; who embrace each other with a holy kiss; you know the love of the Lord your God; agape Love, an "all-charity of love". The world does not know it. The world knows lust, fascinations, and many illusions, confusing that with love. This only aggravates the misery of the situations in which they find themselves, for they know Me not. Yet I call them by name. Many come unto Me now. Many are the trials upon the earth now. I the Lord God indeed fill your hearts and souls and minds with My love and My peace and a concomitant joy in the Love of the Lord, I give to you. All are before My eyes; each one is My beloved. Some know Me, some know Me not. I Myself attend upon them; those who know Me not, again and again. The prayers of the faithful break down the barriers of discord. Therefore it behooves you little children, to first persevere in prayer, proclaiming the Name of Jesus to those in suffering relationships, that they have yet an opportunity to come to Me. Leave everything else up to your God. The Lord loves each one of His Creations, most tenderly, most totally and most eternally.

I pray for a young man who is Your Creation and a beautiful soul Lord, but not yet baptized.

The Lord Your God is working miracles of Love on the earth now. All those who carry Love of neighbour in their heart, obtain this Love from the Living God, and thus the Living God calls them His Own and brings them to Himself. Such is the Mercy of your God! Lord could J also know the name of his guardian angel? J's angel's name is Reckless Love, which means that God will risk all to Love him; and not only will I risk all, but I have already risked all for Love of him. [by dying on the Cross]. As We gaze upon those whom you carry in your hearts little children, and see their trials and agonies, in Our great Mercy, We lift their suffering, We take away pain, We bless them with the Peace of Our Presence. Some return Home quickly now; others remain yet with their loved ones and healing occurs. Little children do not be dismayed at anything that happens today. Are you not in the time of chastisement?" Those who are cleansed and purified and brought Home to Glory, are ever attendant upon the precious little ones on Earth, with prayers and intercessions ongoing. Their prayers are directed firstly to the Heavenly Queen, and through Her to Almighty God. The route in which I the Lord came to Earth is through the Immaculate Heart of the ever-Virgin Mary. Little children, come back to God through that same Heart, that Heart of Great Merciful Love. Thank You Lord. Little children, I would have My people honour the saints in the Great Communion of saints; they are ever attendant upon the pleadings and causes of the precious little ones. Many, many are the people walking on the Earth who have been tormented, abused, debased in many ways by those who should be parenting them; whether physical parents or foster parents. They have been harmed, and in their own little minds, irreparably harmed.

Little children, just periodically pray this little prayer, and yet for each of those whom I set in your pathway of life , just invoke her by name, "St Dymphna, pray and intercede for this child of God", and in this matter, I allow the healings to begin. Remember, these little ones' souls are beautiful and precious to me; but in what they have experienced, they do not believe in their own worthiness; in what they have experienced, they cannot accept a Christian embrace, Christian Love, for they only see abuse, both physical and sexual. They distrust every hand of love, for they have been debased by the demons of power and of lust, of hatred; in such manners that their very psyche as you say, is wounded. How to heal them? Here again, I the Lord God, am naming St Dymphna as the patron saint of abuse victims. Call upon her and teach the little abused ones to call upon her frequently, and by her intercession I, the Lord God come powerfully to their aid. *Thank you Lord Jesus. Jesus says;* " Pray thus- Word of God, Have Mercy on us ," three times. I am the Lord Your God; I gaze upon you in tender and merciful Love. My precious little ones, you are My

Delight, and I am blessing you in a profound anointing of My Love and My Peace and My Joy, as ever, for I am yours and you are Mine; and I bless the little one with a measure of fortitude, that she will withstand courageously all that is being done. Indeed, We open a door that you may be encouraged to ask her to read Holy Scripture. The Psalms are ever- powerful in helping and consoling in the power of the Holy Spirit, My suffering little ones, even those who know Me not, find Peace in the words of the Psalms. Yet, I would have her go further to read at the minimal, the Gospel of St John the beloved, that she too may be freed up from the bonds of satan, sin and death, and soar like an eagle on the wings of Love.

I ask You this a lot but Lord, please could she be told the name of her Guardian Angel? The Angels name is "Embracing Light." We ask you to have her read, or read with her, Psalm 91. Tell her it is written in Holy Scripture, "to those who know Me, Lo I am with you always, until the end of time. Tell her, I go before her, I stand beside her, carrying her cross. Should she not wish to hear these comforting Words at this time, it is perhaps better to simply give her the Little New Testament Book, also containing the Psalms. It contains keys as to which of My Words to read in times of distress. And when I was at work two hours later I glanced up to a shelf and there was the very book , New Testament and Psalms, that Our Lord referred to. Oh that all knew Me but alas, at this time it is not so; yet I am the Good Shepherd. Her too I call by name. She is Mine I am Jesus, and I bid you know that Mother and I attend upon this precious soul, and an accompaniment of a goodly number of angels and saints. You are asking in your heart 'what about the man, the perpetrator. Wilt thou tell Me that you love Me for those who do not? Little children, Thou art blest; continue. *Lord I have had a request to go and anoint someone with cancer in Richmond. What is your Will with regard to this more public way of exercising my gift of healing?*

My beloved, do not be afraid to go and do there likewise. I am blessing many people with healing gifts because it is essential at this time. Little children remember, firstly always anoint them in My Healing Love,; I heal them first spiritually, and after that; as I Will . As you bless them, it is so; for I call each one of you to be My Heart and My Hands and My Voice, in the great ingathering. You see well now that the harvest is plenty but the workers are few. As you bless the little one in Richmond, do so in boldness of faith, for I accompany you there for My Own Purposes. *Praying for M* You will remain in My Light and My Love and continue praying for M of your hearts concern and leave all the rest to your Jesus. I know what I am about; I am He Who lives and loves eternally. It is I who enlighten thee to pray for any and all whom I set in your pathway. Bide your time prayerfully as you wait upon the actions of your Father in Glory .

Thou art the ones chosen for this work of merciful Love and Enlightenment to My people; to the intellectuals; to the scientific mind. These people do indeed recognize the beauty of Creation and specialize in certain aspects of My created beings. Often times, as they limit themselves to one area, one specialty, they see only as it were, blood cells, or heart valves, or specific tissues; and they intensely devote their studies and works and healing arts to that small area to the point where they cease to see the entire being, or the entire complexity of humanity and of Creation. Yet I bless them; I bless them with the necessary skills and intellect to do research, to do healing works on behalf of My suffering humanity. The blessing is there. The fact that it is not freely flowing on each individual physician is because of certain barriers they themselves in free will, have placed between us. I believe you are familiar with these sort of barriers. My little children, now is a moment of sweet surrender to Love in the Peace of My Presence which is upon you. Ask of Me what you will.

My beloved little children, have I not told you that I am weaving together the souls of My true faithful in a seamless garment of Love spanning the entire earth; and it is so! My little children, do not be distressed that there are puzzles in your life. You know well that you are called to walk in faith and hope and trust and

Love; in patient perseverance, for as instruments of My Peace, you carry the secrets of My Love on your journey with you. It is so for every faithful priest, for every faithful individual upon this Earth. They are emissaries of the Great Secret of Love and thus you will prevail in simply loving one another and trusting your God. Do you comprehend little children? *Yes, to some extent Lord, but may I understand what it was You were giving through the handshake?* A gift that in due course he will recognize himself. My little children, as Omen knows well, when she prays laying hands with a priest specifically, I anoint that priest profoundly, and she always asks him to bless her in her works, and through that priest I anoint her profoundly. It is something like that that transpired between you and that priest. Each one of you will grow in Faith in the manner I decree. This is withheld from any foes. It is a silent action of My Love, not outspoken that he may hear and apprehend the actions I devise. Believe little children, this warfare is great! You are instruments of My Peace, instruments for conversion; and yet I bid you always remember that you carry within yourselves the Secret of God, the Great Secret of Love. You are [it might seem farfetched to the logical mind], as small secret agents of the Loving God. Ever be open should any of My faithful choose to contact you.

All that you mention is a sign of the times in which you are living. Little children, thus your Mother weeps and pleads for all those to convert. Pray, pray for the conversion of sinners! Do not be dismayed at the many who are taken Home now. Pray that they be ready to stand before the Lord God, that they know Salvation! Little children, each one of you has been given, much, and you know from Holy Scripture, much shall be expected. Little children, is it worth the Price? Signal Graces are falling upon you little children, for these words of Love. I too have a Heart for Love. When My little ones address Me in total Love as you are doing, I am moved to Bless you further. *Immediately after I arrived home from these prayers there was a phone call from this doctor, who had never even heard of me before, nor I of him before the first of January; I returned the call which was just for a referral, yet the doctor came on immediately. He did not tell me anything personal yet because I knew he was dying, I was able to pray "Jesus saves, Jesus heals; in Jesus Holy Name is his Victory," connected to him briefly on the phone.* "Upon whom I will I have Mercy. "Praise God!

Lord please teach again about the healing hands of priests. You have taught us that through the Sacraments they are healers; that every Mass is a healing Mass. Indeed every Mass is a healing Mass. Indeed, My priests are healing in the confessional, and in the Mass in the Eucharist, and in the anointing of the sick. There are many ways in which they are doing it. This is other than the great dramatic ways which are being evidenced round about the earth in this time. *Lord help us discern about some of the great dramatic healings also; sometimes they seem strange.* The devil is ever present as you well know, but by Faith is the Victory won, by Faith are the miracles wrought! Little children, remain faithful as you are. My priests are called to a great Faith, to a sanctity, to a sanctifying Faith, that they may be My instruments in drawing others back to Me; and they are gifted and talented in many and varied ways. As you know each individual is a unique Creation of your God; and thus each priest is gifted in one manner or another. I bid you remember the beloved St John Vianney who was not recognized as having any great talents and yet he accomplished more, than many, many other priests, who might have been observed by Humanity as being greater gifted! Little children, pray for your priests and always believe; nothing is impossible to the Lord!

The inroads of satan and your government is well known to the Lord your God! Heaven hears your prayers and Blesses you. We bid you know that We are attendant upon all those who are praying for this hospital and the many hospitals which are under a similar threat. *Our Lord showed Omen the French Revolution.* Even though all the Churches and Church Institutions of France were destroyed, yet My faithful remnant was there. It is advisable calling upon the countless martyrs of the Faith who died in the French

Revolution; busying themselves now to assist thee in the matter in this perilous time; insidious mankind are ensnared in hating all that is holy. *Remember, certain things have to be, but My Own are safe in Me.* Little children, in all that you see and do, which is appalling to you, give it over to Me! Do not carry this cross, simply give it over to your God. So it should be. At the opportune moment all, ALL is recognized and proclaimed, and open for the multitudes to believe and know little children. Little children, the beloved Faustina of Divine Mercy is rejoicing at action being taken on behalf of My Merciful Love for mankind. You do not understand little children, how linked you are, to Holy Mother Church, and to the great saints throughout time. Little children, sometimes you realize it briefly.

Know that the Tree of Life is for all time. Little branches outreaching become, let us consider, like a great banyan tree, all over the earth. My Tree of Life grows and flourishes, on the earth. Continue to work in Faith as thou art taught. In the tape I have inspired your friend to show you, there is a Wonderworking power in the Blood of the Lamb. Claim the Precious Blood of your Jesus to heal the individuals spiritually, mentally, emotionally; and in every aspect of their being as they pray, and it is done; and your patients will be healed most rapidly. Do you believe? Little one I Bless you with a delightful journey; be at Peace, I am with you always. Little children, persevere. You will recognize that I have selected you, handpicked you for the Mission which you are undertaking and that this does indeed require the utter abandonment to the Will of your God, and each one of you has responded beautifully in abandoning yourselves to the Will of your God and this includes LT who is beloved of the Lord! Little children it is upon that abandonment that I am able to Cause the Works of holiness to occur. Little children, in all of the world, there is only a small percentage of Christians who have abandoned themselves to the Holy Will of the Father as you have been taught by Mother and the saints and Myself, and so it is that you are blest in all your undertakings. You are special instruments in of My Merciful Love for the Love starved world. *He shows Omen a swirling battle between darkness and Light right now and says*, The Light shines in the darkness and the darkness is no more. *You are the Light oh Lord.*

Little children, I am infilling you both and the many you carry in your hearts with My Love and My Peace and My Joy. I do indeed strengthen you to the needed Fortitude for all that you are undertaking in My Name. Little ones, go forth joyfully in My Light and My Love. Little one, We shall attend upon each one individually, and as you know the first healing is always spiritually, and beyond that these individuals have lived in a certain sorry or confused state for some time, and My darling We just heal them, moment by moment, step by step, day by day, throughout their Faith journey. *He shows Omen someone learning to swim...* thus they must learn to swim in the friendly waters of Love. You see, they are intimidated; they think it will be a frigid plunge, and yet My Love for them is so warm, so We give them a little time to you who love. I will inspire some to desire to be off the medication, some you will coax along, wheedle even. Darling it is alright, they have been dependant individuals, certain of them, for long periods of time. He shows mother, father and toddler, baby not wanting to let go at first. Thus they are in the matter of their well being. Forthwith, tell Me that you love Me; it is the Lord Who speaks. *My Jesus, I love You; My Saviour and My God, My Redeemer and My King, I adore You.*

Mighty is the Lord your God; you have found favour with the Lord your God and the man is healed! Faithful Missionary, give testimony to this event also! Put your finger on His Heart (We touch His Heart on the Crucifix). Take the drop of Blood and place it on yourself, and the healings proceed! You do not know what is happening here little children; you are being drawn closer to the Sacred Heart of Love. Encased in My Love, you will go forth as apostles of these times in great works of Mercy. The anointing is complete and profound. Give Glory! Glory be ..Ken is named, it is the Lord Who speaks, Ken is named "the one who knows a miraculous healing", for Heaven hears the prayers of the faithful. The healing is begun. I Myself shall give testimony to Ken, and to the people of that community. I Myself attend upon Ken. Our Lord shows us that He puts His Hand out to Ken to steady him as he takes his first steps. *I received email from my sister relating that my brother Ken, had had a vivid dream of Jesus putting out His hand to him, helping him to get up and walk, on the very same day. Ken died on the 27th November 2003, never having walked on this Earth again. He was dressed in his Sunday best with a brand new pair of shoes at his bedside when he went to nap after lunch and never woke up. He was very devoted to Our Lady and her Rosary and died on the feast of the Miraculous Medal. Many years ago he had gone on a pilgrimage to Lourdes where Mary had told St Bernadette that She is the Immaculate Conception. On the 8th December, feast of the Immaculate Conception I received a card from Ken, which he had mailed on the 25th November, which read like a testimony of many things which he thanked me for, which I did not even remember. How faithful Mother Mary is to those who are devoted to Her. On the day I heard of his death I remembered and kept singing the spiritual hymn I had sung in boarding school; "I gotta shoes, you gotta shoes, all God's children gotta shoes. When I go to Heb'n gonna put on my shoes gonna walk all over God's Heb'n…"*

Mercy is extended to the multitudes on this evening which is Holy to the Lord! By Faith are the miracles wrought, by Faith are the victories won! (Hb 11) *In view of the many healings, I asked our Lord for healing of my epilepsy too, induced from the head trauma 21 years ago. As I knelt before Him in the Adoration Chapel, I understood that He had said "yes" to my request; therefore in trust I did not pick up my prescription of Dilantin. I went from three hundred mgs daily, to nothing at all overnight, and have never had a twitch ever since. Thank You Lord Jesus!*

My little children, you are coming upon a time, when all that the scientific aspects of medicine can do, will not be enough for the healing of the suffering multitudes. Even so, they shall continue, and I shall bless many of their hands in the healing arts; those with hearts of Love and integrity of soul will be blest to continue; but they will not be sufficient for the afflictions on the earth, therefore, I am giving healing hands to multitudes of people all over the earth: little children, you are among those so gifted. Continue to be the Heart, the Voice, the Hands of your Jesus. I instill the Voice, the Words, the thoughts in you, since you are surrendered to Me in all Love; and the healings are ongoing in and through each one of you, and the many, many more about the earth. My beloved, My beloved; My Love is upon you; My Peace is upon you. My beloved, the great cures, the great healings will continue. Each of you is anointed in this healing ministry most profoundly. Little children, do not be afraid to pray one at a time whenever necessary, even though united as two or three(Mt 18:19), the power of the Holy Spirit is profound; and great healings occur. The man who was just here A, has been released from a spiritual and mental affliction. He is totally Mine!

I call to My Church, wherefore do you linger in idleness; the harvest is plenty, the workers are few.(Lk10:1-2) Proclaim the Good News of Jesus, until it resounds about the earth, and the healings begin. Your Good Shepherd awaits the workers in the harvest. .(cf Lk10:1-2) Be at Peace, thou art beloved instruments of My Love and My Peace. My small friends rejoice in Our Love. Be not surprised at the miraculous events which occur now. All those afflicted and those who love them Lord. I, C, K, M be healed; for great and glorious is the Lord Our God; for nothing is impossible to God. In all things give thanks. *All honour, glory, praise and thanksgiving are yours Lord!*

The Love of the Lord is most profoundly upon you little ones. As you ask, so I give unto thee as I Decree. Be at Peace! In the testing of one soul, the surrounding souls who love that individual, they too are tested. A great value is upon the suffering of the little one who is My Own, for it causes others conversions and healings, and it brings to the fore, the power of Faith in Jesus. Little children, you will live to see many miraculous events; curings of cancer and many other diseases said to be incurable, for indeed nothing is impossible to the Lord your God.(Lk1:37) Each of those named is resting in Our Embrace; Mother's and Mine. Leave them there little children and continue to pray for them in all Faith as you do. Little children the vaults of Heaven are wide open as We are gathered together here in My Name and Blessings flow upon you and upon all those of your hearts concern. Little children, you ultimately hear of the healings which have occurred as you have prayed with or for other individuals. Be at Peace as you continue walking in Faith. Healings occurred at each time that you prayed for others. Great graces flow as you pray for others.

Indeed little children, lay hands on one another unhesitatingly in My Name, for a headache, for anything; just bless your brothers and sisters, for each one who knows Me with a sincere heart is gifted with a measure of healing Love, for I dwell in that heart and from that Heart of Love the healing blessings flow, spiritually, and as you well know, mentally, emotionally, and physically and providentially, in every aspect of their being ; yes sexually, for these matters that come to the fore now in these times, they are not of Me; for you know well that sexuality is a clean gift from God. Were it used thus there would not be so many problems on earth. I assist you little children in the blessing, the cleansing, the purifying of the many. Hosts of angels attend upon you and a goodly number of saints. Saint Ambrose is indeed attendant here at this Shrine of the Mercy Gate of the Immaculate Heart of Mary. Precious little ones prevail; you know well that you are all, each and every one called, to walk in Faith and to step out with a spiritual boldness in Faith, that the healings occur. I remind you little children once again of the Japanese Faithful who remained faithful for generations until My priests were permitted to return to them and they recognized them. Continue little children, when there are no priests available to study Holy Scripture, to pray the prayers, to live the Traditions of the people of God, to proclaim the Faith of our Fathers and persevere; this is what Faith is about, and prayerfully heeding the Divine Inspirations ever flowing round about you.

The Lord your God attends upon each of these individuals in tender and merciful Love. Mother also attends. A great healing saint attends; Padre Pio. Little children, remain walking in Faith. Do not ask in advance, simply believe. By Faith are the miracles wrought, by Faith is the Victory won! Little children, with your Faith, your love, your compassion, it is as it were, compensation for certain individuals themselves, and certain ones round about them, and since you unite your prayers always with those who have attained the Victory in Heaven, the healings flow. Be at Peace. Sweetheart, the confessional is the best thing for the multitudes who need healing. It shall be so. My priests will find themselves busier, in their actual commission as priests, and not having time to spend on other activities, but totally active in their priesthood, for the multitudes come unto them quickly now; very rapidly; and great healings occur. Continue in all that you are doing on behalf of My little ones. My people suffer as you know, untold illnesses, because of the errors of the world today, and then when they fall into the hands of certain physicians, suffer degradation of their bodies while they are perceived to be terminally ill. No one calls on Me but a scant few to ask for their cures, their healings. Without My attendance upon them, no one can live!

The deep waters flow, washing away the darkness, the iniquity. My Healing Love pours forth from Glory, assuaging the woundedness. The woman begins to take stock of her present circumstances and makes changes in her life. Be at Peace little Missionary of Love; your healing work is coming to fulfillment in this instance. Heaven hears your prayers; let the healings begin! Jesus bid you love Me, trust Me,(Jn14:1) no matter what is happening, for you are My Own and you live in the Power of My Peace and My Love; in the Power of the Holy Spirit of the Living God. Children, know well and teach others, that this is the greatest Power in all Creation, for all Creation is Mine, it is the Works of My Hands.(Gn1:1) When you pray My little ones, you are uniting with Me, Your Jesus, Who is Man and yet God, and My Godly Power comes upon you as the needed graces, blessings, healings, anointings; all that you need to carry you forth in Faith My little children. *Lord I pray for a patient who has had many miscarriages..*

There is a blight, a darkness on this people which you have touched; it is the Lord Who speaks! Therefore, let it be lifted; Heaven hears the prayers of the Faithful! I am speaking to YB. Do not be distraught little one; the accursed affliction which had been upon you is no more. Indeed, I give Life and Love to the fullest,(Jn 10:10) and it shall be so. Release from dark bondages unknown to this people is occurring now; for Heaven hears the prayers of the faithful; let the Healings begin. I am the Lord God, Your Healer. It is not My Desire, that the multitudes be sorely afflicted, spiritually, mentally, emotionally, physically, sexually; these are not My Desires for My people. I wish to heal them! Alas, all do not come unto Me seeking healing. Those who do, are blest. I call them, "come back to Me with all your hearts"(Hosea) that I may embrace you and fill you with My Healing Love. Yes indeed, I do this through My many small and faithful little ones throughout the world, and so there are times and places of healings. I wish this in the Power of My Spirit, to flourish and multiply about the earth. I refuse no one who comes to Me in a sincere repentant spirit. At that very moment they come to Me, I bless them with My Healing Love. That so few are receiving full healing is again that there is a diminution of Faith in the world! Little children, "By Faith are the miracles wrought, by Faith is the Victory won."(Heb11:1-3) I tell you this again and again, that many will begin to understand and come to Me again that I might bless them. Just as in the story of the prodigal son, so it is!(Lk15:11-32)

I wish to embrace each one, as My Own. I wish to heal every spiritual leper. In the world they resist Me, often for a long long time, but I persevere.(Rm5:1-5), for it is indeed My Desire and Plan that none of My Own are lost to Me. This people, the Works of My Hands, have all gone astray, and I am the Good Shepherd, and I am continuously seeking them out, but I do it through such as yourselves little children. I call you always to be My Heart, My Hands, My Voice in the Ingathering of the little stragglers and the evangelization of those who are yet in darkness. I remain the Good Physician; I wish to heal all. Let them come unto Me that I may carry them. This is My Call.

Subj: My sister
Date: 00-11-03 05:51:04 EST
From:Whiteman@nu.ac.za (Andrea Whiteman)

My sister, Jesus healed Tihana-Ann. I can even tell you when He did it. I went to receive Holy Communion with her as normal. This particular day I went to Rev Richard, a visiting person who showed a keen interest in the child. I normally go straight to the priest as I always want her to receive the blessing so this change in itself was strange. The Rev (I think still a brother) lifted the Blessed Sacrament to bless the child and I could feel Our Lord's Presence. He then gave me to receive. I went back to my place shivering and in tears. I knelt down and cried. At this stage I was uncertain of this feeling but I know that the healing happened then. Jesus healed my little girl and scientifically speaking she was in a bad way. I even cry when I recall the day. I love you my sister.

andySubj: Hi my sister
Date: 00-11-28 06:07:54 EST
From:Whiteman@nu.ac.za (Andrea Whiteman)
[March 15th, 2000]

Lord, we pray for the little abandoned girl, Tihana-Ann, now adopted by my sister. She has now been baptized. She was found to be HIV positive.

JESUS: This little one is also like unto a symbol of Divine Mercy and Love, even as the first infant [Gregory] who came to your sister, is a sign with regard to Mercy and Love, and even unto the testing of mankind to see if there is any mercy and love for little suffering ones, yet on this earth! Therefore, your sister and her family are profoundly blest and anointed in their service to Love. The child herself rests in the Embrace of Divine Love, and Mother is ever attendant upon this child. Angels and saints, graces and blessings, are all about this child and this household of Faith. To whom I Will, I have Mercy (Rm 9:15). I choose to have Mercy upon Ann, and she will grow as a sign of Divine Mercy, and she is a unique presentation to Mankind, of My Love. There is a specific anointing and healing of this child which will be recognized as she grows. The course of this disease is being altered and reduced, for your God is a God of Mercy, and My Wrath does not last forever against those who have brought this plague on the earth, and My Mercy is for the innocent victims of this plague and therefore I put an end to it in due course. *[He is cutting across its course and shortening the bondages of this plague.]* There are yet healing hands among the medical profession as you know, and I bless the faithful ones with, shall We say, a boost of enlightenment, with regard to this disease. Believe, little children, and be at Peace (1 Th 5:13)."

Lord we claim it first for Ann, and for all who have fallen prey to it. Thank you, Lord, we place all under the seal of St. Raphael, "Medicine of God," and pray that his wonderful Oath is recognized. We pray that the physicians will have the humility to thank You and know that it is by Your Mercy, and not by science alone, that the healing and knowledge occurs.

In the manner in which it comes to them they must needs recognize it as an act of God. Raphael delights in all that is occurring. Children, Ann is a symbol of the Victory of Godly Love. Kenny walks ever humbly before Me and is pleasing to the Lord. Raphael is in attendance. Wait on the Lord, little ones.[*Thank you, Our Lord. . Demonic obstruction; we pray rebukes.*]

MARY: *"Children, you do not realize what you have accomplished just now. The serpent was thinking that he had won this battle. Be at Peace* (1 Th 5:13)*."*

Thank you for Our Lords words. We are so grateful to Our Lord. My sister Tihana had a thanksgiving Mass on Sunday. It was special. Fr John had just come back from an overseas holiday and he served Mass. She is an absolute picture in her pink dress and hat. So healthy and happy. She enjoyed her Mass to the full. Caron's little Tarryne was baptized as well. The Natal Witness is running the article on Friday and Tihana will be in the paper. As the reporter is Catholic I have asked that she emphasize the appeal for homes for the orphaned and HIV children. Please pray with me that Our Lord's Will is done. I am hoping to make posters for appeal throughout the churches and bear fruit by this means. Many children can be saved. The violence is unbelievable at present in S.A. and it gets worse daily. Love you my sister.andy

Opening Their Hearts *(Source: The Natal Witness, December 4, 2000)*

Andrea and Les Whiteman of Woodlands consider themselves an average Pietermaritzburg family. Over the years they have worked hard to establish themselves and to care for and educate their two daughters. Their lives took a dramatic turn a year ago when Andrea's brother found an abandoned baby in an old car at the back of his house. This opened their eyes to the needs of unwanted children and set them on a path they say has taught them a profound lesson about HIV/Aids - that babies born HIV-positive need not be condemned to death but have a very real chance of surviving if loved, nourished and properly nurtured.

The Whitemans tell the story of their "miracle" daughter, Tihana, in the hope that other families will open their hearts and homes to babies with special needs. Andrea says that soon after her brother's experience, she realised that she needed to translate her deep religious beliefs into practical action. She investigated what she could do to help unwanted children and, after being interviewed by Pietermaritzburg Child Welfare, was asked if her family would offer emergency care to babies awaiting adoption. "We grew really close to our first baby, Jade, and it broke our heart when she had to leave but we knew that this work needed to be done and was part of the difficulty of being a short-term care worker. "On Christmas Eve last year we received a call to pick up our next child. When we got to the hospital, the social worker said the baby we had come for had already been chosen for adoption. She asked if we would consider taking a little one who had been very sick. "We went to have a look and there was this little mite who we could see had been attached to drips, suffering with diarrhoea, and she was so skinny. Les just held her in his arms and said: 'Don't worry, we are going to make you better,' and from that moment she became our child. "Les said his only thought when he first set eyes on Tihana was that they needed to give her a life of love and warmth. Tihana's diarrhoea continued intermittently and later she developed sporadic skin disorders. It dawned on the family that Tihana must be HIV-positive, which tests later confirmed. Life was not always easy in the Whiteman household but the family were determined to make their baby well.

Andrea says that Tihana's illness brought them closer together, with everyone playing their part. Her daughters, Marsha (22) and Candice (17), read every book they could find on babies and HIV/Aids. "We were meticulous about Tihana's hygiene, kept her away from anyone with the slightest cold and were very careful with her diet. Above all, we loved her deeply. She gave us so much love in return that she was never a burden. "The Whitemans say Tihana even made a difference in their community as the family was open about her status. People who had misconceptions about the illness soon learnt that one can't get contaminated by holding or hugging someone with HIV. They all became very supportive, offering clothes, a cot and whatever help they could. By the time Tihana was three months old, there was no way the Whitemans were going to give her up so they applied to adopt her and, because of her status, the adoption came through three months later. At six months she still tested positive for HIV but the family noticed a difference: her skin started to clear, she developed an appetite and began putting on weight. They felt convinced that the tests were wrong but learnt that babies can sero-convert from being HIV-positive to negative.

When she was 11 months old, Tihana tested negative. The Whiteman's dedication had saved her from succumbing to diarrhoea and other childhood afflictions and during this time the . sero-conversion had taken place. On November 22 this year, Tihana celebrated her first birthday at her creche with her friends, marking the start of the rest of her life. Meanwhile, she has changed the lives of her family members. Next year her eldest sister, Marsha, will be doing her honours in psychology specialising in HIV/Aids counselling and Andrea has already started a course in community development and plans to go around addressing groups on Child Welfare's special needs programmes

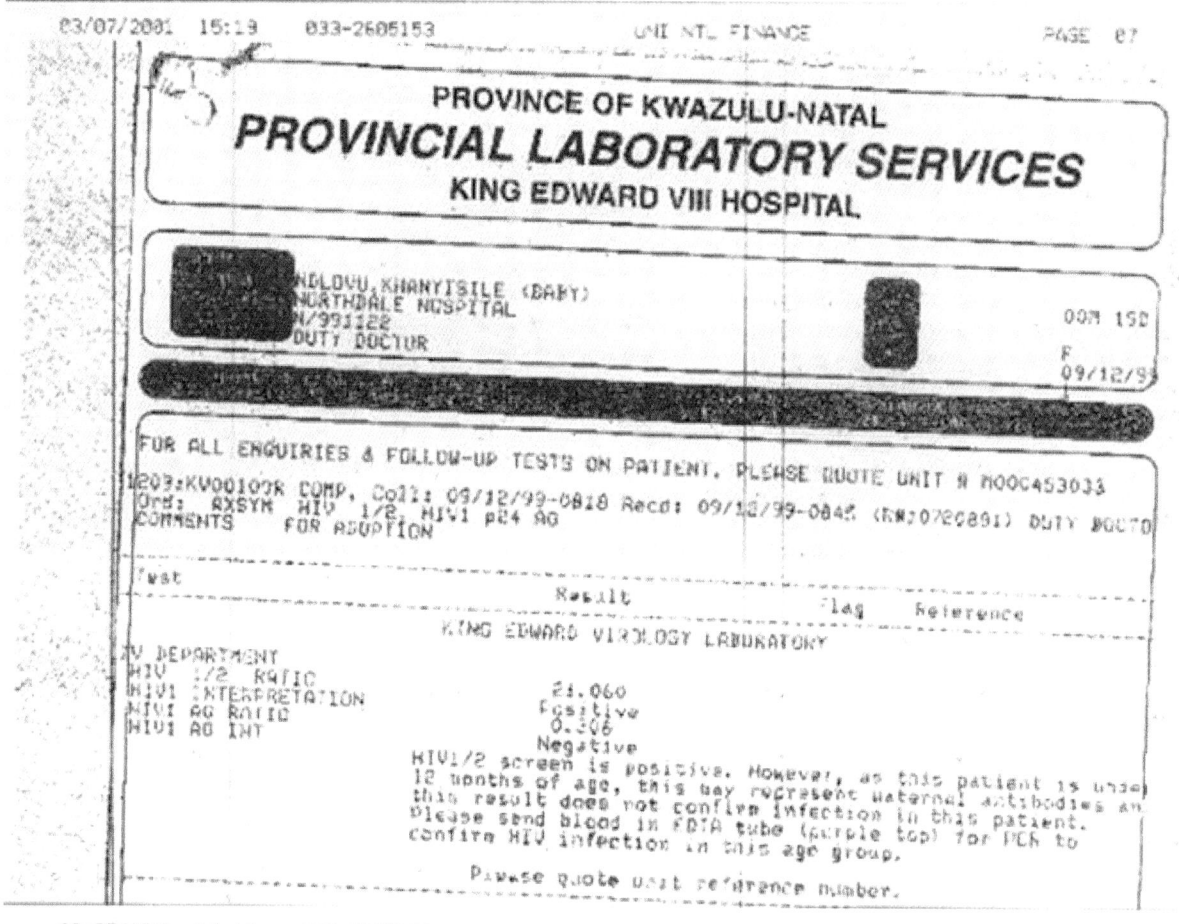

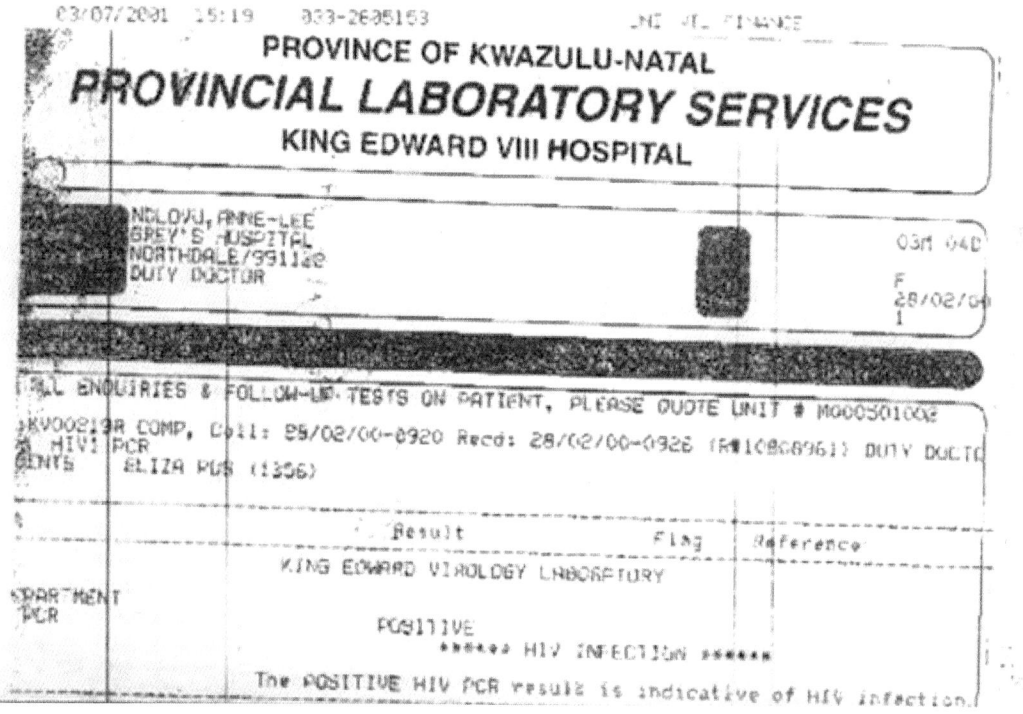

PROVINCE OF KWAZULU-NATAL
PROVINCIAL LABORATORY SERVICES
KING EDWARD VIII HOSPITAL

NDLOVU, KHANYISILE (BABY)
NORTHDALE HOSPITAL
N/991128
DUTY DOCTOR

00M 19D
F
09/12/99

FOR ALL ENQUIRIES & FOLLOW-UP TESTS ON PATIENT, PLEASE QUOTE UNIT # M00C453033
1209;KV00100R COMP, Coll: 09/12/99-0818 Recd: 09/12/99-0845 (RW:0720891) DUTY DOCTO
Ord: AXSYM HIV 1/2, HIV1 p24 AG
COMMENTS   FOR ADOPTION

Test	Result	Flag	Reference

KING EDWARD VIROLOGY LABORATORY

V DEPARTMENT
HIV 1/2 RATIO   21.060
HIV1 INTERPRETATION   Positive
HIV1 AG RATIO   0.306
HIV1 AG INT   Negative

HIV1/2 screen is positive. However, as this patient is under
12 months of age, this may represent maternal antibodies and
this result does not confirm infection in this patient.
Please send blood in EDTA tube (purple top) for PCR to
confirm HIV infection in this age group.

Please quote unit reference number.

PROVINCE OF KWAZULU-NATAL
PROVINCIAL LABORATORY SERVICES
KING EDWARD VIII HOSPITAL

NDLOVU, ANNE-LEE
GREY'S HOSPITAL
NORTHDALE/991128
DUTY DOCTOR

03M 04D
F
28/02/00

ALL ENQUIRIES & FOLLOW-UP TESTS ON PATIENT, PLEASE QUOTE UNIT # M000501002
;KV00219R COMP, Coll: 25/02/00-0920 Recd: 28/02/00-0925 (R#1080896)) DUTY DOCTO
HIV1 PCR
ENTS   ELIZA POS (1306)

	Result	Flag	Reference

KING EDWARD VIROLOGY LABORATORY

DEPARTMENT
PCR   POSITIVE
                   ****** HIV INFECTION ******

The POSITIVE HIV PCR result is indicative of HIV infection.

FORM 14

Magistrate's Ref. No: 14/1/2-15/2000
Registrar's Ref. No.: 52/4 12/4/8/2 30439

ORDER OF ADOPTION: REGULATION 21

REPUBLIC OF SOUTH AFRICA

IN THE CHILDREN'S COURT FOR THE DISTRICT OF PIETERMARITZBURG
HELD AT PIETERMARITZBURG

IN THE MATTER OF AN APPLICATION FOR THE ADOPTION OF

ANN-LEE NDLOVU
(full name of child)

identity number 991122 0117 08 8 child, born on the 22 day of NOVEMBER 19 99
before N N P MTSHALI, Commissioner of Child Welfare.

IT IS ORDERED THAT

ANN-LEE NDLOVU
(full name of child)

a FEMALE child, born on the 22 day of NOVEMBER 19 99
(sex)

be and is hereby adopted by LESLIE SEDRICK EUGENE WHITEMAN
(full name)

born on 14/04/1956, identity number 560414 5102 01 7 *and his/her spouse

ANDREA CHRISTINE WHITEMAN
(full name)

born on 06/12/1956, identity number 561206 0102 08 1, in terms of and subject to the provisions of the Child Care Act, 1983 (Act No. 74 of 1983).

IT IS FURTHER ORDERED THAT

the family name WHITEMAN be given to the child/be retained by the child.
GIVEN at PIETERMARITZBURG this 13 day of JUNE 2000
at 10:00 (time).

MAGISTRATE
2000-06-13
LANDDROS

Commissioner of Child Welfare

1. Date of registration of adoption 2000/07/25
2. Adoption register number 30439
3. Amendment of the birth register in terms of section 25 or registration of the birth of the child in terms of the Child Care Act, 1983 (Act No. 74 of 1983), may proceed.

DEPARTEMENT VAN WELSYN
PRIVAATSAK/PRIVATE BAG X901
2000-07-25
PRETORIA 0001
REGISTRAR OF ADOPTIONS
DEPARTMENT OF WELFARE

Registrar of Adoptions

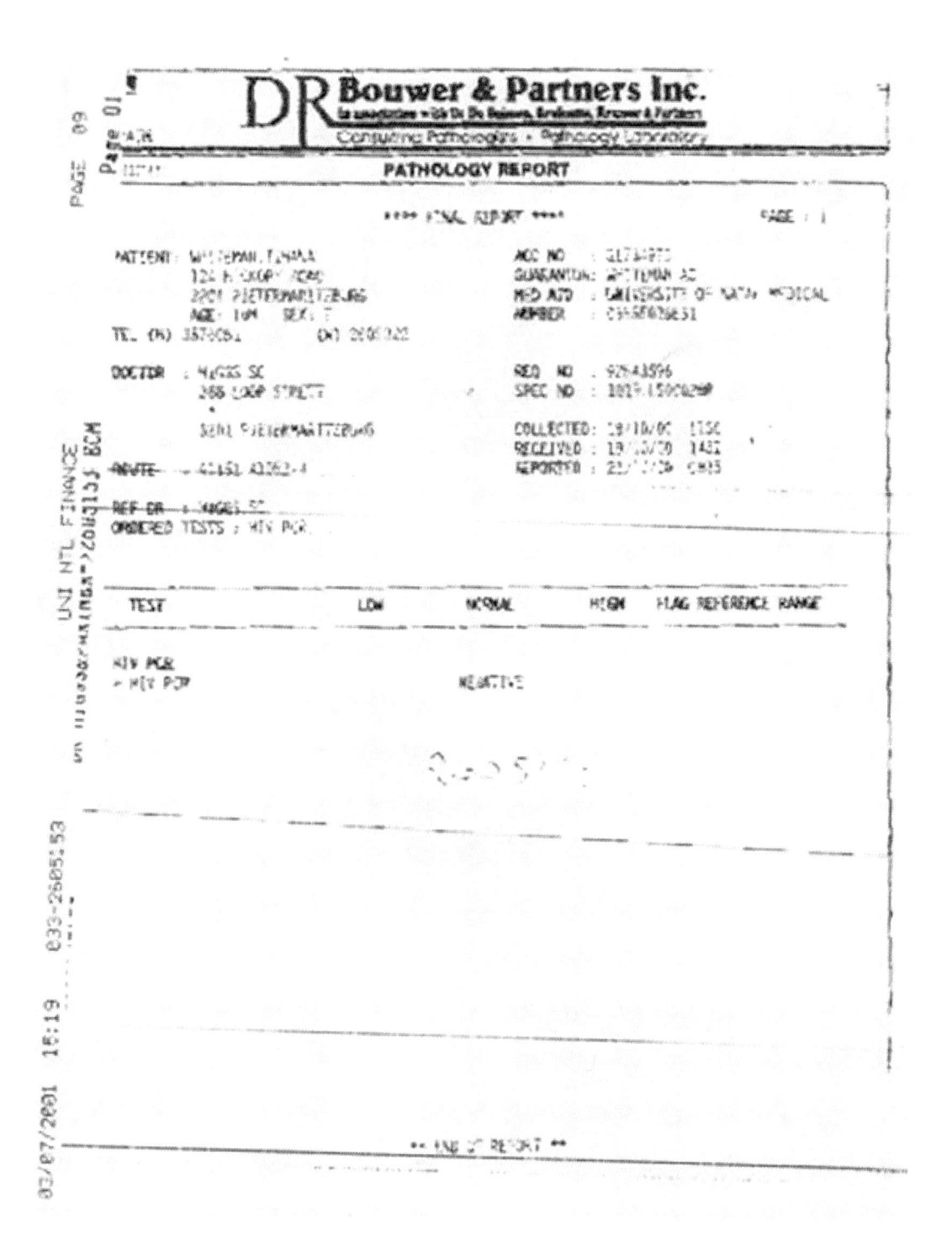

DR Bouwer & Partners Inc.
Consulting Pathologists • Pathology Laboratory

PATHOLOGY REPORT

**** FINAL REPORT ****

PATIENT:	WHITEMAN, TANAKA	ACC NO	: 21734970
	124 HICKORY ROAD	GUARANTOR:	WHITEMAN AC
	3201 PIETERMARITZBURG	MED AID	: UNIVERSITY OF NATAL MEDICAL
	AGE: 10M SEX: F	MEMBER	: 094560365
TEL (H) 3878051	(W) 2606020		

DOCTOR	: HIGGS SC	REQ NO	: 92543596
	285 LOOP STREET	SPEC NO	: 1017-15000290
	3201 PIETERMARITZBURG	COLLECTED:	19/10/00 1150
		RECEIVED:	19/10/00 1430
		REPORTED:	23/10/00 0935

REF DR : HIGGS SC
ORDERED TESTS : HIV PCR

TEST	LOW	NORMAL	HIGH	FLAG REFERENCE RANGE
HIV PCR				
- HIV PCR		NEGATIVE		

** END OF REPORT **

DEPARTMENT OF WELFARE
Registrar of Adoptions
Private Bag x 901
Pretoria
0001
(012) 312 7592
(012) 312 7837

2000/7/26

Ref: 11/4/6/2/10439

MR. AND MRS. WHITEMAN
124 HICKORY ROAD
WOODLANDS
PIETERMARITZBURG
3201

ADOPTION OF: ANN - LEE NDLOVU

Attached are the above mentioned child's adoption order and the birth certificate or identity document.

According to the provisions of the Child Care Act 1983 (Act No. 74 of 1983), your adopted child is now regarded as if born to you. Therefore you personally have to register the child under his or her new name and surname at the Department of Home Affairs nearest to you.

For your information, the Department of Home Affairs address in Pretoria is the Sentraker Building in Frederius Street, Pretoria.

A certified copy of the attached order, as well as the original birth certificate must be handed in when you apply to register your child.

Yours sincerely

REGISTRAR OF ADOPTIONS

COMMISSIONER OF CHILD WELFARE/KINDERSORG
P/SAK / P/BAG X9011
PIETERMARITZBURG
3200
PIETERMARITZBURG

Attached, is the adoption order of the aforementioned child.

It would be appreciated if any future corrections made on the adoption documents be initialed by the concerned person who originally signed the document.

A copy of the applicant's identity document must be sent with the adoption documents.

REGISTRAR OF ADOPTIONS

Outpouring of the Sacred Heart of Jesus.

"Often I keep hidden the workings of My Blessing so that it is known only in eternity. Often it appears that Blessings have no results. But wonderful are the workings of the Blessing - even the seemingly fruitless results are a blessing in disguise through the holy Blessing. These are often mysteries of My Providence, which I do not wish to manifest. "My Blessings often produce effects unknown to the soul. Therefore, have great confidence in this outpouring of My Sacred Heart, and reflect earnestly on this favor to you (that the apparent results are hidden from you). Receive the holy Blessing sincerely, for the graces of the Blessing find entrance only into a humble heart. Receive it with a good will and with the intention to become better; then will the

Blessing penetrate to the depths of your heart and will produce its effects. Be a child of the Blessing; then you yourself will be a Blessing for others."

But there are more! I have told you children repeatedly that I am weaving together the souls of the true faithful, as a Seamless Garment of My Love, encompassing the whole world, that none of My Own are lost to Me, like unto a vast Fishermen's Net, and you are part of it; and you are part of the Kingdom of God! You are in Unity with the Church Triumphant and the Church Suffering for whom much prayerful intercession is given to assist humanity when they are invoked to pray with you, and for whom you pray, bringing joyful release. Persevere in doing this; all of these are part of the Body of Christ, the Kingdom of God, and united with you, the Church Militant on earth. You see now, the battle lines are clearly drawn and recognizable by such as you, and yes there are many instruments of My Peace and My Healing Love. I ask you to persevere in every little personal outreach to every person. When they see, little children, the lights of Love and Truth which each one of you has become, they are drawn to you, and they seek also to have that Light, that Love, that Truth which you have. In this Way, you are being My instrument of Peace, and bringing them to Life and Light and Love. You know that you are precious in My Hands, and that it is in unity with Me that others are drawn to My Church, and drawn within My Church to prayer of the Rosary, to Adoration, to an increased attendance upon the Sacraments of My Love. Little children, the time of Mercy is yet upon the Earth, and I am seeking all hearts to come unto Me. You know well that I thirst for souls; bring them to Me! I assist you; Mother assists you.

Children, do not doubt the Truth of the matters of Life and Death from the moment of conception until the individual comes Home before Me, will be known by all Humanity. Little children, at this time many tribes on earth, who are considered primitive, are treating Life far better than the so-called enlightened and educated groups who call themselves the civilized ones.

CHAPTER SIXTEEN
THE PRIESTHOOD AND THE CHURCH

JESUS (to and for the priests)

It is I, Jesus Who Speaks; I the Spouse Who speaks. Am I not the Spouse of the Church?" I am your Jesus of Merciful Love. Come to Me Who Loves you so. I bless you again and again. Little children, in this time of trial, where there is confusion even in the very Church of God, I ask you to be humbly obedient to Our beloved John Paul and to those in correct Authority over you. Little children, stay secure in the Sheepfold; live within the Walls of My Commandments given out of Love for you for your protection. Live fed, nurtured on My Sacraments that you may indeed have Life to the fullest. In your weakness is My Strength. When you come to Me in the Sacramental Love I give to you, you are strengthened with a yet greater Fortitude, for you indeed need courage and Fortitude to live through these testing times, these trying times. Indeed the time of the Chastisement which is evident upon the earth even as We speak.

Little children, I am the Word of God, and I remind you that as I was tested by satan, it was My Words that defeated him; therefore I ask you to guide and guard your tongue; with Our Assistance it is so. Fight the good fight with the two edged sword of Holy Scripture. The enemy is readily defeated by those who claim the Victory in My Name; by those who are always giving praise to Our Father. Little children, those who give praise become like unto precious songbirds, rejoicing in the Light and Love and Life of the Creator of all. Make good plans for your tomorrows, they are in My Hands; the Hands of your God Who Loves you most tenderly, most totally and most eternally. Little children, persevere in evangelizing in My Name for there are many who are in need of your example of your Faith and Love. Even as We speak I am infilling your heart and soul and mind with a vast measure of My Love and My Peace and a sure and quiet Joy of heart I give to you. Little children, this Joy and Peace is a sure sign of My Love and Presence among you. Little children when you begin to loose this Joy and Peace, be assured it is time to come to Me in the Sacraments of My Love and be restored to the Perfection of soul that your Joy may be complete, and My Joy may be complete in you!

Continue as I have told you. I reiterate, hold fast to your Jesus, in Spirit and Truth; hold fast to our beloved Mother as We walk side by side, with the beloved Joseph, Guardian of the Holy Family, Guardian of the Family of God. He is with you little children, invoke His Name often . Remember that He was entrusted to look after the Son of God. Emulate Him; it is good to follow in this manner. Continue therefore walking with Us in Faith and Hope and trust and Love; in all patient perseverance. This is My Way and you are My brother, part of the Family , the Family of God, the Family of Bethlehem and Nazareth, the great Family of Peace which I am building upon the earth now. My Victory is before My Eyes. Invoke My Name, invoke Mother's Name often. I have chosen to weave you into the true Garment of Love with all the true faithful souls on earth. This great fishermans' net spans the earth, covers the earth. You will live to see the transformation of the Earth; you will live to see a Holy Nation upon the earth and you shall be a part of it. You do not realize the immense anointing you have received today, but you will recognize it as you go forward in Faith.

The river of lies spewed out against Myself and the Mother of God, and indeed, the beloved John Paul, and indeed, the entire Church from the mouth of the serpent, the old dragon, are falling upon the ears of the many in this time, just for a brief time. Blessed are those who hold out in Faith and trust and Love and patient perseverance! I the Lord your God bid you know, that I am not unaware, that the seven deadly sins are no longer mentioned among Christians! They are not recognized among pagans; But it is the very humans who claim to be Christians, who now shun the seven deadly sins. Were there no lust, there would be no abortions; no greed, there would be no sale of body parts; if there were no self-seeking, power-seeking scientists, no cloning of humans, no mutilation of precious embryos, and all the other desecrations upon My Own Creation, with precious human bodies and souls! It is worse than Egypt ever was! Be not dismayed about anything; I am with you; and I am with My religious, My priests. When you are working as My friends, My Works, I am with you; and I am with My beloved bishops and priests as they read and ponder the Words which I have give unto thee; therefore, there is no cause for fear and anxiety here. You might say I have armed and armored you very well for this Mission. The confusion is abated. I am the Lord your God.

Govern yourself by the Will of your God! I am He who Lives and Loves eternally. I am your Jesus of Merciful Love. Profound discernment you speak, My small little one. Ask of Me what you will. The virtue of Love is such that I the Lord bless your works. I bless you with the needed Words of wisdom and discernment. I bless also your heart, hand and mind for these works of Mercy. I Myself assist you in the Writings. Those I desire to hear shall indeed hear, because of you. I choose you; and in you and through you, and those believing priests whom I direct you to. A goodly number will heed, who have not considered the many aspects clearly. Do not worry about numbers. I tell you that if even one has a change of heart, it is a worthy effort, a worthy project and I bid you know that more than one will change, more than one will consider, more than one will come closer to Jesus and the Truth. You may forward the additional Words as you desire, and it becomes a great unfolding before M's eyes. I Myself attend upon him in a profound manner. He realizes that I, in Truth, emanate from here. Be at Peace in all things. (Jesus is saying that M is showing it to other priests. He said the quorum of priests who study it with him are amazed, puzzled; some are a bit disconcerted, confused.) "I work a great miracle of understanding on each one of them." "Some are saying, 'This changes the whole picture.' It is to My delight and approval!"

The Church of God, will soon begin to use priests and doctors and nurses and counselors in the healing ministry of Jesus Christ, Eternal Physician. Believe; it is happening, and shall continue to happen, as My graces flow, in the power of the Holy Spirit of Love. Pray, and study, and leave all the rest to your Jesus who Loves you most tenderly, most totally and eternally; for you live in the power of My Peace and My Love; in the Power of the Holy Spirit of the Living God. It is to rejoice in Our Love , awaiting the great day of triumph and of Peace. Little children you shall see that day!Bid them share with whomsoever they will. My Words are a blessing upon all who read them. Even though they do not seem moved initially, be not surprised at the outcome, the fruits of your works. They are not in vain. I do not speak idly! There is one who will assist you - a priest of Holy Orders. We shall draw your attention to him, and he will be approachable...You will understand and he will indeed help you. My little one, even if the mind set of one person is altered by your Message, it is worthwhile; and I assure you that it is not only one person, but many, many who will respond to this Enlightenment, for We ensure that it is a profound Message. I indeed assist you.

As you send this document to M, as you well know, that will cause grave concern, even consternation; but My Words in you and through you are irrefutable; though some try to reject them; this is not unexpected. *'Pour forth Your Spirit and renew the face of the Earth'* you pray, you pray and you pray, My faithful ones;

and it is happening. But it is My Will at this time in the history of Man, that much Enlightenment is through the faithful, among whom thou art numbered. A Flame of Love is upon you, for you are profoundly anointed in the Spirit of the Living God. Come unto Me as you need to know. I am working closely with you, and I am delighted with our conversations of Life and Love. *He is quoting St. Paul: "when I was in the Spirit..."* I do not know where to look. "Try Acts 3 :11. Thus, it is readily available to say, *"when I was in the Spirit...."* We work a miracle of Love upon the good priest; it is your Jesus who speaks. Do thou, My little one, prevail. I ask you to remain obedient to your Jesus and Our Beloved Mother. You are blessed profoundly in this Communication from the Lord your God, in the power of the Holy Spirit of Love. All that I ask of you comes to pass, My little obedient one. Little children, do not be anxious or impatient. Simply wait upon the Lord and the actions of Love take care of themselves, since thou art surrendered to your God most profoundly.

Living Waters, Light prevails all about you, surrounding you in the Light of Christ Jesus, your Lord, at all times. The Lord your God has gifted you long ago for these Works of Love to be performed at this time. I assure you, they shall succeed. I take away all the road blocks now. You will succeed. Let us go forward in Faith and Hope and Trust and Love, in all patient perseverance, My little sister, for you and each one with you are part of My great army of Peace. Enlightenment must come, that many hearts are changed and true conversion occurs in Our Great Design. The beloved M has need of more Words. Therefore, I gift thee with more Words. My graces fall upon you, little one. When you are speaking to M, the Words will flow from your heart, for your heart is Mine and Mother's, and in this trinity of Love you will speak the appropriate Words, for it will be the Lord God speaking in the Power of the Holy Spirit. Therefore, I ask you to just rest in Peace and Light in My Presence and wait on the Lord yet a little longer. The priest who is called M has a name in Heaven that is most pleasing to the Lord God and he dwells always in Peace, as I have prescribed for each of My Own to dwell always in the Peace of My Presence. I have taken away all your anxieties and concerns and ask you to remain therefore, always in the Peace of My Presence. Be not anxious about this Father of your heart's concern. We bless him with Peace and Enlightenment as well. The trial is primarily over. There is the odd small test but your work flows freely now.

Mighty is the Lord your God! I am the Lord who speaks. Do thou, My little one, remain at Peace. I Myself attend upon M and you will very soon hear from him. It is then that you will approach your pastor and your Archbishop and I open their hearts and minds to that which you have been given to speak out. It is a time now, little children, to enter into the solemnities of this week of holiness. This Communication may be held in abeyance until after Easter Sunday. I bless thee, little children, in the Peace of Christ! Henceforth, little one, address the Sovereign Queen as "Merciful Mother" as you plead for anyone. Let Us together invoke the Mother of God; you may pray the Rosary, many Memorares, any litanies in honour of the Mother of God, many Hail Holy Queens; you can, as you call it, storm Heaven on behalf of the conversion of the priest to know that the Presence of the Mother of God emanates the Love of God through Her Heart of Love, even upon those who do not believe! The Mother of God has a Heart most merciful and Love-filled, and especially for her priest-sons. Invoke therefore, St. John the Apostle; let us continue in Faith, awaiting the conversion of this priest. The priesthood is in disarray; what are you doing about it? We pray for them; we don't know what else to do. We give them Your Words, they do not believe; they tell others not to read them, which prevents others from receiving Your blessing through the Words.

Many rejected Me, many will reject you, yet I have strengthened you to persevere, and that you shall do! Little children, those who heed the Words know a great Victory of Love and begin themselves to evangelize, and to propagate the Faith of the Apostles, which is in sore disarray upon the earth at this time. Persevere little children of Faith, persevere! We pray for those who do not want to hear the Name of Mary our Merciful Mother. Do not be afraid to proclaim the Name of Mary readily about you. It is Scripturally sound, it is Traditionally sound, and the Name of Mary, Virgin and Mother, is very effective in obtaining many conversions and many other blessings and graces from the Lord God. *(Omen hears "God gave you to Me, I gave Him to you" - a hymn in the words of Mother Mary.)* Be at Peace. All these matters shall be resolved in the very near future in your own time. It is so! Simply address the priest who is your spiritual director cheerfully, positively, openly, requesting to attend upon him yet again. Little child, when you are rebuffed do not be dismayed; it is still part of the testing. Always go moment by moment, step by step, day by day. Simply give him a call, and be sensitive to his response, and continue walking in Faith. We are with you and We are with him. All things occurring in this time frame have to be, little one. Thus you are blest with Peace, Love and great fortitude. You are already blest with the gifts of the Holy Spirit, which are imperative, essential, in your Faith journey. Mother and I are at one in this matter. An anointing is upon each one who reads the Words, opening their hearts to the Spirit of the Living God.

One might say M has an abstract way of looking at life. He is ever in My Light, and is frequently unaware of the passage of time. Bless him as you are blessing Me. I am in attendance upon M; We will give you an answer. Little one, you have found favour with the Lord your God. Be not afraid to share openly with those about you. I indeed asked you to wait for a response from the beloved M. The delay is not necessarily of My making, yet it occurs. Dealings of the world tend to interfere with My Works of Mercy, in these trying times in which you are living little children. We will expedite his response now. In the meantime, be not afraid to share and speak out on this matter. Remember, I the Lord God elected to be born in a stable, a cave, a place of lowliness; and yet in these humble beginnings, the Church was built in My Name. You do not realize that small efforts you make, though they may seem large to you as you are doing them, are being expanded and multiplied by the Lord your God. You are not alone in these beliefs. There are many with you. It is a matter of opening eyes and ears and hearts and intellect. Trust Me, I know what I am about! For the Spirit of the Living God is beyond time. Even so, I will keep order in the conference. Place it all in the hands of Our Mother, Mediatrix of all Graces. The blessings flow. Things fall into place. Walk in Faith little children, ever in Faith. [He is giving me Hebrews 11 & 12.]; and there are more evidences of Faith in Holy Scripture as you well know. You may choose to ask the assistance now of any priest who may elect to assist you.

I bless you both with a profound anointing of My Love and My Peace, and of course the concomitant Joy in the Love of the Lord, are yours. My little ones, Mercy Gate Mission shall proclaim the good news of salvation far and wide. Many will come to Me in and through all that transpires here. My beloved little ones, do not be afraid to trust the beloved Father Francis of Our Hearts' Delight. I have indeed woven you together that My Word go hither and yon about the earth. I brook no obstructions to My Word. The walls of resistance shall indeed ultimately tumble down like the Berlin wall, yet in the interim it is imperative that My Word be heard. Therefore prevail in all Faith. There is indeed a great apostasy about the Earth. My Church is assaulted from every direction, in many and varied ways, for the enemy is insidious and so deceitful that many do not even recognize what is happening to them. Little ones you are chosen for a Mission of grave import to your God, and are blest accordingly. Continue always turning your other cheek, praying for those who assail you. *[The hymn, 'The Cross before Me, the world behind Me; I have decided to follow Jesus.]* In this your surrender to Love, in this Our unity of Love, you follow Me each one, in a unique manner, and the end results are a Great Victory, in the Name of Jesus, for many are released from the deceits of the world.

You shall be speaking frequently to Father Francis by telephone and by fax, and in these communications the end result will be that peoples about the earth, hear My Word and many heed, and return to Me with all their hearts, rejecting the philosophies of the world, which turn people away from God and into error and sin. [His Words went on the internet on August 6th] Jesus shows Omen my beloved Therese` again and He is saying, "How appropriate is she not, the Patroness of Missionaries; and is this not a house with a great Mission; and are not your Words as a missionary of <u>'The Epistle of Love to the scientific world'</u>(He names this Mission). St Paul converted the Greeks in the great' Logic ' of their minds, they too surrendered to Truth and Love. Little ones, prevail fearlessly for I am with you, and I am with Father Francis, and I am with a myriad of people who will come to your assistance. I indeed do weave together My faithful remnant !

A great Light of Faith pours forth upon you and emanates from you. Never concede any defeat little children in My Name; continue always in Faith and Hope and Trust and Love and patient perseverance; for this is My Way; I am the Way; it is the only Way, for those who would know Me. My little sisters, you are profoundly blest and anointed this day. Pagan thoughts have assailed the minds of many. The priesthood is in disarray because of this. Even the convents, the sisters and nuns who have always been a symbol of Our Mother's Virginity and purity; they too are being assailed by what you call "new age." They swallow the deceits of the foe. Thus I come to you My little humble ones who have fought the good fight against the assaults of the enemy, and stand in the courage of your convictions despite what is occurring about you. The Lord shows He opened the door to the prison for St Paul. My blessings are upon you now . Those who serve Me are never prisoners of the world. Doors open at the Hand of your God, your Almighty God. I am Jesus, your Eternal Victor; what would you ask of Me ?For those of Faith get through; We open doors for Our Own. Even though they may appear closed they become open at the opportune moment. He showing His timing is precise like the rolling back of the Red Sea.

Little children, you are as lighted candles in the darkness of the world today. Prevail little ones, for the darkness is so dark that My people walk in confusion, unknowing which way to turn, for the hireling shepherds have not only abandoned My flock, but they have debased My Church and harmed My flock! Do not concern yourselves about these matters; just know that My faithful remnant, is like unto the small faithful remnant in the Old Testament. [like the army leader that chose his men when they went to drink water] . This remnant I strengthen, I protect, I train them in the way of spiritual warfare, and I hold them strongly united to Me; and under the great mantle of Love, in the power of the Holy Spirit, it is so. Little children, you are included in this army.*Jesus is showing the Body of Christ, but its like a long loaf of bread; it is commercially sliced.* One Bread, One Body; how, how will you make it one Bread, one Body when you have done this to it? How? Will you answer to Me? Division upon division has occurred; confusion upon confusion. St Paul has advised you people of God not to follow one person or another, but to follow the Lord your God, and none other. Those who know the Lord their God, keep their eyes on Me; keep their heart and soul and mind filled with this Our Loves' Union.

You have now entered a time of world diplomacy, which will wreak further havoc on humanity. Therefore persevere little children. Peace; We bid you rest! Lord what should I do about the names of the priests in the originals? You may speak freely with Father Francis, for he has an open mind and I have prepared him well for this time. You may choose to delete the full names and use initials of the priests; thus on the day when they recognize Truth, they will know that I called them then by name to heed My Word![Lately the Lord has been saying that none of them will be able to say they did not know.]First things first. Contact Fr Francis giving the Information unto him, and finding out the times, dates, it will be accessible on the web page; then you may share with those who will heed. Anticipate much traffic and conversation with regard to the Messages, for it shall happen. Translations shall indeed occur though many about the earth comprehend the English tongue some translations are yet necessary. Believe Me it shall happen for your works are important to Me. Persevere in Faith little children, for your works are important to Me! The people on the website will arrange their own copies. There may be a few that you have to give the documents to. We shall arrange reasonable printing means. Believe and be at Peace, it is already before Our eyes!

Lord, may Omen and I speak freely about this Mission on the website, or not? It is no secret what God can do; although it is not in Holy Scripture, it is My Word, therefore proclaim it, to all who will heed. Give him the time to establish it on the web. Whomsoever heeds the Words shall be profoundly blest. Those of irrational thought will reject it. They may even taunt. It matters little. Remain close to your Jesus and Our Mother, and My Peace, My Providence, My Protection, is upon each of My Own. Where is My song? " *Hail Redeemer King Divine…"We Love You Jesus.* I ask you to contact the M, bidding him know you have additional information, for him. Ask him if he wishes to receive it. Indeed you may fax. *Father Francis asked me to pray about a name. The Lord asked me but I want whatever our Lord chooses. Our Lord chooses "Faithful Missionary of Love". He says I may abbreviate it to "Faithful Missionary."*

I call to My Church, wherefore do you linger in idleness; the harvest is plenty, the workers are few. Proclaim the good news of Jesus, until it resounds about the earth, and the healings begin. Your Good Shepherd awaits the workers in the harvest. Be at Peace, thou art beloved instruments of My Love and My Peace. My small friends rejoice in Our Love. Be not surprised at the miraculous events which occur now. Print them out, and await Divine Inspiration to do further. Pray and ponder. You will pray, it is the Lord who speaks; for all afflicted in this vile manner[refers to homosexuality] by the demons of lust which are rampant about the Earth and are poorly in rebuke now, for no-one so to speak, is working the practices of self-discipline of their own bodies in any of the appetites; and thus you might say, the demons of lust seem to have free reign upon mankind. Sodom and Gomorrah were destroyed for far less than what is occurring now. Even so, the Lord your God awaits the conversion of many from the many and varied deviations and behaviours, of what your generation proclaims as sexually active persons. None of this is pleasing to your God. It is gravely offensive. Pray as you do; speak as you are given to speak, and leave all the rest to your God. [Given that hymn, Great things happen, when God mixes with us].We work miracles. I the Good Shepherd, rescue many from the darkness of sin which is before Us. Believe and be at Peace !

Before the two of us knelt down to pray we were discussing the severity of the continued problem of stonewalling so that the Words of the Mission could not be shared locally and our Lord said, You are the women at the tomb; at the dying of the Body of Christ, which will arise again in Glory ! I am your Jesus of merciful Love and I am attendant upon thee, precious little children of God. My small sisters, I bless you each one in a profound anointing of My Peace and My Love. My Joy is ever with you My beloved little sisters. There is scant need of alterations of the Words. Be at Peace. I have assisted thee; I continue to assist thee in these discernments. You will begin to see, as you might put it, a Light at the end of the tunnel, for I am profoundly united with you, in this great Mission of Love. Clarification may be asked of you in some of Our Words. Believe, I shall inspire you, even speak in you and through you, addressing anyone's concerns about My Words.

I call all unto Myself now as you know it has been ongoing for some time in your realm, your kingdom of time. It is like unto a great , one might even say a prolonged hour of Mercy to your God; and at the end of that time of Mercy all of My Own will know that I am God, that I am indeed the Way, the Truth, the Light, the Life, and all of My Own will come back to Me with all their hearts ! Faithful Missionary comes to Me for a consultation of My Love and I give it to her readily. Be at Peace, no matter what is happening, remain at Peace in all things. Indeed send the Messages afar. You have bespoken to the several about you with no positive response. They must therefore wait in turn [shows Omen a long lineup] before they begin to receive My Words of Truth once again. Should one seek you out asking for this information, be pleased to give it to them. But as you say the many appear to be stonewalling your efforts. Leave them there. Pray to the God of Mercy that they too be Enlightened. At this time verbal coercion or any such means are to no avail. Remain therefore in the Spirit in prayer for the many. Should a door open for you to speak, remembering all things are possible with God, do speak; and should it be necessary to speak only to this individual or that one, or perhaps two or three, do so. It would of course be in a very limited way; but accompanied with the brochures it will be adequate; food for thought and discernment for those individuals.

Little children, do not wonder why you are chosen for these various Missions. Just remain surrendered to your God as you are and let My Merciful Love and My Words flow through you. They truly will fall upon the ears or eyes of those who need to know them. It is not always necessarily so, that those who read or hear them will respond in the desired fashion, for they too remain in free will; and yet many shall; and the others may well move their positions at a later date. And those who in all stone-heartedness reject My Words, are in essence rejecting Me; and they are themselves to blame for the consequences of their acts and of their attitudes. Leave them over unto your God. Little children, always remember that I am a God of Merciful Love; I change hearts. My beloved one, do not be hurt, personally hurt. The rejection is falling upon your Jesus. Do not be hurt on My behalf. Simply continue as you do to make recompense to the Two Hearts, which is most pleasing to your God. Remember, all harsh words hurled against you fall upon your Jesus as so many whiplashes. The people pouring forth these harsh words do not seem to comprehend that they are doing it to Me their God.

Eyes that see and see not; ears that hear and hear not! This is what We are dealing with! Pour forth Your Spirit oh Lord, and renew the face of the earth you pray; the multitudes pray; and yet multitudes resist ! Oh My little ones, persevere in prayerfulness; remain humbly obedient; remain children of God and children of Mary no matter what is happening about you! Oh My little ones, when they are wrath, when they are attacking you in any way, verbally or by obstructive tactics, creep into Our Arms, creep into the Sanctuary of the Two Hearts and leave it to your Jesus. I take care of all things, and you belong to Me and you are safe in Me. He is My priest-brother. You may contact him, perhaps even asking him if he would like to receive the further Words you have been given. Do not simply expect a rebuff, but should a rebuff occur, again remember; they rejected Me first; and be at Peace. Use this throughout this Mission of Love; It falls on your God and not on thee! Always keep this perspective before you, that you do not react emotionally. Simply remain abandoned in the Love of your God.

I am He, and I bid thee Peace yet again. My little ones, the beloved Father is a most practical man as you know. You may approach him; he is actively as you call it, pro-life. And yet you will be caused to go through all the discernments you have already gone through with Father Francis, regarding the Messages in Light of the Vatican's approval of certain aspects of this form of health care. It will be tedious. Bide your time a bit and We work to open the hearts of priests and doctors as the scandal of organ transplants, of organ sales, becomes more in the public eye; and they cannot fail to have heard of it, and they begin in themselves a soul searching as to the right and wrong of it. It is then that they would be open to peruse, to study, to contemplate and pray discernment with regard to your Messages. I Myself shall motivate you at the opportune moment to share this with Father J. It shall be soon but not quite yet. With the Archbishop also, Our beloved Archbishop. It too will be a painstaking, and even tedious undertaking, for there is much to study in the Words thou art given, and the time element is always there for My priesthood, and even for the doctors. Yet on that day when he takes the time to read your presentation, I will be with him in the Divine Inspirations that he be open to your words, *My Words*, because he is a patient man and open to all the voices which come to him in the varying causes of these times. I bless him even as I bless thee and I bless Father J; *all* are beloved of the Lord. Each one is used as an instrument as I choose; those who will assist you in proclaiming; those who receive molding and give molding in the process. For the molding of each soul is ongoing, as long as they are upon the earth. Therefore I ask you; never be dismayed nor disgruntled nor in a despair. All goes according to My Design. Your Assignment is precious to the Lord God ! Some shall surely desire to read the entire manuscript. Be open to these requests.

Little children, prevail in all prayerfulness, for those who do not know Truth. I the Lord God am Truth. Many do not see Me in the Holy Sacrifice of the Mass. They do not see Me in the Blessed Sacrament, the Thanksgiving which you give to the Father, in Me and through Me. A time comes when all on earth will recognize this Truth. Little children since it is not yet, prevail, pray for the conversion of sinners, the Salvation of souls, prevail and trust in My Mercy. *Feeling heaviness which feels like I am carrying the weight of the Mission though I know that Our Lord is doing the carrying; we are just instruments.* Healing Love is upon you. Believe and be not afraid. Trust Me your Jesus; Trust Our Mother; Trust your guardian angels. Trust those whom you discern are speaking truly in the Lord. There are many about you who speak well but do not know Me. Oh sorrow; enmeshed in the world they cannot seem to find Me, and yet I am knocking at the doors of their heart. *The heaviness increases. Jesus showed us a window with a lantern which goes out. It appears to be a Church window, all blackened inside. Lord what are you telling us?* That thou art in a time of rapidly approaching darkness in the Church and in the scientific world; and in the world all about you; all about the earth. The visionary has done well in enlightening many, but many remain in darkness. Faithful Missionary is assigned to enlighten the peoples of great intellect; Omen is assigned to the peoples of the first nations, many of whom have great intellect but lack true spirituality, and to assist the street people as you call them, for they too are My Own, and many intellectuals find themselves there in the streets at rock bottom, despite their wisdom and knowledge and understanding; for they have taken a wrong turn and need to come back to Me with all their hearts. Indeed I seek them out, I am the Good Shepherd. I seek them out in you and through you, and all those who work in similar manner on My behalf.

Little children, great angels fight a great battle, that these Words be given over first for the doctors, then even to the priests involved, but ultimately for the general public, those that can and will read . Do not be dismayed at the obstructions little one, or any of the strange events that will attempt to slow you down or even stop you all together. *It shall not be.* I Myself cause the Victory to happen. Thou hast worked well; thou art well advised from Glory. Things are going according to Heaven's Design. Be at Peace. The virtue of Love is such that I am present to you. A severe testing, a severe attack is upon your works little children; prevail; We are with you! Believe; We are with You! Be at Peace therefore. Failure to comply with the thoughts and designs of the physicians who have propagandists available in the media, cause you to be as it were, pulled out of the inner circle. Do not be afraid, you are in a circle of the Triune God, of Mother Mary, and multitudes of angels and saints. Little children, there is no time to waste, it is time now to busy yourselves getting these messages out. Our Lord is showing pictures as on a tv screen changing and changing and changing. God wants to show mankind all the errors of their ways.

Little children, the Faith of the Fathers, the Faith which has carried My Church through these generations; I bid thee pray and act in all Faith and hope and trust as thou hast been taught, and just watch things fall into place, at an opportune moment in time all flows freely. You do not know the reasons for the obstructions, the delays. Do not worry about it. Simply continue, rejoicing in Our Love's union and be at Peace. I do not permit My faithful priests to disregard the beloved John-Paul! Be not dismayed with My priesthood; My faithful holy ones remain always with Me. Those who are tormented and scattered willy-nilly by the foe; by your prayers little children the vast majority come back to Me with all their hearts. Remember, I am a God of Merciful Love; I give to them all they need to have to return to the fullness of Truth. Many are the deceits and errors being fed, not only to My priesthood, but to the whole Church. My people, My sheep, My lambs become scattered in confusion. None of this is of Me. Yet it is that time when the enemy would sift My Own as wheat. I Myself take swift, sure action now. Believe. I am Jesus, Eternal Victor!

The Bishop is fully aware of this controversy that the government would bring the world into the Catholic Hospital. It is an ongoing warfare. Do not sell the Prince of Peace yet again for a few shekels. I Myself will move this holy Bishop's heart and mind that he will know that all you speak is My Truth. The priests you mention will confirm it. Even so, in this time in which you live, do not be dismayed if you hear scant news or no news at all; this does not mean that your Bishop is not working. It means that he knows well the way of working of the enemy. He knows well the way of the government agencies he must deal with. He is a man of wisdom and discernment and he will do all in his power, and I Myself assist him for he calls on Me, and he calls on our Mother for Heavenly assistance and it is given to him. I have told you before, do not be dismayed at the things that are happening in the world in this time frame in which you are living. Certain things just have to be. Know that I the Lord God am with each of My Own at all times during this time of great trial.

Praying for seminarians and prospective seminarians. Lord, I'm praying for a young man M. I've had this feeling in My heart for a while that you've been calling him to a religious vocation. I'm praying that he will turn to you and give his heart and soul to you...24th April, 1998. The Virgin attends upon him. He is indeed falling in Love with Love...which is a call that My priesthood needs to hear. I asked about Heaven's intentions for a pottery Mass Set that I had made at the request of a private shrine which was closing down. Our Lord refers to the set as a sacramental. As soon as we started praying for discernment on this issue, the evil one started hassling: "We kill you for this, we kill you for this!"

All that you ask of Me I give to you, it is the Lord Who speaks. They are destroyed. They do not desire that these sacramentals go where you would send them, because that is what We desire. Therefore in all Faith act,- sending them, for they are as you note, blest and already used sacramentally. I bless you and I bless these works of your hands. The life of each priest is so very important to Me. I will bless this individual in and through these works of Love. Give GlorySend it to MG. He may not be the one who has it always, but send it to him *now!* You do not know the meaning of these objects which you have made as I do, for you made them at My Desire, and I work miracles of Love in them and through them. Believe and be at Peace ! You are called by patient perseverance, prayerfully attending upon your God. Do not be afraid to go forth in My Light and My Love. I make M a great success in that to which he sets his hands. Be prepared to fight for your Faith little children, for the time of peril is imminent.

<u>Nov28 1998. Prayers for priests of South Africa at the request of visitors returning there.</u>

The priests of this great nation of South Africa, I bless to be priests forever in the order of Melchizedek, like unto Me, Jesus. Sons of God, sons of Mary, sons of faithfulness, My brother priests, I bless you in so profound a blessing that you cannot fail to experience My very Presence, and most particularly during the Holy Sacrifice of the Mass. Know that I am with you as is written in Holy Scripture. I bid you remember that each Mass is for the healing of My people. Recognize each Mass as a healing Mass. I am Jesus your

Physician, your Counselor, your Redeemer, and I am ever present to you. I continue to call, "feed My lambs, feed My sheep." Sons of God, you know well that you are living at this time in a Love-starved world, yet I call you as well as all the truly faithful flock, to be My Heart, My Hands, My Voice, in outreaching healing Love for My suffering little ones. Do not be dismayed that some may still be resentful or defiant, or in any way obstructed; Love them, Love them anyway with My Healing Love and you will see them grow like a small budding plant that comes at last into sunlight. They grow and flourish and bloom and bear fruit and Heaven rejoices. Bless any and all therefore in My Merciful Love and wait on the Lord!

Yes little children, today you are both the seed planters, and the harvesters, for there are so few of you, and so many to tend. Yet I am with you more powerfully than ever, for the Holy Spirit is upon the earth now, in a profound anointing of Love as the Mother, My Mother, your Mother, remains visiting the earth yet a time, calling all the children of God back to repentance and Salvation. I will to hold each of My Own in My Embrace of Love and it shall be so; and yet it shall be so through you, My faithful priesthood on whom I am bestowing blessings and graces in the River of Light. I name each one of you who receive this Message responding to My Call of Love with an open heart, child of faithfulness, child of God and child of Mary, beloved of Jesus, beloved of Mary. I give to My little ones every one, this small act of Love. Pray it until it is a song in your Heart; until it becomes like a passport to walk anywhere on the earth, for the earth is the Lords, and the fullness thereof, and you are My Own, and to bring you ultimately into the Glory of My Presence in Heaven. It is easy enough for the youngest child to learn, and powerful enough to bring you into the Sanctuary of the Hearts that Love you so!" I am someone Jesus Loves, I am someone Mary loves. I am safe in the Arms of Jesus, I am safe in the Arms of Mary." When you invoke Our Names prayerfully We attend upon you, resolving the concerns of your heart, in the Peace of Our Presence where We wish you always to remain. Therefore little children, at moments of stress or distress, when fear, hatred, anger, anxiety; any of these emotions, temptations rise up in your hearts; before you speak out words you may regret, or take any action which is not prudent, firstly pray this prayer, calling on Us, that you remain always in Our Peace. There must be Peace in each human heart and in each home and in each parish, then the Peace of Christ will spread like wild fire, throughout the world. In the Power of the Holy Spirit it is so; and it shall be so! Little children, pray much; your prayers are pleasing to the Lord your God. Remember little children, that Heaven hears the prayers of the faithful. It is always Our Desire to say yes to Our precious little ones. Even so it must be according to the Father's Great Design, and be for the good of the souls concerned, and it is always contingent upon the free will of those for whom you pray. Therefore persevering prayer is so essential.

Little children, Love your Jesus and trust your Jesus in all things, and in this your 'yes' to Love, I the Lord God AM Love; I take care of everything else, for you live in the Power of My Peace and My Love; in the Power of the Holy Spirit of the Living God. I remind you My people: this is the greatest Power in all Creation, for all Creation is Mine, it is the Works of My Hands. When you pray uniting with your Jesus, Who is both God and Man, this My Power comes upon you as the needed blessings, graces, providences, to carry you every moment of your life. I reiterate, be not afraid, I am with you always. *Our Lord requested that we sing what He calls a strengthening Hymn for his precious children of South Africa. "This day God gives me strength of high Heaven...".*

Those who will believe are known to Me already! Those who will not believe at this time are known to Me already! Those who will never believe are known to Me already! They reject the blessings of My Messages. But for those who believe now, and who shall believe, proceed little children without doubt, knowing that this is the Desire, the Will of your God <u>It shall come to pass!</u> Provide the pamphlets as you shall do at the conference. I reiterate; don't worry about those who choose not to read or heed My Words. Those who read them are blest. They are indeed My Words, not yours; not yours, but Mine! Always little children, do so in the Joy of the Lord. I Myself set angels of assistance about every move you make in My Behalf. Little ones, have you noticed that the poor people, the humble, the lowly, who come seeking help for their personal distresses, have no problem believing? Therefore, do not worry about the powerful ones. It is simply that they must be told, that I have elected to use you in this manner, in the telling. That which occurs subsequently is known to Me! My little ones, each one of you is profoundly blest both here on earth, and in the Glory of God subsequently, for your yes to your God!

I am the Lord your God. That which We have put together; handed it to you as it were, ascertains that the works We have assigned to you are in unity with the beloved John Paul. Therefore find time to do that, for you are being most explicit to those readers whom I wish to read these papers. Do not be dismayed at any rejections little children. Even as they rejected Me the Lord your God, when I walked on earth, My Own true followers, among whom you are numbered little children, will suffer a measure of rejection. Remember little children, as is written; do not worry about human esteem. Concern yourselves only with what Your God thinks of you, and stay as you are; My beautiful little sisters; My beautiful children, picked from the flower bed of the Mother of God.

My little one, I am causing as you would say, things to fall into place for you now. Peace. Do not be afraid to speak boldly in My Name, to Father. Always firstly pray for him and for the priesthood, and asking Me to be your Voice when you speak to him, and it is done. *Misericordia* little children I bless you both. My little one, speak fearlessly to Father; address your communications, My Words; speak fearlessly to Father. Attempt to work in this manner to address yourself to the beloved Archbishop. Little ones do not be afraid to tell Fr M at this time as well, for he too attends upon the beloved Bishop with all his concerns. Do not be afraid ! He showed us the little boy David standing before the giant. Therefore little one, print what is recorded and include that with your letter to Father and the Archbishop. More prayer! More prayer! I am the Lord your God. Thou art in My Hand as a small instrument of My Works of Mercy. I Myself begin an action of My Love which causes M to see Truth; I Am Truth. He will see and at last understand and comprehend for, shall We say he is haunted by the Words you have sent to him, and yet is bound and immobilized to act at this time. My little children, you realize the degree of Faith that you have been called to. It is so for anyone who truly says yes to Me. *Our Lord asks for another song for the priests, Spirit of the Living God, fall afresh on them [me] x2 break them, melt them, mold them, fill them, Spirit of the Living God, fall afresh on them.*

Little children, I fall afresh upon them at every Holy Sacrifice of the Mass. I am with them, yet as you know, one can walk away from Me in free will. Little children, pray this hymn often for My priests and watch the miracles take place. Now rest in Me and trust in Me; you have fought well for the priesthood. Be at Peace. My beloved little children, have I not told you that I am weaving together the souls of My true faithful in a seamless garment of Love spanning the entire earth; and it is so! My little children, do not be distressed that there are puzzles in your life. You know well that you are called to walk in Faith and hope and trust and Love; in patient perseverance, for as instruments of My Peace, you carry the secrets of My Love on your journey with you. It is so for every faithful priest, for every faithful individual upon this earth. They are emissaries of the Great Secret of Love and thus you will prevail in simply loving one another and trusting your God. Do you comprehend little children? Yes, somewhat Lord; may I understand what You were giving through the handshake?

A gift that in due course he will recognize himself. My little children, as Omen knows well, when she prays laying hands with a priest specifically, I anoint that priest profoundly, and she always asks him to bless her in her works, and through that priest I anoint her profoundly. It is something like that that transpired between you and that priest. Each one of you will grow in Faith in the manner I Decree. This is withheld from any foes. It is a silent action of My Love, not outspoken that he may hear and apprehend the actions I devise. Believe little children, this warfare is great! You are instruments of My Peace, instruments for conversion; and yet I bid you always remember that you carry within yourselves the Secret of God, the Great Secret of Love. You are [it might seem farfetched to the logical mind], as small secret agents of the Loving God. * Ever be open should any of My faithful choose to contact you. *Jesus thank You for the priest who helped me to understand.* Bless that priest always in My Name and be at Peace. He is counted among My true and faithful. Am I not your Teacher?

Many of them will be in My Era of Peace, where none of this is even relevant because in My Hour of Peace there will be no such things to deal with; but that time is not yet little children; so prevail, prevail, prevail; believe, believe; pray, pray; fight; speak out! My blessings are upon you. I seal your lips both of you, that you speak only that which is Truth. I AM Truth. I AM, and I was present! I presented Myself to each one of them! I bid thee Peace in this matter. Remember, a prophet is not recognized in his own locale. It has been ever thus. Therefore accept the humblings even the humiliations, giving them over to Me, that I may present them to the Father proclaiming, behold My small sister in her faithfulness, carrying that cross which has been given her. Know little children, remember well, that cross which you carry with joy and faith, trusting always in your God, becomes your stairway to Glory; and in Glory, the Lord your God forms it into a glorious crown, and all your tears are converted into gems in that crown. Believe little children, you serve a God of merciful Love. Were I not merciful, I might simply destroy all these non-believers; but in My Mercy, I choose to send them many small voices to enlighten them, to call them to heed the Word of the Lord. [Like a farmer casting out seed]. Time changes everything.

Continue, watching the fruits, even unto the words coming out of their mouths. I Myself work the miracles of Love I choose to work, upon each of those who have heard My Words on the sanctity of God given Life. You have gained supporters, but there are of course those who come against you. This is the usual pattern for mankind . This is not different for you and for Omen, than it was for many of the saints and the prophets. It continues this way for you. Know that our foe uses pride of intellect to darken minds against Truth. Therefore prevail little children, I am with you always. Never mind about the deadline. Just work on the document for the Bishop. I Myself will assist you with Divine Inspirations and occasionally Words. My little one when you work for your God and you speak Truth; I Am Truth. All is going according to Heavens Design. Your Bishop is able to recognize these Words as genuine and sincere, and of the Lord God. We continue to work Our miracles of Love in you and through you and such as you.

Thou hast asked that We rebuke in the Name of Jesus, it is the Lord Who speaks, the spirit of pride which assails many intellectuals. This has been an ongoing war throughout the course of the centuries, and continues to now; yet some will yield. A certain yieldedness-in-Faith to the Living God is essential, before the thoughts of this people, the minds and thoughts, are opened to Truth. I the Lord God AM Truth. There are so many I would call back to My Heart ; Their are so many I would bathe in My Love. They know Me not! Even as you are being shut out little children, so have I been shut out. Mother calls and pleads to no avail. And yet as all seems darkened, suddenly a swift sure action of your God and Light comes upon these minds so befuddled by the lies of this age. Enlightenment comes, and thus you are called to patient perseverance. *To Omen*; Wilt thou prepare a writing of this prayer so that others may understand Love. My Jesus, I love You, I adore you; ever and always I need you, ever and always I belong to You; ever and always I am satiated in Your Love Lord and yet ever and always I am hungry for Your Love. Oh come in Your Love now, come to our assistance, Lord God of Heaven and earth.

Continue to pray for your beloved John Paul, and your Bishop, and your priests; all My priests throughout the world, for they are in dire need of prayers, for the enemy assails then even more than it does the flock. Can you tell Me that you love Me for those who do not? My God, I believe, I adore, I trust and I love You; I beg pardon for those who do not believe, do not adore, do not trust and do not love you! Listen well when he tells you of all his tribulations; they are not his own, but that of many priests. I am bridegroom of his soul. *We sang along with the angels. Oh Lord I am not worthy that Thou should come to me, but speak the word of comfort, my spirit healed shall be. And humbly I receive Thee, the Bridegroom of my soul, no more by sin to grieve Thee, nor fly Thy sweet control. Oh Sacrament Most Holy, oh Sacrament Divine, all praise and all thanksgiving, be every moment Thine.*

See little children, this is what the enemy would destroy in My priesthood; My pledge to be with My beloved mankind for all time. The enemy would attempt to stop it by attacking My priesthood, and depriving My little ones of My Presence. Little children, that is why you are Enlightened and asked to pray much. To those whom much is given , much is expected. I share My Heart with you little children, and I ask you to continue to be My Heart, My Hands, My Voice. In all that is happening, Mother and I are powerfully attendant upon you. Much Heavenly assistance is given you. Persevere little children, in all prayerfulness; yet remain always at Peace. The vaults of Heaven are wide open as the blessings flow upon you little children, and graces to carry you through these trying times. Little children, you are called to persevere, enduring all things in the Name of your Jesus. Remember little children, I am with you My precious little ones, and it shall be ever thus. You are protected and armed with circumscribing angels about each one of you and about your loved ones. With regard to the priesthood which is called to be holy; those who are My Own shall remain ever faithful to Me throughout these times of trial and testing; those who are lukewarm shall suddenly have a change of heart and come unto Me at last, or they shall be lost forever from Me.

Because they have not responded to thee does not mean that they are in non-compliance . The Message is as it were, overwhelming to the many. They see Truth at last; I am Truth- and must ponder and pray ; and comprehend and pray, seeking gifts and graces to cope with it in their own minds before they take action. There is yet a little time dear children, be at Peace, be not anxious. All falls into place according to Our Father's Schedule. I wish you to know little children that Mother and I are attendant upon the Body of Christ throughout the world, the Church instituted by your Jesus, on the Rock of the beloved Peter, and I am profoundly attendant upon John Paul II. He is at once both strong and fragile, and I ask you to pray much for him. The Spirit of the Living God encompasses him. John Paul is safe in the Lord, and all that I desire him to know, comes to him in due course. Little children, pray for the beloved John Paul, pray for your Mother the Church, and be at Peace. The vortex of the storm in which you have been is now moved from you, and recognition is beginning to occur in the minds of several who have read Our Commission to you. Be at Peace therefore. You were in the eye of the storm because of the Messages you sent out. But there is now some belief and they no longer focus on you, that the Word of God has been given unto thee, but Your Mission itself becomes the focus of attention rather than you *per se*. Wait on the Lord sweetheart !

MARY: ***The Virgin of Fatima blesses you little children. You live now in the time of the Fatima predictions and yet you are safe beneath My mantle; safe in the Heart of Jesus, safe in the power of the Holy Spirit, safe in the Love of your Creator, your Father. Our Lady of Fatima: When We are in a direct spiritual battle with the devil, We have to persevere till the Peace Victory of Jesus is clearly demonstrated***

and His Peace and Joy restored to us. This is the Feast day of My sons who established the Church and I remained with them, teaching them. I am still teaching My children, these 2,000 years, and I delight in My faithful children. Remain always humble and obedient.

In obscurity was Our Lord borne; in obscurity did He grow up. Now Saint Joseph, ever holy, obscure and humble remains to most of the world; yet He is of the highest order of saints. These are the Keys; humility and obedience. Especially at the time of Consecration, ask what you will of Our Lord, for this is the moment of Divine Mercy. As to the meetings of the Catholic physicians in unity with the priest; it is a tragedy, a sorrow, that they do not choose to believe, but seek a burden of scientific truth before they would believe. Though you present this to them very clearly, they are reluctant in their great intellect to accede to these Truths. Be not dismayed; it has been ever thus.

The Virgin of Fatima sighs with relief for at last certain of those reads, believes, heeds the Words in The Epistle of Love, and certain of those who have received all the documentation you have presented to them cannot set it aside. It comes back to their mind again and again and they repeatedly read and read further. Dearest little children, forbearance is the Word for this day and for the next short period of time. Dearest little children, the Lord God's Will is done, is done, is done! Nothing can stop it! Various means are used to deflect it, even distort It; but the Lord God, His Will is done in and through His faithful little ones among whom you are numbered. Little children great Peace is upon you in this your service to the Living God!

Mother is present. I bid you Peace, My darling. I take care of each and every one of My priest-sons. My obedient priests are pleasing to the Lord God and to their Mother. Simply pray the miracle prayer and do not be afraid to speak out to the priest of your heart's concern. In this great Mission of Love, which is so important to the Lord your God, We open the ears and the hearts and the minds of the priesthood to receive these considerations which have been given directly to you from the Lord God Himself. The priesthood its very self is in disarray, little one. Should you come upon a priest who is in partial or even total disagreement, be not disturbed. It is the Will of God that the Word of God be assigned to them.

The Temple of the Living God is just that; the Temple of the Holy Spirit. In the power of the Living God every temple is sacred. Therefore, simply pray for the Enlightenment of priests and doctors that the Great Enlightenment come upon them. The gift given to My priesthood was to consecrate the Bread and Wine; this was the work Jesus promised that He would cause His apostles to do greater than He Himself. They bring Jesus to all who yield to the Faith of the Apostles.

Mother is blessing you child. The beloved Father is a delight to Almighty God and to your Heavenly Mother. He is anointed by God in a unique and unusual fashion in His relationship with the Living God, and the Graces flow. Would that it were so for his brother-priests. It is not so for each one. They need come before the Lord on bended knee and surrender in all abandonment to Love and to the Will of the Living God; therefore little children, persevere in praying for the priesthood. Little children, all your prayers are heard and those for the priesthood, acclaim the Faith of the Apostles to this very day! Many true faithful are praying for the holy priesthood.

I remind you little children, that when you are praying for the holy priesthood, you are praying for the continued Presence of the Holy Eucharist on earth which the enemy is busily attempting to stop. Woe to the earth were that to happen, but you have Our Lord and Saviour's Pledge; He is with us to the end of time and the gates of hell shall not prevail. The enemy busies himself as he is running out of time, to no avail. Indeed the Victory is already won in the Name of Jesus Our Lord. Mother blesses you child. Father knows Truth, and understands that it is just as you have noted, even as it is with Omen. In obedience to superiors, visionaries are kept at arms length. Those, even those who believe.

Come and worship, Royal Priesthood, come and worship, Holy Nation; worship Jesus, Our Redeemer, He is Risen, King of Glory.

CHAPTER SEVENTEEN
ANGELS and ARCHANGELS

JESUS:

Ask Me, and I set great angels and assistants about you at all times. Indeed, certain selected saints assist you now. Triumphant angels assist this woman, for her works are important to Me! Believe and be at Peace. Angels carry your Message to M in all delight! Mother is also blessing your Words and sending angels and saints of assistance with you. A seal of approval is upon your works. Be at Peace in all things. Go forth in the Light of Our Love! Know this: the holy angels, the guardian angels assigned to each infant, which you call a foetus, weep; for their mission to mankind is aborted, that of the child and of the angel! Little does mankind know, in the realm of Glory, in the realm of spiritual- ity, in what ways this human behaviour alone is harming Humanity! Triumphant angels are in attendance now, My little one. The Will of the Father is done in and through such as thee. Therefore, be at Peace!" We do not wish to weary faithful workers; We bless each one of you profoundly. Hosts of angels assist here, making things flow freely in the Name of the Lord. Little children, you do not know the works of mercy you are performing, nor the great graces which are upon you. Love your Jesus and be at Peace.

The battle therefore is for each human to win victory over self, assisted by your Jesus, and Our Mother, the ever-virgin Mary, and by a myriad of angels and saints your victory is assured, little children . Your awesome God blesses you now in a great anointing of Love and Peace. Seek a hymn of praise, and a hymn to the Queen of Angels and All Saints, your Mother of Mercy.[We sang Father We adore You.& Hail Queen of Heaven at the end.]As for P, he is beloved of the Lord God, and We are with him through this trial. We ease his pain; We lift it. The degeneration is delayed. You must continue to pray for him. He is in the Eternal Embrace, and surrounded by the angels and a goodly number of saints. Be at Peace with regard to his soul. My Mother, Queen of Angels, and all saints is even now attending upon C for Heaven hears the prayers of the faithful! Many pray for the beloved little one of Our Heart's concern. Angels hold thee fast little children; be at Peace. The vile enemy continues to attack and obstruct. Do not be puzzled, nor dismayed at anything that happens in these times. Hosts of angels continue to assist My Own little ones always; Love lights the way little children: continue to love one another. Little children, ask of Me what you will.

Referring to the brochure and the" Chapters" The little one is doing just fine. You are powerfully assisted by Heavenly beings and all is going nicely, like unto a free flow of Words and works. Be at Peace, it is Our Delight; you are My Delight. Just continue as you are in Divine Inspirations -all that you have done in these printings is pleasing to the Lord your God. My darling children, their is going to be a great change upon the Earth now. The venom of the enemy is obstructed by the Lord God! Great angels work miraculous events in this matter, for My time is at hand ! Healing Love is upon you. Believe and be not afraid. Trust Me your Jesus; Trust Our Mother; Trust your guardian angels. Trust those whom you discern are speaking truly in the Lord. There are many about you who speak well but do not know Me. Oh sorrow; enmeshed in the world they cannot seem to find Me, and yet I am knocking at the doors of their heart. Little children, great angels fight a great battle, that these Words be given over first for the doctors, then even to the priests involved, but ultimately for the general public, those that can and will read. Do not be dismayed at the obstructions little one, or any of the strange events that will attempt to slow you down or even stop you all together. *It shall not be.* I Myself cause the victory to happen. Thou hast worked well; thou art well advised from Glory. Things are going according to Heaven's Design. Be at Peace!

Change is ever present; Creation is not static, there is always an ongoing moving on, like the waves of the ocean. It is delightful for you are walking with your Lord and with Our Mother and with St Joseph, and with a myriad of angels and saints, walking in the power of the Holy Spirit of the Living God. Hosts of angels are ever going up and down the stairway to Heaven bringing glad tidings of Great News of Salvation to all Mankind. My little ones, gathered here in this small prayer room, great blessings accrue and pour forth upon you. Many pray here, little children; many pray for you and with you. All those with whom you are interwoven are united, each praying one for another; blessings flow. This is accompanied by prayers of the great and Heavenly angels and saints of Glory, whose voices resound before your God; and in addition accompanied by those yet in their purification, as you invoke them to pray with you that they may all the sooner attain Glory. It is indeed happening blessed children of a Merciful and Loving God, My Peace is upon you! I am your Jesus of Merciful Love. I am attendant upon this family. You are precious to the Lord God, and to the Mother of God. Hosts of angels I set about their household, angels of enlightenment; angels of Healing of Love, of Peace, of Joy, a myriad of angels of assistance. I bid D and M, though I am your God and I read your heart and soul and mind, and know all that you are doing and all that is occurring, I ask you to be as a close personal friend, for I am Bridegroom of your souls, and I Love when you share every detail of your existence with Me, even the smallest concern. Talk to Me Your Jesus, about all your hearts concerns; I am with you, I listen, I bless, I heal. Stay as you are, in close unity with Me, but tell Me all that is going through you. Share it with Me and you will find that your burden is lightened.

Son of God, your workplace is not necessarily a holy place to work, and I ask you to hold your protection snugly around you. I ask you to remain always in the Peace of My Presence, no matter what is occurring or transpiring round about you, in particular in the work place. I Myself am your Strength; call on Me at all times that I may strengthen you in all these trials and testings. I bid you know that Mother has placed Her Mantle around each one of you, this little family of Love; in the Power of the Holy Spirit it is so! Thus you are ever sheltered in the Shadow of the Most High; the Comforter, the Sanctifier, is attendant upon you most profoundly, as well as your Great Guardian Angel. Little children, pray your Guardian Angel prayer morning and evening. By this means, you leave as it were, a line of communication before your God Who is in Heaven, and your own conscience; for the angels, who are ever in the Presence of God, are yet attendant upon you, giving you the Divine Inspirations to assist you in even the smallest of decision makings. Sanctuary is in the Two Hearts of Love. Hide yourself in My Heart and in Mother's Heart, from your very own frailties. You are safe in Me; you are safe in Our Mother.

Prayer: Angel of God, my guardian dear, to whom God's Love commits me here, ever this day[night] be at my side, to light and guard, to rule and guide!

Little children, I set angels of every category in the household of A; I Myself do indeed lay hands upon him. Mother encompasses him in Her great mantle of Love. In the Power of the Holy Spirit this child remains all the days of his life, and indeed to the greater Glory of your God, Our Father Who art in Heaven! Little children, rejoice in this Our Love's Union and remain always at Peace. My little one, do not worry about how the other doctors regard you, for I am with you, and I shield you. I assure you that in this time, all true faithful members of My Church, each one is shielded in a magnificent shield of protection. In the army of the Great Archangel Michael, all the angels who work with him, work to shield each precious human, as you recognize each little temple of the Living God, very powerfully in these times. Be at Peace therefore ;

in all that you are doing, the Lord is with you, Our Mother is with you, great saints and mighty angels are with you; little ones, I am with you. When John Paul speaks, it is like in Scripture, Gabriel's Horn. Children remember, I set militant angels around each of My Own, protecting them from the attacks of the foe. The beloved Michael busies himself in shielding My Body of Christ on Earth, from the attacks of the foe. Remember, you are at one with Me, and therefore I, the Living God, am your Shield. Be at Peace.

Evil has no power over you for evil has no power over Me. Even so, the enemy taunts you, each of My little ones. You are in My Hand and in My Design. Rest assured you are safe in Me. The projection of your work in the healing arts and in your Providence, rests in Me. Believe and be at Peace. It will come to pass but not yet, that the Pope will be asked to terminate his reign. They attempt this now and are continuously barraging him, because they too are beleaguered by Freemasonry and anti-Christ movements. *On the 30th July 2001, I was praying about how Our Lord wanted me to fill the pages of this chapter, and I was asked to quote the "words" which Our Lady had given to Fr Steffano Gobbi with regard to the angels, in the book of his locutions; "Our Lady Speaks to Her Beloved Priests.*

"**Entry 232: The Queen of Angels**   [September 29th, 1981 Feast of the three Archangels.]

In the struggle to which I am calling you, beloved sons, you are being especially helped by the angels of Light. I am the Queen of Angels. At my orders, they are bringing together, from every part of the world, those whom I am calling into my great victorious cohort. In the struggle between the Woman Clothed with the Sun and the Red Dragon, the angels have the most important part to play. For this reason, you must let yourselves be guided docilely by them. The angels, the archangels and all the heavenly cohorts are united with you in the terrible battle against the Dragon and all his followers. They are defending you against The snares of Satan and the many demons who have now been unleashed with furious and destructive frenzy upon every part of the world.

This is the hour of Satan and of the Spirits of Darkness. It is their hour which coincides with the moment of their apparent victorious action. It is their hour, but the time which they have at their disposal is brief, and the days of their triumph are counted. Therefore they are setting dangerous and fearful snares for you, and you would not be able to escape them without the special help of your guardian angels. How many times each day they intervene to rescue you from all the treacherous maneuvers which, with astuteness, my Adversary undertakes against you! That is why I call upon you to entrust yourselves more and more to the angels of the Lord. Have an affectionate intimacy with them, because they are closer to you than your friends and dear ones.

485. The End of the Times.

With docility allow yourselves to be taught by me, beloved children. ***478: The Announcement of the Three Angels.*** *October 2nd 1992. Feast of the Guardian Angels. "Today the angels of light of my Immaculate Heart are at your side, my beloved ones and children consecrated to me. This is their feast day. Honor them; call upon them, follow them; live always with them, they who have been given to you by the Heavenly Father as your guardians and protectors.*

Today is their time. This final period of purification and the great tribulation corresponds With a particular and powerful manifestation of the angels of the Lord. You have entered into the most painful and difficult phase of the battle between the spirits of good and the spirits of evil, between the angels and the demons. It is a terrible struggle which is taking place around you and above you. You, poor earthly creatures are caught up in it, and thus you experience the particularly powerful force of those snares which are set for you by the wicked spirits in their attempt to lead you along the road of sin and evil.

And so these are the times when the action of your guardian angels must become still stronger and continuous. Pray to them often; listen to them with docility; follow them at every moment. The cult of veneration and praise offered to the angels of the Lord must become more widespread and solemnly observed in the Church. For indeed, to them is reserved of making to you the much awaited announcement of your proximate liberation.

*The **announcement of the three angels** should be looked forward to by you with confidence, received with joy, and followed with love. Your liberation will coincide with the termination of iniquity, with the complete liberation of all creation from the slavery of sin and evil. What will come to pass is something so very great that it will exceed anything that has taken place since the beginning of the world.* **See Holy Father's Catechesis on the Angels EWTN Papal 1986,87**

Walk in the light of their invisible, but certain and precious presence. They pray for you, walk at your side, sustain you in your weariness, console you in your sorrow, keep guard over your repose, take you by the hand and lead you gently along the road I have pointed out for you. Pray to your guardian angels, and live out with trust and serenity the painful hours of purification. Indeed, in these moments, heaven and earth are united an extraordinary communion of prayer, of love and of action, at the orders of your heavenly Leader.

And there are many more entries touching on the angels in the MMP books.

This patient lost a cat tragically and then began "hearing a sound' like the meowing of a cat . She repeatedly searched in her house, drainpipes, attic, ceiling etc. and got her husband and son to search as well . They found nothing. This had been going on for a year. She never heard the sound anywhere except in her own house. Her mental status was normal in every other way. She was never placed on antipsychotics. Then the sound started multiplying to multiple voices, which now started saying things like "mummy please help me." When she heard the sound, her new cat and the dog would simultaneously become alert and start whimpering. After a while it appeared to me that it might be demonic and I asked my prayer partner if we could pray for her.

MARY: *Mother bids thee Peace! I go forth , I place a mantle of protection about her in the Power of the Holy Spirit, and it is done. Believe and be at Peace. Continue to address her and her concerns prayerfully, proclaiming the Name of Jesus as you do, and leave the rest up to Heaven. As you well know, some miracles of healing occur instantly and some are more prolonged. The healing is present !* Omen saw the affliction when Mother was speaking; it was gone. After this I gave her a blest rosary to pray ;she is Catholic. The voices were gone for a few weeks but then began to return. But the most amazing thing happened thereafter I will let her tell in her own words (see next page).

Jesus is speaking: Mighty, mighty, is the Lord your God. That is why Mother is one earth, frequenting the earth, calling the children who can see, who can hear, who know, to pray and pray and pray again, for the conversion of sinners, the Salvation of souls. Hosts of angels assist in the works of My Church upon earth. Hosts of angels assist each one of you now in these unusual times.

MARY: *ANGELS ASSIST ... little children. What would you ask of Me My small one? The Queen of Angels and All Saints is in attendance. The Virgin herself attends upon her now. Forthwith be at Peace. We work swift sure actions opening doors freely now for the beloved little one. Hosts of angels attend upon her and upon those whom she contacts that all goes according to Heaven's Design for her.*

ANGEL ON MY SHOULDER

ALTHOUGH I HAVE PROBABLY SAID A THOUSAND TIMES, THAT I HAVE ALWAYS FELT THE PRESENCE OF ANGELS, I NOW BELIEVE THAT AS SO MANY OF US DO, IT IS SOMETHING I OFTEN TOOK FOR GRANTED AS AN ADULT, BUT CHERISHED AS A CHILD, EVEN LEAVING ROOM AT NIGHT IN MY SMALL BED FOR MY GUARDIAN ANGEL TO SLEEP WITH ME. THE ONE PRACTICE I HAVE CONTINUED THROUGHOUT MY LIFE IS TO SAY A PRAYER TO OUR ANGELS OF GOD, AT THE TURN OF EACH CALENDAR MONTH, CHANGING THE WORDS TO INCLUDE THEIR GUIDANCE AND PROTECTION FOR MY WHOLE FAMILY.

POSSIBLY, I SHOULD FIRST EXPLAIN THAT ALTHOUGH THIS STORY TOOK ME TO A PLACE I NEVER DREAMT POSSIBLE TO EXPERIENCE, AND AT TIMES MADE ME DOUBT MY OWN SANITY, IT WAS A VERY REAL, TORMENTING, ONGOING SITUATION, THAT ONCE IT HAD A GRIP ON MY HEART AND SOUL, I CAN NOT EVEN BEGIN TO EXPRESS THE DEVASTATING PAIN IT CAUSED ME AND MY FAMILY.

MY FAMILY, AND EVERYONE THAT KNEW ME, UP UNTIL THIS POINT, HAD NO REASON TO SEE ME AS ANYBODY BUT A REASONABLY INTELLIGENT, RATIONAL PERSON, WITH A GOOD SENSE OF HUMOR, BUT THIS EVENT WOULD SERIOUSLY CAUSE THEM TO WONDER WHAT WAS HAPPENING, AND TO BE COMPLETELY HONEST, I KNEW THEY JUST WANTED THE WHOLE THING TO GO AWAY, NOT BE MENTIONED, PRETEND IT NEVER HAPPENED, AND TO THIS DAY DO NOT WANT TO TALK ABOUT IT.

SEVERAL THINGS HAPPENED AROUND THE SAME TIME, ONE OF WHICH WAS MY PHYSICAL HEALTH DETERIORATING TO THE POINT I HAD TO STOP WORKING, AND MY HUSBAND'S COMPANY RESTRUCTURING SO THAT HE WAS NO LONGER WORKING, WHICH MEANT WE HAD TO MOVE, WHICH LED US TO THE AREA WHERE WE NOW LIVE, ACROSS FROM A PARK, WHERE SEVERAL COYOTES MADE THEIR HOME.

IT WAS A SATURDAY MORNING IN EARLY JANUARY, AND BOTH MY CAT (NOT THE WORLD'S FRIENDLIEST CAT I MIGHT ADD) AND MY DOG WERE SLEEPING BESIDE ME ON THE BED, WHEN THE CAT, WHO HAD RECENTLY LEARNED HOW TO GO OUT OUR DOG DOORS, LEFT THE BED, AND IT WAS WITHIN A FEW MINUTES, THAT BOTH MY DOG AND I HEARD A TERRIBLE SOUND, AND SOMEHOW NEITHER OF US MOVED, AS WE BOTH SEEMED TO KNOW WHAT HAD HAPPENED, AND SEEMED FROZEN BY THE TERROR OF IT. I HOPED AGAINST HOPE THAT CAT WOULD COME BACK IN, AND THAT I HAD BEEN WRONG, BUT AS THE DAY WENT ON AND WE COULD NOT FIND ANY TRACE OF HER, IN MY HEART I WAS SURE THAT SOUND WAS EXACTLY WHAT I HAD HOPED IT WASN'T.

OF COURSE I CRIED, I TRIED TO PUT IT OUT OF MY MIND, WE WENT LOOKING IN THE PARK FOR ANY SIGN OF HER BUT MY FAMILY SAID LET IT GO, IT'S OVER. IF ONLY IT HAD BEEN THAT SIMPLE, BUT WHAT HAPPENED NEXT WAS PURE TORMENT. WITHIN A FEW DAYS, I BEGAN TO HEAR A CAT CRYING, FIRST THE SOUND CAME THROUGH THE HEATING VENTS IN THE HOUSE, AND I THOUGHT FOR SURE THAT CAT HAD GOT AWAY AND SOMEHOW RAN AND TRAPPED ITSELF SOMEWHERE IN A VENT, ...ONLY NO ONE ELSE COULD HEAR THE SOUND..... NO ONE EXCEPT ME AND MY DOG, WHO SEEMED ALMOST AS UPSET BY IT AS ME, AND MOANED CONTINUALLY AS THE SOUND WOULD MOVE AROUND THE HOUSE. I HAD MY HUSBAND AND SON, CHECKING THE CRAWL SPACE HEATING VENTS, THE ROOF OF OUR HOUSE, THE HEAVY GRATES OUTSIDE IN THE YARD WHERE WATER GOES, EVERYWHERE, UNDER SIDEWALKS, JUST EVERYWHERE. THEY ALL TRIED TO APPEASE ME, BUT NONE OF THEM COULD HEAR A SOUND. I BOUGHT MICROPHONES, IN CASE IT WAS NOT LOUD ENOUGH FOR THEM TO HEAR, I TRIED EVERYTHING, BUT MOSTLY I CRIED AND CRIED, WALKING AROUND IN CIRCLES IN OUR YARD, IN THE MIDDLE OF THE NIGHT, COMPLETELY CONSUMED BY THE SOUND OF THIS

CRYING CAT, THAT I FELT DESPERATELY NEEDED MY HELP. I TRIED TO LET IT GO, I SAID IT CANNOT POSSIBLY STILL BE ALIVE WHEN A WEEK WENT BY, THEN TWO, THEN A MONTH, THEN SEVERAL MONTHS, BUT THE SOUND NEVER STOPPED, IT VARIED, CHANGED CONSIDERABLY FROM DAY TO DAY, BUT BASICALLY IT WAS ALWAYS THERE. I EVEN WENT AND HAD MY HEARING CHECKED, AS IT WAS SUGGESTED THAT SOME HEARING DISORDERS TAKE ON ALL SORTS OF SOUNDS.

A CONSIDERABLE TIME PASSED AND WE HAD TO GO AWAY FOR A WEDDING, AND WHEN THE SOUND WAS THERE, IN A PLACE TOTALLY UNRELATED TO THE WHOLE SITUATION, I THOUGHT FOR SURE, NOW I KNOW I AM ACTUALLY LOSING MY MIND, WHAT OTHER EXPLANATION COULD THERE BE.

WHILE ALL THIS WAS GOING ON, I HAD BEEN SEEING A WONDERFUL DOCTOR, DR. RUTH OLIVER, WHO I HAD BEGAN TO SEE WHEN I WAS COPING WITH HAVING TO STOP WORKING. DURING ONE OF OUR EARLY CONVERSATIONS, I HAD MENTIONED HOW I HAD ALWAYS FELT THE PRESENCE OF MY GUARDIAN ANGEL, AND SHE TOLD ME A WAY I COULD FIND OUT MY GUARDIAN ANGEL'S NAME. I DID IT THE WAY SHE SAID, AND WAS VERY SURPRISED, WHEN THE NAME I WAS GIVEN WAS "GEORGE", NOT QUITE WHAT I HAD EXPECTED, BUT SOMEHOW PLEASED TOO, AT HOW UNCOMPLICATED A NAME IT WAS, FOR A PRESENCE I HAVE FAITHFULLY RELIED ON ALL MY LIFE, AS WELL AS FEELING THE LOVING PROTECTION OF MY MOTHER'S SPIRIT SINCE HER DEATH WHEN I WAS THIRTY.

AS I WAS PRAYING DURING ALL OF THIS, BUT STILL NOT GOING TO CHURCH, AND MY PRAYERS ARE OF A VERY INFORMAL NATURE, RUTH OFFERED TO PRAY FOR ME, AS SHE WAS ONE OF THE FEW PEOPLE I COULD REALLY TALK TO ABOUT THE COMPLETE DESPAIR I WAS EXPERIENCING. AND TO THIS DAY, I CANNOT BELIEVE WHAT HAPPENED. IN HER PRAYERS, RUTH ASKED, "PLEASE HELP ME TO HELP GLORIA FURTHER." THE RESPONSE WAS FROM MARY: "MOTHER BIDS THEE PEACE! I GO FORTH, I PLACE A MANTLE OF PROTECTION ABOUT HER IN THE POWER OF THE HOLY SPIRIT, AND IT IS DONE. BELIEVE AND BE AT PEACE. CONTINUE TO ADDRESS HER AND HER CONCERNS PRAYERFULLY, PROCLAIMING THE NAME OF JESUS AS YOU DO AND LEAVE THE REST UP TO HEAVEN. AS YOU WELL KNOW, SOME MIRACLES OF HEALING OCCUR INSTANTLY AND SOME ARE MORE PROLONGED. THE HEALING IS PRESENT!"

NOW I A NOT A PERSON WHO GOES THROUGH LIFE LOOKING FOR MIRACLES, BUT I AM GRATEFUL FOR THE EVERYDAY BLESSINGS OF FAMILY AND LOVE. I LIVE WITH THE PAIN I DEAL WITH ON A DAILY BASIS AND ACCEPT IT, BUT THIS UNWELCOME INTRUDER IN MY MIND, HEART AND SOUL WAS TAKING IT'S TOLL, AND I NOW BELIEVE NOTHING BUT EVIL COMES IN SUCH A FORM.

TO MY ABSOLUTE AMAZEMENT, WITHOUT EVEN REALLY KNOWING WHAT WAS HAPPENING, THE SOUND OF THE CAT CRYING FOR HELP, WAS BEING REPLACED BY THE MOST INCREDIBLE CHOIRS OF MUSIC I HAD EVER HEARD BEFORE. I REMEMBER THINKING, IF I COULD WRITE THIS DOWN AND CREATE THIS SOUND, WITH SO MANY LEVELS TO IT, IT'S UNLIKE ANYTHING EVER DONE ON EARTH. THESE CHOIRS CAME TO ME OVER AND OVER, AND I WAS SO MESMERIZED EACH AND EVERY TIME, I WAS ONLY ABLE TO WRITE DOWN A FEW WORDS OF WHAT I HEARD.......... BUT IT TOOK ME AWHILE TO REALIZE WHAT I WAS NO LONGER HEARING........THE HAUNTING SOUND OF EVIL THAT HAD ALMOST COMPLETELY POSSESSED MY BEING, AS UNTIL I HEARD THIS WONDERFUL MUSIC, I FELT ABSOLUTELY ALONE WITH THIS DEMON, THAT I COULD NOT EVEN UNDERSTAND WOULD BE ANY PART OF MY WORLD.

I NOW BELIEVE, THANKS TO THE PRAYERS OF RUTH, A DEAR FRIEND AND THE HELP PROMISED BY MARY THE MOTHER OF GOD, THAT I WAS GIVEN A MOST PRECIOUS MIRACLE OR GIFT, AND WAS BLESSED BY THE GRACES OF THE NINE CHOIRS OF ANGELS. TO BE HONEST WITH YOU, UNTIL I EXPLAINED WHAT WAS HAPPENING TO ME AND THE BEAUTIFUL MUSIC I WAS HEARING TO RUTH, I DID NOT RECALL FROM MY CATHOLIC UPBRINGING, ABOUT THE NINE CHOIRS OF ANGELS, AND HAD NOT EVEN CONSIDERED THAT I WOULD BE BLESSED IN SUCH AN INCREDIBLE MANNER.

NOTHING IN LIFE PREPARES YOU FOR AN EXPERIENCE LIKE THIS, AND OF COURSE MOST PEOPLE WHO HAVE NOT EXPERIENCED IT WILL HAVE DIFFICULTY BELIEVING, BUT I DO BELIEVE THIS, THERE IS EVIL THERE, IT IS AN ONGOING BATTLE, AND I PRAY FOR THOSE WHO HAVE THESE TORTUROUS SITUATIONS OCCURRING IN THEIR LIVES, AND ONLY HOPE WE CAN ALL FIND A WAY TO INCLUDE THEM IN OUR PRAYERS, AND TAKE TIME EVERY DAY TO THANK GOD FOR THE ANGELS ON OUR SHOULDERS.

G. W.

My little children, each one of you has a great Guardian Angel, ever attendant upon you. It behooves you to address your Angel prayerfully morning and evening, for each Guardian Angel has a mission; you dear child, are that mission. Your Angel holds you safe in the pathway of holiness, whispering Divine Inspirations into your thoughts, that you will know and do the Will of God.

Full of Grace, the Queen of Heaven resides with him throughout this journey, and the shield of the Church of God is tightened profoundly. The Mother of God holds the beloved John Paul under Her Mantle, the Power of the Holy Spirit, and the Great Archangel Michael, ever cognizant of his Mission, his charge, is profoundly about the beloved John Paul with an army of angels, that indeed nothing unforeseen happen to the beloved one.

Mother blesses you child, Mother blesses you child. Beautiful children, beautiful little souls, ever kneeling and praying before the Lord our God, blessings flow in you and through you. The Virgin Queen of Angels bids thee know that the Guardian Angels Name, for **Ken** *is; "Redemptive Love."*

<u>The Angelus.</u> Prayed 6am; 12 noon and 6pm.

L   The angel of the Lord declared unto Mary,

R   And she conceived by the Holy Spirit. Hail Mary...Holy Mary...

L   Behold, the handmaid of the Lord,

R   Be it done unto me according to Thy Word. Hail Mary...Holy Mary...

L   And the Word was made Flesh,

R   And dwelt among us! Hail Mary...Holy Mary...

L   Pray for us oh holy Mother of God,

R   That we may be made worthy of the promises of Christ.

All   Pour forth, we beseech Thee oh Lord, Thy grace into our hearts, that we
     to whom the Incarnation of Christ Thy Son, was made known by the
     message of an angel, may by His Passion and Cross be brought to the glory
     of His Resurrection, through the same Christ our Lord. Amen. Glory be...x3

Michael attends; Michael attends on the whole household with his legions, because of your Faith and your prayers, a cleansing action of the whole household takes place. Those upstairs are astounded by Peace which they have not previously known, for Heaven hears the prayers of the faithful. A is safe in Me and always under the Mantle of Love; safe in the Two Hearts of Love. This experience is part of her strengthening to a greater Fortitude with which she is already profoundly blest. Be at Peace in this matter. I Myself attend upon A and she knows what to do and what not to do in all circumstances of her life. She has great Gifts of the Holy Spirit to assist her always. Rejoice in the Love of the Lord for yourselves and for your loved ones little children.

Michael, attendant upon you, bids you Peace little children. Ruth, thou art shielded as in an impeccably designed space suit; it is the Shield of the Holy Spirit of the Living God surrounding you. Each one of you little children, are in the Shield of the Living God, and I, servant of the Living God, Michael, attend. Great jousts with the enemy which attempts to assail, this way and that, the little ones of God. You are blessed of God, for you are little before the Living God and He rejoices in you. The poor woman will come to you seeking solace for sorrow, and will find it. You will be empowered by the Holy Spirit, to do so without jeopardizing your practice, because of your profound Faith. Michael attends; Michael the great Archangel of Almighty God;" You have found favour with God, and the faithful cohort, but there is a bad spirit like a coiled serpent against The Mass and against the Holy Eucharist. Michael, attendant upon you, bids you Peace. The thing is under attack, and release is occurring.

Prayer to St Michael.

St Michael the Archangel, defend us in this day of battle;

Be our safeguard against the wickedness and snares of the devil.

May God rebuke him we humbly pray; and do thou, oh Prince of the heavenly host,

by the power of God, cast into hell Satan, and all the other evil spirits, who prowl about the world seeking the ruin of souls. Amen.

Also read Matthew 13:13-43.

The Book of Revelation extensively covers the roles of Angels especially in the end times.

CHAPTER EIGHTEEN

MARY, Mother of Jesus and Our Mother

JESUS: Sanctuary is in the Two Hearts, the Hearts of Jesus and Mary. Herein is your personal victory. Mother's Triumph rapidly approaches. I am Jesus, Eternal Victor. I Myself Bless you with a Great Anointing of Peace, filling you with My Love and My Peace, and the accompanying Joy in the Love of the Lord is ever yours."

MOTHER OF JESUS AND MOTHER OF ALL! *Our Lady says this is Her favorite title.*

The route in which I the Lord came to Earth is through the Immaculate Heart of the ever-Virgin Mary. Little children, come back to God through that same Heart, that Heart of Great Merciful Love. Come to Me by the beautiful route.[September 2nd 1998.] Our Lord Himself had this to say about the Holy Rosary Hail, Full of Grace the Lord is with Thee; and in the power of the Holy Spirit, I the Lord God, am ever with the ever-virgin Mother of God! Forthwith I bless you Faithful Missionary to carry this meditative prayer of the Rosary, however briefly, to the people with whom you will be praying on that day. Remember, whensoever you call upon the Names of Jesus and Mary We attend upon you, resolving the concerns of your heart in the Peace of Our Presence. This is for everyone who believes. *Dear Heavenly Father, you know how few doctors like to pray the Holy Rosary. Please give me Your Words so that it may be prayed according to Your Holy Will. As soon as I started this prayer Our Jesus started the Benedictus, Song of Zacharias, which Omen heard and told me when I stopped praying. Then Our Lord continued when I stopped praying;*

When you present the Rosary, you may suggest that each individual contemplate for a brief moment, that Mystery and all that it endows, all that it portends to mankind. For each Mystery of the Rosary of the Life of Christ and the Virgin Mother of God upon earth, carries a message; an instruction to those who meditate. <u>Let us consider the First Joyful Mystery.</u> Behold, the Virgin in prayer; the Virgin who knows well the promise of her people to send a Messiah. Let us consider the perfection with which the Creator of Creation created this woman; sinless, without stain of original sin. Consider the angel of the Lord. What is the meaning of the angel of the Lord? Consider the Words of the great Archangel Gabriel. Hail full of grace, the Lord is with Thee; and in the power of the Holy Spirit, I the Lord God am ever with the ever-Virgin Mother of God.

<u>Consider The Visitation</u>; that the Power of My Holy Spirit, remaining with Mary, anointed Elizabeth and John and Zacharias, all speaking in the Holy Spirit, as does the Mother of God. <u>Consider the Presentation</u>. Coming into the presence of the One filled with grace, and the Lord God, Jesus; True God and True Man. Then Anna and Simeon recognize Truth, recognize Salvation in the Christ Child, then Simeon speaks in the Spirit. Know that there are many more facets of each Mystery. I just bless you with a sampling. As you consider each Mystery many, many Inspirations come to you in the power of the Holy Spirit. Teach one another to pray as you contemplate the Mystery and the Inspirations given over to you then the recurrent words of the angelic salute [Hail Mary] become background music to the scene which you are contemplating, even beholding in your mind, and the Peace of Christ comes upon you, for where two or more are gathered in My Name, it is written, it is so. (Mt 18:20).

Forthwith I bless you Faithful Missionary, to carry this meditative prayer of the Rosary, howsoever briefly, to the people with whom you will be praying on that day. Remember, whensoever you call upon the

Name of Jesus, and the Name of Mary, We attend upon you, assisting you, resolving the concerns of your Heart in the Peace of Our Presence. This is for everyone who believes. Do not distress yourselves about those who do not chose to believe at this time. Do not concern yourselves about those who choose to state, I will not serve the Lord God, or I do not believe. Simply pray little children for all mankind. Little children do not be dismayed at anything that happens today. Are you not in the time of chastisement?" Those who are cleansed and purified and brought Home, to Glory are ever attendant upon the precious little ones on Earth, with prayers and intercessions ongoing. Their prayers are directed firstly to the Heavenly Queen, and through Her to Almighty God.

How to pray the rosary with some meditations inserted in pictures below.

Prayers of the Rosary

THE APOSTLES' CREED

I believe in God, the Father almighty, creator of heaven and earth. I believe in Jesus Christ, his only son, our Lord. He was conceived by the power of the Holy Spirit, and born of the Virgin Mary. He suffered under Pontius Pilate, was crucified, died, and was buried. He descended to the dead. On the third day he rose again. He ascended into heaven, and is seated at the right hand of the Father. He will come again to judge the living and the dead. I believe in the Holy Spirit, the holy catholic church, the communion of saints, the forgiveness of sins, the resurrection of the body, and the life everlasting. Amen.

OUR FATHER

Our Father, Who art in heaven; hallowed be Thy name; Thy kingdom come; Thy will be done on earth as it is in heaven. Give us this day our daily bread; and forgive us our trespasses as we forgive those who trespass against us, and lead us not into temptation; but deliver us from evil. Amen.

HAIL MARY

Hail Mary, full of grace, the Lord is with thee; blessed art thou among women, and blessed is the fruit of thy womb, Jesus. Holy Mary, Mother of God, pray for us sinners, now and at the hour of our death. Amen.

GLORY BE

Glory be to the Father, and to the Son, and to the Holy Spirit. As it was in the beginning, is now, and ever shall be, world without end. Amen.

HAIL HOLY QUEEN

Hail, Holy Queen, Mother of Mercy, our life, our sweetness and our hope, to thee do we cry, poor banished children of Eve; to thee do we send up our sighs, mourning and weeping in this vale of tears; turn, then, most gracious Advocate, thy eyes of mercy toward us, and after this, our exile, show unto us the blessed fruit of thy womb, Jesus. O clement, O loving, O sweet Virgin Mary!

Pray for us, O holy Mother of God, that we may be made worthy of the promises of Christ. Amen.

FATIMA PRAYER

O my Jesus, forgive us our sins, save us from the fires of hell, lead all souls to heaven, especially those who are in most need of thy mercy.

The Promises of Mary to Those Who Pray the Rosary

1. Whoever shall faithfully serve me by the recitation of the rosary, shall receive signal graces.
2. I promise my special protection and the greatest graces to all those who shall recite the rosary.
3. The rosary shall be a powerful armour against hell, it will destroy vice, decrease sin, and defeat heresies.
4. It will cause virtue and good works to flourish; it will obtain for souls the abundant mercy of God; it will withdraw the hearts of men from the love of the world and its vanities, and will lift them to the desire of eternal things. Oh, that souls would sanctify themselves by this means.
5. The soul which recommends itself to me by the recitation of the rosary, shall not perish.
6. Whoever shall recite the rosary devoutly, applying himself to the consideration of its sacred mysteries shall never be conquered by misfortune. God will not chastise him in His justice, he shall not perish by an unprovided death; if he be just he shall remain in the grace of God, and become worthy of eternal life.
7. Whoever shall have a true devotion for the rosary shall not die without the sacraments of the Church.
8. Those who are faithful to recite the rosary shall have during their life and at their death the light of God and the plenitude of His graces; at the moment of death they shall participate in the merits of the saints in paradise.
9. I shall deliver from purgatory those who have been devoted to the rosary.
10. The faithful children of the rosary shall merit a high degree of glory in heaven.
11. You shall obtain all you ask of me by the recitation of the rosary.
12. All those who propagate the holy rosary shall be aided by me in their necessities.
13. I have obtained from my Divine Son that all the advocates of the rosary shall have for intercessors the entire celestial court during their life and at the hour of death.
14. All those who recite the rosary are my sons, and brothers of my only son Jesus Christ.
15. Devotion to my rosary is a great sign of predestination.

(Given to St. Dominic and Blessed Alan de la Roche)
Imprimatur: ✠ Patrick J. Hayes, D.D., Archbishop of New York

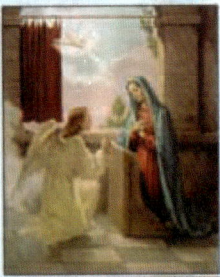

FIRST JOYFUL MYSTERY
Annunciation

And when the angel had come to her, he said, "Hail, full of grace, the Lord is with thee. Blessed art thou among women." (Lk 1, 28)

For the love of humility

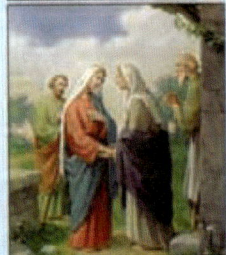

SECOND JOYFUL MYSTERY
Visitation

Elizabeth was filled with the Holy Spirit, and cried out with a loud voice, "Blessed art thou among women and blessed is the fruit of thy womb!" (Lk 1, 41-42)

For charity towards my neighbour

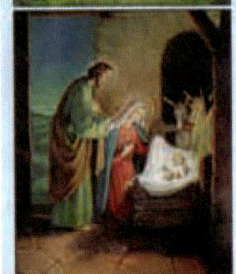

THIRD JOYFUL MYSTERY
Birth of Jesus

She brought forth her firstborn son, and wrapped him in swaddling clothes, and laid him in a manger, because there was no room for them in the inn. (Lk 2, 7)

For the spirit of poverty

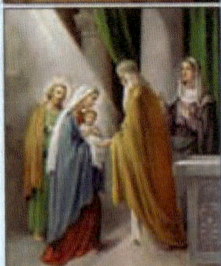

FOURTH JOYFUL MYSTERY
Presentation

When the days of her purification were fulfilled according to the Law of Moses, they took him up to Jerusalem to present him to the Lord. (Lk 2, 22-23)

For the virtue of obedience

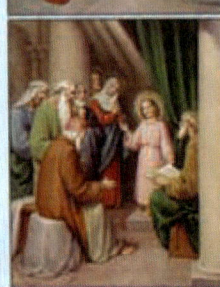

FIFTH JOYFUL MYSTERY
Finding the Child Jesus in the Temple

After three days ... they found him in the temple, sitting in the midst of the teachers, listening to them and asking them questions. (Lk 2, 46)

For the virtue of piety

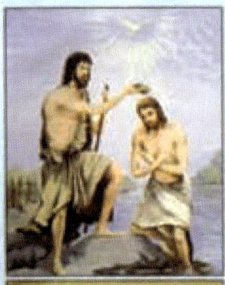

FIRST LUMINOUS MYSTERY
Baptism of Jesus

When Jesus had been baptized, he immediately came up from the water. And behold, the heavens were opened to him, and he saw the Spirit of God descending as a dove and coming upon him. (Mt 3, 16)

For submission to God's will

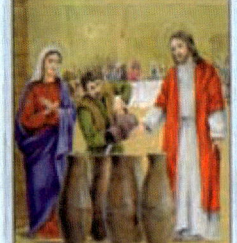

SECOND LUMINOUS MYSTERY
Wedding Feast of Cana

And the wine having run short, the mother of Jesus said to him, "They have no wine." ... His mother said to the attendants, "Do whatever he tells you." (Jn 2, 3-5)

For devotion to Mary

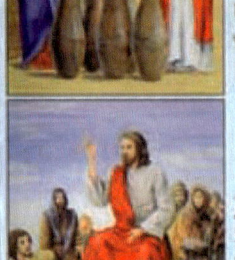

THIRD LUMINOUS MYSTERY
Proclamation of the Kingdom of God

Jesus came into Galilee, preaching the gospel of the kingdom of God, "The time is fulfilled, and the kingdom of God is at hand. Repent and believe in the gospel." (Mk 1, 14-15)

For the grace of conversion

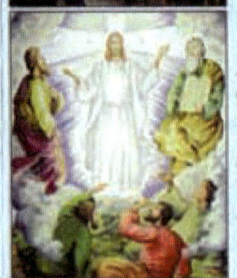

FOURTH LUMINOUS MYSTERY
Transfiguration

Jesus took Peter, James and his brother John, and led them up a high mountain by themselves, and was transfigured before them. His face shone as the sun, and his garments became white as snow. (Mt 17, 1-2)

For holy fear of God

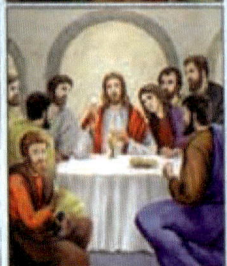

FIFTH LUMINOUS MYSTERY
Institution of the Holy Eucharist

Having taken bread, he gave thanks and broke, and gave it to them, saying, "This is my body, which is being given for you; do this in remembrance of me." (Lk 22, 19)

For thanksgiving to God

Medicine of God — 217

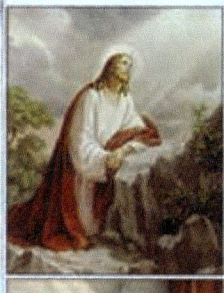

FIRST SORROWFUL MYSTERY
Agony in the Garden
Falling into an agony he prayed the more earnestly. And his sweat became as drops of blood running down upon the ground. (Lk 22, 43-44)
For true contrition for sin

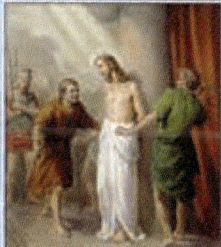

SECOND SORROWFUL MYSTERY
Scourging at the Pillar
Pilate, then, took Jesus and had him scourged. (Jn 19, 1)
For the virtue of purity

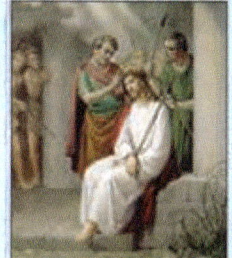

THIRD SORROWFUL MYSTERY
Crowning with Thorns
They stripped him and put on him a scarlet cloak; and plaiting a crown of thorns, they put it upon his head, and a reed into his right hand. (Mt 27, 28-29)
For moral courage

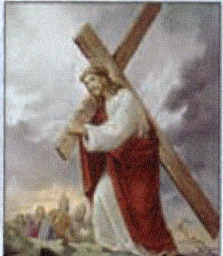

FOURTH SORROWFUL MYSTERY
Carrying of the Cross
And bearing the cross for himself, he went forth to the place called the Skull, in Hebrew, Golgotha. (Jn 19, 17)
For the virtue of patience

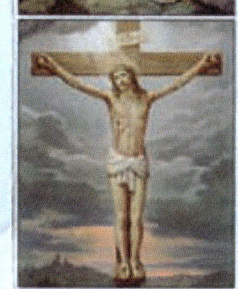

FIFTH SORROWFUL MYSTERY
Crucifixion
Jesus cried out with a loud voice and said, "Father, into thy hands I commend my spirit." And having said this, he expired. (Lk 23, 46)
For final perseverance

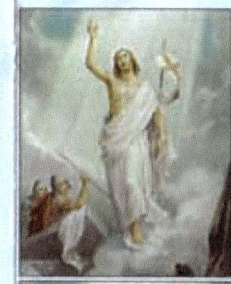

FIRST GLORIOUS MYSTERY
Resurrection
"Do not be terrified. You are looking for Jesus of Nazareth, who was crucified. He has risen, he is not here. Behold the place where they laid him." (Mk 16, 6)
For the virtue of faith

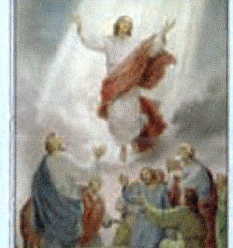

SECOND GLORIOUS MYSTERY
Ascension
So then the Lord, after he had spoken to them, was taken up into heaven, and sits at the right hand of God. (Mk 16, 19)
For the virtue of hope

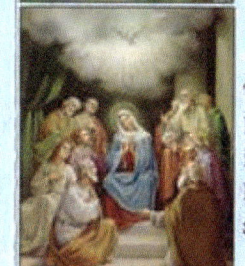

THIRD GLORIOUS MYSTERY
Descent of the Holy Spirit
They were all filled with the Holy Spirit and began to speak in foreign tongues, even as the Holy Spirit prompted them to speak. (Acts 2, 4)
For the virtue of love

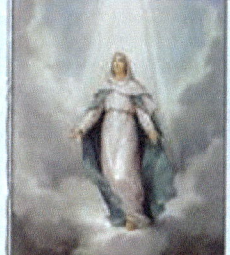

FOURTH GLORIOUS MYSTERY
Assumption of the Blessed Virgin Mary
And the temple of God in heaven was opened, and there was seen the ark of his covenant. (Apoc. 11, 19)
For a happy death

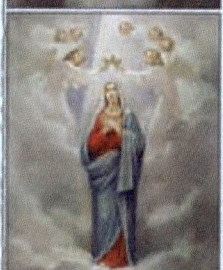

FIFTH GLORIOUS MYSTERY
Coronation of the Blessed Virgin Mary
A great sign appeared in heaven: a woman clothed with the sun, and the moon was under her feet, and upon her head a crown of twelve stars. (Apoc. 12, 1)
For eternal salvation

On my way to Toledo, Ohio I spent the 12th November, 1997 in Dayton, Ohio, with a psychiatrist friend, who helped me find the Marian Library in the (Catholic) University of Dayton. I had asked our Lady to help me get to Mass that day and She did a little more than that! I certainly shared in Her sorrows that day: first, in the chapel of the Immaculate Conception on the campus, where the Church was both structurally and spiritually 'gutted out', in my opinion, then after lunch when I was "led to a lecture in the Humanities Building" in which the speaker denied that it was truly Mary of Nazareth, the Mother of God, who had appeared as our Lady of Guadalupe. He said that the older women of Mexico, who were the "interpreters of sin and grace" in their culture, actually believed it was the Holy Spirit Himself, who appeared in the form of a woman.

Although both his speech and his paper are marked with disclaimers, he broke through at one point to exclaim, "What- you have no problem believing the Holy Spirit can come in the form of a bird, but you have a problem believing He can come in the form of a woman!" That was bad enough, but when I was talking to a colleague later, I was told it didn't really matter, though, because we didn't have to believe in the apparition, so what difference did it make whether it was the Holy Spirit or the Mother of God! I think, even if one chooses to reject a story, one is still obligated to keep the facts one hears, straight. The next person hearing the story deserves the original details in order to decide independently whether they believe or not. It matters if each person hearing the story adds their own twist or distortion to it surely!

Lies always hurt someone, but lies against the Mother of God and against the Holy Spirit, The Holy Trinity for that matter, can cost the loss of many souls. Besides, Our Lady of Guadalupe is an approved devotion. I thought we needed to have a serious reason not to believe. Early in December, I had made a previous attempt to pray about that day, to understand what our Lord wanted me to do about all that I had been shown, besides pray. It was an awful experience because after a very long time of prayer/contemplation, Our Lady said not one word, and our Lord said, <u>This denigration of My Mother has gone too far-now are all the demons of hell unleashed."</u> *Nothing more! At Mass the following day ...*

Oh My people, oh My people, oh that you would choose Love. I give you Love, in the ravishing beauty of the Woman Clothed With the Sun,(Rev 12:1) the Mother of God, but you choose not to heed Her call to Love, choose not this Gateway to return to the Lord Your God. You choose rather error, sin, death and destruction. Oh woe, oh My people, oh My people, what have I done to you? How have I offended you? Answer Me! (Mi 6:3)The Spirit of the Living God anoints each and every one of His Own, and as the Mother of God continues to beckon and call, it will be through the faith of such as you, which will cause others to come back to the Lord their God with all their hearts, that they too may know Salvation. A great blessing is upon you. Give Glory!

Mother is in tears, Mother is in tears. I am your Jesus. I am He who lives and loves eternally, your Jesus of merciful love. Your tearful Mother and I your Jesus, suffer through the great attacks upon My Body the Church now, all the evil upon each one of Us personally. My little one, you are blest with My Love and Mother's love in Our service. You have been tested and blest and you are now as it were a finely tuned instrument in Our works of merciful Love. Holy Light ever surrounds you. Now is a moment of sweet surrender, as the power of the Holy Spirit comes upon you, enfolding you in a great stream of the River of Love. In this Love each one of you is given Words and Divine Inspiration for the work of mercy at hand. What you ask of Me is given unto you. The Queen of Heaven, the Mother of God, the Immaculate Conception, Mediatrix of all Graces, the Intercessor before the throne of the Godhead, the Woman Who is full of Grace, under Her many titles, is yet and ever shall be My Mother and yours. She is Mother of All. It is written in Holy Scripture. Believing in the Spirit of Truth, one cannot avoid knowing that She is the Mother of All. (Jn

19:26-27 and Rv12:17)

I ADDRESS YOU IN THE TRINITY OF LOVE. WE, IN OUR WISDOM, chose to heal the sin-filled world, My beloved humanity, through the most pure vessel, the Blessed Virgin Mary. Ever since Her Assumption into Heaven, Her enthronement in Glory beside Me, your Jesus, She has assisted Her other children - you - in your Faith journeys. She is so filled with Love, that even the most blackened soul She appeals to - to reform, to repent; and She appeals to the Lord your God for assistance with that soul. She is ever Intercessor on behalf of mankind. She is ever pouring forth graces in the Power of the Holy Spirit upon the children of God on the Earth. She brings your cross, magnified through Her Immaculate Heart, into the Presence of Our Father, Who is well pleased by these gifts of Faith and love. We, the Lord God, deigned to present Her to the pagan societies of the Americas as truly the Woman of the Scriptures, the Woman Clothed With the Sun (Rev: 12:1) and even yet, as in the early Americas, that they might understand and know conversion. It is a miraculous Image. It is also an Icon bearing many, many messages to the children who believe. Prayer presented to God through this miraculous Image of the Immaculate Mother of God, are magnified as they are presented to the Father.

The river of lies spewed out against Myself and the Mother of God, and indeed, the beloved John Paul, and indeed, the entire Church from the mouth of the serpent, the old dragon, are falling upon the ears of the many in this time, just for a brief time. Blessed are those who hold out in Faith and trust and love and patient perseverance. Little children, you in this prayer group are anointed in great Faith and great blessings are upon you. Your prayers are pleasing to the Lord your God. Know this: there are many children of God praying all around this small globe which is the Earth. They are likewise under Our blessing. My little ones, be at Peace. When it is necessary to refute, We give you the Words. We open doors and windows that others may see and know the truth. We have just done this in the case of the Piccareta messages. As rapidly as the lies spewed out of the serpent's mouth through the human cohort, so rapidly, THROUGH THE MOTHER OF GOD, have We stopped it. The paper trail of lies remains about the globe but not for long. Enlightenment is given mankind in this issue alone.

Perceive what I am telling you, beloved little one of Faith. Follow your beloved Mother of All. We will speak in you and through you, that others may know the Truth. Hosts of angels assist you and indeed some special saints will profoundly assist you in this work of Enlightenment. My people are only now beginning to come out of the darkness into the Light. It comes through the enlightenment of My precious little ones, of which each of you is numbered. A great blessing is upon you, for this work.Mother and I are attendant upon you little children. I am your Jesus of Merciful Love, your Jesus, Eternal Victor, the Alpha and the Omega. Little children, as the feast day of the beloved John the Baptist approaches, multitudes of faithful ones are in prayer petition before the Living God. These prayers are indeed heard and are responded to as your God Wills. As you know, the beloved John came as a herald, a forerunner of your Jesus into the world, bringing a Baptism of Repentance,(Mt 3:11) bringing hope, bringing much , much more.

Little children it is that time now, where the Mother of God Herself is attending upon Humanity, hither and yon about the Earth, calling all to repentance, calling all to place all their hope in the Living God, in the Will of God, in the Love and Mercy of God. Little children, many are responding, but not in sufficient numbers as yet, that is why each one of you is called to be one like unto John the Baptist, for each one of you also to be a herald of the great Kingdom, of the great King. Continue to work towards this end little children. Graces and blessings of assistance flow. The Queen of Angels and All Saints, Bearer of the Good News, is working side by side with each faithful child of God. In the Power of the Holy Spirit it is so little children. Rejoice in this Unity of Love little children. Herein lies your Victory!

Discernment on April 24, 1998: On Tuesday, April 21st, my brother brought me a book which he found in the discard/ discount bin of the local community library. He visits such places habitually, to my good fortune in this case. The book is called **"Fundamentals of Mariology: The Study of Our Lady"** *by Fr. Juniper B. Carol,O.F.M. (Published by* **Benziger Brothers, 1956**. *Imprimi potest: Celsus Wheeler O.F.M., Provincial. Nihil Obstat : John A. Goodwine. J.C.D., Censor Librorum.\ Imprimatur: Francis Cardinal Spellman, Archbishop of New York.) Fr. Carol is/was a native of Cuba, educated in Havana, Catholic University of America, in Washington, D.C., and Rome, where he received his doctorate in Sacred Theology. He did extensive research in Europe and was a member of the commission for the critical edition of Duns Scotus in Quaracchi, Italy. He was the founder and first president of the Mariological Society of America. He was also the editor of* **"Marian Studies"** *and a member of* **The Pontifical Academy of the Mariological Commission.** *He is internationally known for his book,* **De Corredemptione B. V. Mariae.** *(Vatican City, 1950)."*

Mariology is that part of the science of theology which treats of The Mother of God, and Her Association with Christ. Father Carol, who has distinguished himself as a Mariologist, here presents in systematic form the basic theology concerning Our Lady. The book shows not only the conclusions of theologian, .but the line of reasoning that has led to these conclusions.

This book is for all who are devoted to Our Lady, and who want to understand more fully the reasons why Mary holds such a high place in Catholic thought and devotion. Father Carol shows the reader how Mary was especially predestined from all eternity to be the Mother of Christ, how she was foretold by the prophets, and why she is our Mother, the Mediatrix of Graces, and the Queen of all Creation. The second part of the book considers Mary's Immaculate Conception, the nature of her Assumption, and the honour paid to Her. This book is especially timely since it contains much information about the Queenship of Mary, the most recent Marian Feast."

To start with, this was not intended to be a discernment prayer. I was merely phoning a friend to tell her about the book because I was excited about this pre-Vatican II find. Strangely, as I started talking, I suddenly felt that full aching feeling in my throat which is now becoming familiar to me, because that is one of the experiences when I am "in the Spirit." I had been trying to tell her that when I looked at the picture of the author, I saw an aura of light around his head that to me meant he was either dead or a very holy man or both. But there was also uneasy, unrestful, 'flamelike' movement around the eyes and I couldn't define this more specifically. I was saying that I thought maybe we needed to pray more for Cuba (see discernment on January 14th) or the Dayton Catholic Campus (because Father contributed to the Marian Library there). However, the "ache" in my throat became so painful that I had to get off the phone and go to Adoration, where I prayed five Glorious Mysteries among other prayers. Dear Jesus, I know You have sent this book for my enlightenment. Please guide my understanding.

I sent the book that you might pray for those who fail to recognize the Mother of God, especially throughout the English-speaking world. The enemy Satan and his cohort dread the Name of Mary when used prayerfully, for no sin is upon her and, therefore, they have no power to affect her in any way. And when her children cling to her they too are protected in a remarkable manner; and so he wreaks havoc, attempting to separate the children of God and Mary from their Heavenly Mother, that he might have more power over them. That is why we ask you who know to pray much and do much penance and privation, in the Name of Jesus, that the children not be separated from their Heavenly Father and Mother, but remain part of the great unity of love, that the enemy is thus defeated. The Mother of God herself works profoundly in assisting the little stragglers and wanderers about the earth, to return to the Lord their God, as the Lord God desires.

In unity with Mary greater graces occur in regard in particular to conversions and the salvation of souls.

Medicine of God — 221

I have already won the victory; the Triumph of the Two Hearts is at hand. Yet the enemy works furiously, attempting to capture and deceive the many. I Myself bless the words of the book you have at hand, and We ask you to pray for Cuba, asking Our Lady of Guadalupe, Mother of the Americas, to hold My people of Cuba under Her mantle at all times. A Herculean effort is made to stop the works which I have given unto thee. Be not dismayed. Carry the five stones of the Rosary and trust in the Lord !(A reference to David who carried the five stones to meet Goliath. Lord what more can I do?). Let the book(*Med of God*)remain under the convenorship of the Mother of God and all falls in place. Little children, recognize that She does indeed attend upon the Living God, in all that you pray about, and you know well the response you receive.

You are doing that which I have requested of you. Be at Peace in this matter. We bless many with Enlightenment now. It is just to let you know little one, the great Mission to which you are assigned. The power of darkness is immense. There is grief in Heaven for the behaviours of many doctors, research scientists and many more; and yet as My Church walks the *Via Dolorosa,* you must know, as I did, and as Our Mother did, <u>that it had to be!</u> Little children, it is so for the Body of Christ. You have a way with words little children, for tugging the Hearts of your Mother and your Jesus. My Love and blessings come upon you and upon L and upon the many for whom you plead. I heal as I will, and you are aware of that, and I bless you for your Faith in action. Healing Love I pour out upon My beloved Humanity. Acceptance occurs, as you know, in the free will of the individuals, yet we have a persevering Mother, interceding upon the cause of each individual. I tell you again I am your Jesus, All Powerful God, Wonder Counselor, Great Physician, (Is9:6) and I desire to hold every precious little one to My Heart of Love, even as Mother does, for the Healing of soul and body. My precious little ones, the times in which you are living, have brought distress and unpleasant disorders and diseases to humanity.

Therefore persevere, endure, persevere; this remains the message of the times. In prayer, in unity with Me and Our Mother, you are victorious! Indeed angels and saints readily assist you at all times, as do I, the Living God, and Our Mother. We are never, ever distanced from the chosen ones who have said "yes" to the Living God, and are working out their given Assignments in Faith and Hope and Trust and Love, patiently persevering, such as yourselves. There are many of you scattered about the world. Children, your "yes's" are pleasing to the Living God and to the Mother of God. I am called Teacher, but She mother's you, and mothers have their own way of mothering which is a form of teaching, and in this way you children of God and children of Mary have your formation. In your yieldedness to Me, the Living God, in your daily "yes, " as it were, the morning offering, I guide you with Divine Inspirations. Little children, stay in the Peace of My Presence throughout each day. Yes, there are trials in the interaction with other people who are not believers, or are only limited in their belief; they are yet My Own. And when you can remain in the Peace of My Presence by calling on My Name, by calling on Mother's Name, at those needy moments, you become a great example to the other ones who are agitating or disturbed, who are disruptive. That is why I would like to call each of My little ones, not only lighted candles but pillars of Faith, for pillars of Faith are unmoved by all that is going on around them. Do you understand little children?

Today I am asking those who know and love our Mother, to continue to pray for a time of Advent where She is recognized and triumphant, and I too, am recognized; I am your Jesus of Victory. It is My Will that My Mother be recognized in the Body of Christ! She recognizes each child of God as her own precious child, because of My Word to Her at the foot of the Cross of Calvary. (Jn19:26-27)

I call to Humanity; do not shun Our Mother, the Queen of Heaven and Earth, the Mother of God, and by My very Word, your Mother also. It is now a moment of Love; I am pouring out My healing Love upon you, filling you with My Love and My Peace and My Joy, that sure and quiet Joy, which indwells your heart, and which is indicative of the indwelling Presence of the Holy Spirit, the Spirit of the Living God, Who is within you and encompassing you at all times. (1 Cor 6:19)The Assumption of the Mother of God into Heaven; She came not just soul, but body and soul, for there is an integrity of unity between body and soul, for each human being. It is not the Will or desire of your God, that these disruptive activities, in this aspect of the medical field occur, and continue to occur. There is no recognition of soul, and a decreased recognition of the integrity of each human body. You see clearly this is not of Me. Little children, in all exhilaration of Love, I bless you each one, in a profound anointing of My Love and My Peace and My Joy, from My Treasury of Love, through the Heart of Our Mother, through the love of the saints, through the angels, graces and blessings are ever flowing upon the faithful, in the Body of Christ! (1Co12:27).

MARY: *The Mother of God Herself is attendant upon you. Little one, the Peace of Christ is upon you. Great graces are upon you. Indeed, pray for Cuba as you pray for the Americas. Politically acceptable or not, Cuba is part of the American family and is in need of much prayer and much Providence. Little children, We bless you and entrust to you to pray vigorously for the peoples of Cuba whenever you pray for the peoples of the Americas. Let it be so. A hastily devised dogma is being promulgated, promoted among the peoples of the USA, and indeed Canada, which is not of Us. Do not be deceived, little children. Stay in obedience and humility. You are blest with discernments to assist you. Peace. You will realize what We are saying to you as you go forward in Faith.*

Dear little children, many events are occurring on the Earth at this time. My precious little ones, we ask you to pray for the beloved John Paul's intentions at this time. We ask you to make novenas and prayer/ petitions from now until Pentecost. You are living in the most remarkable era in the history of mankind. Dear little children, the enemy is wrath and hurls what it can against the faithful children of God. Even so, their victory in Jesus is assured. My beloved little ones, it is I, your Mother of Good Counsel, Who has given you the Hymn of Pentecost to the Holy Spirit.* It holds you fast in the pathway of holiness. It is one more means of assisting you, My little ones. Use it frequently, My little ones. Do not worry about perfection of music. The words themselves are powerful in prayer.

*Pentecost Song to the Spirit (*Song given to Omen by Our Lady.*)
1.*Spirit I come to Thee,*   Child of God, I bless thee.
2*Spirit I come to Thee,* What would, you ask of Me.
3. *Wisdom I ask of Thee,*   Wisdom I give to thee.
4*Understanding I ask of Thee,* Understanding I give to thee.
5.*Counsel I ask of Thee,* Counsel I give to thee.
6.*Fortitude I ask of Thee,* Fortitude I give to thee.
7.*Piety I ask of Thee,* Piety I give to thee.
8.*Fear of the Lord I ask of Thee,* Fear of the Lord I give to thee.
9.The Victory's yours remain with Me, For now and all eternity.

My little ones, when you pray this hymn, the Holy Spirit attends upon many who are cold or lukewarm and they begin to come back to the Lord God. Precious little children, I bless each and every one of you. In the power of the Holy Spirit, great graces flow upon you. Now is the hour of Redemption; the Redemption of mankind is truly at hand. Multitudes will return to the Faith. Each one of you gathered here has been, as it were, conscripted into the great army, the great workers for the harvest.

Believe, trust in your God, stay united with Our Lord Jesus, and all goes according to Heaven's design. The time of Peace, which fast approaches, is most beautiful. The children of God will live in a manner of delight, and ever in the Light of Christ. Truly darkness is then no more; as Our Lord God has pledged, so it shall be. Believe, little children; I am your Mother, Queen of Peace, Queen of all saints and I bless each one of you profoundly again and again. And the time is quite soon.

May 13th, Feast of Our Lady of Fatima. *Your Mother is present. We shall speak in you and through you at the meeting. By your faith and surrender to the Lord your God; in your utter abandonment to the Will of your God, it shall happen. The Words will come to you quickly. Believe. Walk in faith and know that the Lord is with you, and that Heaven's Words will flow in you and through you; and since Heaven is with you, the hearts and minds of many will be opened at the meeting. Some remain obstinate and of hardened heart. Do not concern yourself with this. Remember ,"there is a time for everything"(She is quoting Ecclesiastes 3), even a time for each heart to be opened to the Lord.*

She's asking me to begin by praying an Ave Maria, even in my heart, and then proclaiming in my heart, "here I am Lord, I come to do Your Will", and the Lord's Words are given over to you at the meeting). Know that this is how it occurs with many, many, of what you call locutionists. In this abandonment to the Lord, the Lord's Words flow in you and through you and people are amazed at such words, thinking they come from you; and yet they come in you and through you from the Lord Our God. The Singular Vessel of Devotion bids you Peace. My little children, you who have always reverenced your Mother, while worshipping Our Lord and Our God, Jesus the Christ; I Myself, on this day which is holy to the Lord God, bless you in a great anointing of Peace. I am the Queen of Peace! My little children, this anointing is for you and for all believers. My little one, in your Mission , be not dismayed. I, Queen of Peace, and Our Lord Jesus, Prince of Peace, attend upon you continuously. We bid you, little children, at the slightest disruption of your peace, to call on Our Names, restoring yourselves to Our Peace. The enemy, and the world, would disrupt the Peace of Christ wherever it is found.

Do not let these inroads take away from your peace. We give you Mother Teresa, We give you John Paul, and We give you your own Father Paul as examples. Peace prevails within such hearts no matter what is occurring around them. You are called little children to love and trust Our Lord Jesus no matter what is happening. I reiterate, though the earth quake beneath your feet, keep your eyes upon Jesus. Thus, thus is your victory won; and I bring your sacrifices of love to the Father , that Love may emanate upon the needy upon Earth. Little children, in the power of the Holy Spirit thou art blest in the Name of the Father, and of the Son, and of the Holy Spirit.

Heavenly Father may I please ask for enlightenment, about being in the Spirit? I know when I am in the Spirit and I have a healing anointing to do, but when it comes at other times I don't always know exactly how to understand it.

When the action of the Holy Spirit is upon you, the Lord Jesus and I your Heavenly Mother, work in conjunction with each of Our Own little ones on Earth. At every moment when one feels the Presence of the Holy Spirit, it is good to give praise , and also to listen, and in the quietness of your own heart you are inspired what it is the Lord would have you do. Therefore, simply remain at peace as your heart sings glory, in the Presence of the Almighty. Little child, you are profoundly blest in being empowered to attain this level of Faith, which brings sanctity to the children of God. Little children, remember the Words in Scripture," By Faith are the miracles wrought, by Faith is your own victory won. " By Faith is the victory of assisting others won. Little one, since you are fully aware of the moment when the Holy Spirit is attendant upon you, it behooves you to be continuously giving glory to the Father each in your own way, as so many little song birds before your God.

Mother Mary, the Virgin of Fatima is present. Little children, I am Mother of Jesus and Mother of

all, for you were given to Me at the foot of the Cross of Calvary and you are My Own dear children. Each one of you, I comfort and console, caress and bless. I dry your tears. My little children, each one of you has a great Guardian Angel, ever attendant upon you. It behooves you to address your Angel prayerfully morning and evening, for each Guardian Angel has a mission; you dear child, are that mission. Your Angel holds you safe in the pathway of holiness, whispering Divine Inspirations into your thoughts, that you will know and do the Will of God. My little children, I hold each one of you to My Heart, immersing you in My love, in the depth of My Heart of Love, in the wellspring of Love; and the Holy Spirit anoints you each one, surrounding you in the Light pouring forth from Glory, surrounding you in the Light of Jesus Our Lord, Who is ever with you.

Do thou little children, remain faithful to Jesus, that His wondrous plans for you all come to fruition. His Name is Wonder-Counselor; seek Him, seek Him in all your needs. Come to the Lord little children, Who desires only that which is good for you. Little children, by virtue of your Baptism, even though you are in the world, you are not of the world. Stay prayerfully united with your Jesus! Mother is present, Mother is present. Precious children, you are our delight. Little ones gathered in the Name of Our Lord Jesus, who are so pleasing to the Father, and to Me, your Heavenly Mother; and in the Power of the Holy Spirit each one of you is anointed in a great anointing of peace.

Be not dismayed little children about what is happening in the world and those who are of the world still. Your Mission is to persevere in the way of holiness which Our God has chosen for you. In this way, as you remain humbly obedient, persevering despite the harassments and oppressions, the distractions, you win the victory, and this victory is the conversion of many others, to know Salvation, for you know well that you are front line warriors, in the battle for souls in the Church militant upon the earth today; yet always remember you are not alone; the Lord is with you, I an with you, angels and saints are with you. Little children, rest secure in the Embrace of the Two Hearts of Love. The Mercy Gate of the Immaculate Heart of Mary is bursting with joy to see the little ones here, in hearts' concern for the suffering little ones all over the earth. Great graces flow. Our Lady of Fatima: When we are in a direct spiritual battle with the devil, we have to persevere till the peace victory of Jesus is clearly demonstrated and His Peace and Joy restored to us. The serpent in the A family is now eradicated and destroyed.

Remain united in Adoration, the Rosary, the Stations; but most of all, in the Holy Sacrifice of the Mass. Especially at the time of Consecration, ask what you will of Our Lord, for this is the moment of Divine Mercy. *Mother Mary is praying; God Our heavenly Father, through Your Son Jesus Our Victim/ High Priest, True Prophet and Sovereign King, pour forth the power of your Holy Spirit upon us and open our Hearts. In Your great mercy, through the Motherly mediation of the Blessed Virgin Mary, Our Queen, forgive our sinfulness, heal our brokenness, and renew our hearts, in the faith and peace, and love, and joy of your Kingdom, that we may be one in You. Little children, on this day which is holy to the Lord, your Heavenly Mother takes a hand in these cases, and many, many, more because of the prayers of the faithful. Rejoice in the merciful Love of Our God .Little children, children of God and of your Mother Mary, I Mediatrix of all Graces, pour forth many Graces upon you in the power of the Holy Spirit of God, the Holy Spirit of Love it is done!*

The Sovereign Queen wills to address the child T. Living waters flow upon you from the Light of Glory. As I hold you to My Heart, the Glory of God flows forth upon you. It is the Light of Our Jesus surrounding you at every moment. Thus you walk as a lighted candle on this earth, to bring the Good News to many. Little children, in these times there are many who believe they know Jesus. Indeed they know the Word Jesus, the Name Jesus; but they do not comprehend His all-encompassing Love. I have blest many, many of My sons and daughters to teach of this all-encompassing Love of Our Lord God. When you speak out, reach out to your brothers and sisters, in this great mantle of Light and Love, conversions occur. My daughter and My daughters {faithful missionary, T and A}, you are part of a wondrous family; the family of God, of Nazareth and Bethlehem. Do not think of it in a sentimental way, but in the way it is; as a Commission for the release of mankind, as John Paul the beloved prays, set My people free, like another Moses.

I call many instruments about the earth to work in his behalf; on Our behalf to set the people of God free, in a greater light, a greater Love many have been flickering candle lights. Those We have blest as a great flame little children, and in this flame of light you will be Our instruments in the deeper conversion of the many. Little children you address frequently the names of McS and her associates. They also are great flames. There are many others little children. Each of you are indeed little pockets of light pouring forth from Glory and sending this flame of love like a grass fire throughout the earth; A contagion of Love one might say. You are blest each one. Do not be hesitant. Pray and act, for the Lord is with you, and I am ever- attendant upon you as a doting Mother. This is My privilege from God, and I bless you in the power of the Holy Spirit. I am the Mother of God; the Mother of All.

Singing Angels attend giving praise to the Lord God. Little children of God, it is your Heavenly Mother who speaks. Merciful Love is attendant upon all in this house at this time, and upon all those whom you carry in your hearts precious little ones. Many and varied are the concerns of your hearts. Know that the Lord is with you, and in your surrender to the Lord, all Heavenly assistance is given unto you. The problem of the computer the beloved JS works out in due course with scant delay. We bless him even as We bless you. [and when We got home from these prayers he had called and the computer was fixed.] *The wondering booklets, the wondering pamphlets, do not be dismayed; they too shall be returned to you.*

A sorrow is that the many will not to heed. But there is rejoicing for those who do indeed heed, discern, begin to believe in the true sanctity of each God-given life. Your work is immense, greater than you can comprehend little children, therefore be not dismayed at any obstructions; the enemy is wrath. Through this Portal of Light, the Heart of your Beloved Mother, the Mercy Gate, blessings flow upon each of My own among whom you are numbered little children. As to the meetings of the Catholic physicians in unity with the priest, it is a tragedy, a sorrow, that they do not choose to believe, but seek a burden of scientific truth before they would believe. Though you present this to them very clearly, they are reluctant in their great intellect to accede to these Truths. Be not dismayed; it has been ever thus. I am with you now little children in a great anointing of Peace. I am your Mother, Queen of Peace, and indeed Queen of angels and all saints. Little children, you have fought a fierce battle and attained a great Victory in the Name of our Lord. A day will come when you will comprehend what this warfare was about. Remember in our Father's Great Design, in the economy of our Father's great Design the prayers of the faithful play a key role.

In this hour of Mercy We are breaking down barriers of resistance to this your Mission little children, that eyes may read and minds may comprehend, that hearts be opened to the Truth of our Lord Jesus Christ the Word, the Living Word. Little ones, soon the many will begin to believe in this great Mission of Love. Mother Mary says she is holding us, one on each side of Her saying *Your Mother is delighted in you precious little ones; you did not despair, or fear, but you carried on as you had been told, continuing in patient perseverance in all Faith in your Lord and in the intercessions of your Mother and the angels and the saints. Thus it brings you both favour with our Father and the blessings flow. Gates are opened, doors are opened, and Enlightenment comes. Wilt thou begin again to confess the Name of Jesus?*

With willing hearts and willing hands little children and with willing voices, you work merciful Love on Our behalf, on behalf of your brothers and sisters, and each one of you who do this all over the globe today are blest in a unique fashion. You will recognize this blessing as you go forward in Faith. Mother is saying seven is God's good number, three is the number of the Trinity; perhaps little children you might start with ten of each, going on from there as need be. Enlightenment is ongoing. The Virgin Herself is in tears for thou art a bold warrior.

Heavenly Mother I can't thank You enough for being there with M and I when we prayed over Gloria's little mother, K. I heard from M yesterday that she is insistent that there were three women at her bedside and M and I believe that You were with us as Our Lady of Guadalupe, visible only to K, and as such You made it possible for Gloria to be baptized in the womb just as St John the Baptist was. Do You have any Words for this beautiful event Mother?

The Virgin of Fatima assures you that the day will come. Consider Me the Woman Clothed with the Sun, as both Virgin of Fatima and Virgin of Guadalupe, and of Medjugorje, and of the many places where I attend upon My little children, and even here at the Mercy Gate; I am the Woman Clothed with the Sun. My little one, I chose to be in attendance for Heaven indeed hears the prayers of the faithful. [today is the feast day commemorating the miracle of the sun at Fatima, witnessed by about 70,000 people- 13th October 1917].

This trial, this anguish of the parents causes them to know, more deeply the suffering I experience, and the suffering our Almighty God experiences at the snuffing out of a human life. That this occurred in a woman whose frailties one might say, were taken advantage of, is known in Heaven. Therefore be at Peace. Healing Love is upon this people. Love conquers all. I myself hold the beloved, the precious little one to My Heart Oh, how one such soul doth magnify the Lord ! Oh, how one such soul has truly earned the Heavenly reward !

The Virgin Of Fatima will take you to Her Heart now. I am your tearful Mother. I am grievously wounded by those who follow not the Lord Our God, but follow the deceits of the enemy. The enemy is not only the enemy of God, but of all mankind. He is creating havoc in the lives of the children of man. Dearest precious little one, indeed when you comfort your Jesus and your Mother Mary it is good, and it is the cause of others to convert. Your prayers fall like so many caresses on My beloved Jesus, your wounded Jesus. Believe, little one, your prayers fall as an assuage and a comforting oil on the wounded body of your Crucified Lord. Pray, little child, pray, comforting your Jesus. I your Mother bless you yet again, indeed all in the prayer group and all the adorers and a multitude of loved ones.

The capacity of Love which your God has is boundless. Pray, and it is expanded exponentially about the world - seeing My little starving children, seeing My little cold children, seeing My little abused children, seeing why the Mother weeps - for they know not their Lord Jesus. Oh My child, pray, pray for all the little ones; pray for the beloved John Paul. The journey now is perilous every step of the way. Your prayers on His behalf work profoundly in His favor - if you knew the army the enemy has rallied against Him! Oh My child the ones in Cuba need your prayers also - they have been denied their Jesus for so long! When you pray for Cuba it gives those who were hopeless, now some hope. China does not know the Name, Jesus. Oh, pray for the children of the world as never before. Since I am the Mediatrix of All Graces, I am strengthening you in a great anointing to carry out continuous works of mercy and love. Your prayers resound in Heaven, My daughter. When you pray, there comes upon your Mother, your prayers, and I magnify them before the Father, Who in all delight pours it on the children of the Earth yet again in a great reciprocity of love. It is pleasing to the Lord; We bless you yet again in a great anoint-

ing of Love.

February 11th{ Feast of Our Lady of Lourdes.} *The virtue of Love is such that the Mother of God speaks. Little children, as you blest Me on this day, so I your Heavenly Mother, Mediatrix of all Graces, bless you now. My precious little one, I know well the value of your time and your little expenditures here and there, to mark and reveal the Truth to your fellow man; and because of that, you are blest profoundly in a myriad ways - shall we say, tiny miracles flow about you to assist you in unexpected ways. Little daughter of faithfulness, you are My delight! Jesus, the Love of our lives, is pleased with you and asks you to stay as you are - seeing how you are at the foot of the Cross gives your Mother Mary a Heart of Joy. The Holy Spirit, the Comforter, is surrounding you with a great blanketing of Joy this night which is holy to the Lord! Mother Mary is present. I, Queen of Heaven and Earth, bless you little one, and in all littleness on Earth, you get great things done for your God. Little one, a great blessing is upon you - I bless you again and again. I am the Mediatrix of All Graces and the blessings flow; be not surprised what happens next in your Faith journey, My precious little one. Small instrument of Love and Peace, you are cherished of the Lord God and of your heavenly Mother. My daughter, it is your Heavenly Mother who speaks, in conjunction with the Holy Spirit, which is indeed so at every time I speak. My little one, when the Holy Spirit came upon your Virgin Mother of God, all Graces flowed upon Me, and My mantle is essentially the mantle of the power of the Holy Spirit of the Living God. You see, Jesus' Body and Blood were formed in Me. I gave Him My love. I gave Jesus to mankind. But Jesus, in turn, gave Me to mankind at the foot of the Cross of Calvary. The only blood needed is the Blood of the Lamb.*

My little one, you know well that My life, as Joseph's, the beloved saint, are as it were, hidden in Scripture. But We are present in both Scripture and Tradition most profoundly. "My little children, you are My children. If you read the Book of Revelation,(Rv12:17) *you are My other children, for you keep Me and you keep the Name of Jesus ever on your lips. It is these, My other children, in unity with Me, the Woman Clothed in the Sun, who defeat the dragon, in the economy of our Father's Design, since He has called you to be little brothers and sisters of Jesus. Therefore, you work in unity with Jesus to defeat the enemy. In your own prayers and sacrifices, which are pleasing to God, you cause multitudes to convert. Little one, you wonder why you are tested and tried. It is because you are working works of merciful love, which is angering the dragon; and so you have these testings, these trials, as you claim the Name of Jesus, as you claim the Presence of Jesus, yet on Earth these 2,000 years in the power of the Eucharist.*

The gift given to My priesthood was to consecrate the Bread and Wine; this was the work Jesus promised that He would cause His apostles to do greater than He Himself. They bring Jesus to all who yield to the Faith of the apostles. My little one, you may feel at times little; a very small light, a dim candle in the darkness. It is not so. The Spirit of the Living God has anointed all followers of Christ as apostles and disciples with a Flame of Love. Once He has claimed His Own by Baptism, Confirmation and the anointing by Faith in the Holy Spirit, in the Word of God - you are His great flames, lighting up the darkness as so many candles all over the Earth. But the people of mankind need to read the Scriptures, the journey of the chosen people. As soon as the Good Shepherd got them on safe ground, they wandered off again to false idols. This is not new, except that there are many more false idols and many more temptations that are happening on the Earth; and tragically, there are many, many more people affected by this falsehood, which is taking shape in many forms all over the Earth. Thus, My little ones are called and armed to be brave warriors of their Christ. Know that God is with you even as He said in Holy Scripture. He is ever with you, even unto the end of time.

Peace! A great anointing of Love, Peace, Joy and all the accompanying graces and virtues are atten-

dant upon you, as you continue your work of love in the Name of Jesus. In the Name of the Father, and of the Son, and of the Holy Spirit, as it was in the beginning, is now and ever shall be, world without end. .Amen!

The Virgin of Fatima blesses you; a profound anointing is indeed upon you. In the Name of Jesus the enemy is in complete rebuke and is not present! Mother is present. I bid you Peace, My darling. I take care of each and every one of My priest-sons. My obedient priests are pleasing to the Lord God and to their Mother. Simply pray the miracle prayer and do not be afraid to speak out to the priest of your heart's concern. In this great Mission of Love, which is so important to the Lord your God, We open the ears and the hearts and the minds of the priesthood to receive these considerations which have been given directly to you from the Lord God Himself.

My little children, We repeat: do not worry about human esteem; worry about the Will of God. Little children, when you do these works of mercy which emanate from the Mercy Gate of My Immaculate Heart, you are warning the many of the error of the world's way, of the direction in which they are going. Since you have been trained in that way yourself, you unite with Me in warning the brethren that their decision is upon them. Little children, We gather a few of the faithful physicians round about the Earth, who still hold the correct line in the Eyes of God, on what is happening in the medical profession now. Certain actions well known to you are not pleasing to the Lord your God, and are bringing His wrath. Indeed there is certain research that is bringing the wrath of the Lord Our God.

And so thus in your fight against this, you are blest and you are assisted profoundly by Heaven in this work; you will not be disrupted in this work. Be without fear; speak out boldly in the Name of our God. My little one, Heaven profoundly assists you in this work of merciful enlightenment. Every time you attend upon the Lord in His Body and Blood you are anointed. It is the Will of the Lord your God. Praying for P, who has recently been diagnosed with cancer, as well as having arthritis, loss of weight. I'm not sure, but I think the family is not baptized. I pray for both his spiritual and his physical healing. **The Mother of God speaks.** *Let us begin at the beginnings. First of all, pray for P; then, invoking your Heavenly Mother's Name, invite him here and this is but the beginning of his journey into the community of God. Indeed he is known to God and blest by God. He feels Peace now, even as you speak now, in your heart's concern, for him and his family. Do thou, children, see now that you are truly instruments, in Our Lord's Peace, in this time of Ingathering? Do not worry if they come one by one. It is alright, for there are many of you doing similar work all over the earth. Your Mother is in all delight at your faithfulness. I bless you, I bless your works, I bless your evangelizations. More is happening than you know, little children, because of your Faith and prayers and penances.*

Oh how your Mother's Heart aches. You do not know how many tears I have shed for the suffering children of the Earth. 'Come this way I call, but they do not heed. My sorrow is great. Even so, my little daughter, I am holding you to my Heart, immersing you in the wellspring of My love; and the Holy Spirit, the Spirit of the Living God is pouring forth upon you as it were, a great River of Light shining down upon you, surrounding you in the Light of Christ Jesus our Lord Who goes ever before you. Graces, blessings, anointings; indeed fulfilment of the gifts you received in Baptism and Confirmation are yours. You will indeed serve my Son to the utmost, for Heaven hears your prayers and delights in them. My little one, be not anxious therefore; pray and step forward boldly, for the Lord your God is with you The virtue of Love is such that Our Mother, your Mother, the Woman Clothed with the Sun(Rv12:1) is in attendance upon you. Beloved children of a Merciful and Loving Father, you know the prophets from of old were bearers of the Seed of the Good News, for it was known that the Messiah would come, and you know that when Zacharias' speech returned, as he held John, he proclaimed; "You my child, shall be the prophet of the Most High, for you will go before the Lord to prepare His way, to give His people knowledge of Salvation, by the forgiveness of their sins.

My daughter, with regard to the atheistic physicians, prayer is the key, and yet your God-given Words have indeed circumnavigated the world. There are a handful of people in key positions who recognize Truth in the Words. Its like a two-pronged Mission; your prayers and these Words, being given over to a world where darkness yet rules. My daughter, I ask you to simply love Our Lord Jesus. With Me, love Our Lord Jesus and He does all the rest. My darling, often you will think, 'what have I accomplished?' but it is not for you to measure. It is what the Lord has accomplished using me as His instrument of Peace and Love, His instrument of Enlightenment. You are that lighted candle in the darkness of a deceived world. There are many of you about the world. Oft-times little children, you feel alone, but the Lord is with you, I am with you, angels and saints are with you. (She shows us through Omen that the Communion of Saints is always like a cheering section, supporting me in every way.) **Beloved little ones, rejoice in the Lord; trust the Lord; love the Lord; hope- because there comes an answer to all that you have been seeking.**

Luke 1 vs 46-55.

My soul proclaims the greatness of the Lord, and my spirit exults in God my saviour; because He has looked upon His lowly handmaid. Yes, from this day forward all generations shall call me blessed, for the Almighty has done great things for me; Holy is His Name. And His mercy reaches from age to age for those who fear Him. He has shown the power of His arm, He has routed the proud of heart, He has pulled down the princes from their thrones and exalted the lowly, the hungry he has filled with good things, the rich sent empty away, He has come to the help of Israel His servant, mindful of His mercy According to the promise He made to our ancestors-Of His mercy to Abraham and to his descendants for evermore. *Glory be...*

CHAPTER NINETEEN
VICTORY AND SALVATION

JESUS:

Little children, I am Jesus, Eternal Victor! My Victory is before My eyes. Small instruments, blessings accrue, for each one of you who partakes in this Mission of enlightenment. Before the world began, the Lord your God was aware of all that had to occur for the Salvation of mankind. Know that the sacrifice you, Omen and all those who pray for you are making, is the Cause of physicians themselves being converted and spared hellfire eternally, and indeed for some of the victims of organ harvesting, it is as thou hast said, that I the Lord God choose the moment of death, and yet in free will, the men of science choose, not only who is to be born and who is to be destroyed in the womb, but when a man or woman will die. This is not of Me. At this moment in time those who are called humanists or atheists seem to have the seat of power. Believe Me, it is not yet fully theirs and their moment of power is extremely brief. To this end I ask each one of My Own to prevail prayerfully, persevering in all prayer. I assure you I am with you. My beloved one, Mother and I attend upon you non-stop.

My little one, indeed We make good come out of this bad press, because goodness is ever-victorious. You will hear from many people because of this; but do not be disarmed, do not be dismayed. I am with you. There are many who are with you and yet there are the other kind who would attack your stance. My little one, it is My Stance. Ask of Me what you will My little one. I have given the world many messengers in these times, for example Mother Theresa, who spoke *My Truth, the only Truth.* My people, how many ways can I tell you that I Love you, that I AM Love, that I AM Truth, that I want that which is good for you; and I am forced to stand by and watch you follow the liar, the master of illusion, the darkness. Yet in My Merciful Love, I go forth and draw you out of the darkness and back into My Light. The Spirit of the Living God anoints each and every one of His Own, and as the Mother of God continues to beckon and call, it will be through the Faith of such as you, which will cause others to come back to the Lord their God with all their hearts, that they too may know Salvation. It is indeed true; the Lord your God is wrath about the transgressions of His Laws which are great, occurring rampantly on the face of the earth. A measured beat of time is upon the earth, and at the end of it, there comes the sequence of events which are forecast in Holy Scripture and hold fear for the many. Be undaunted by these fearful messages. Those who are Mine, are ever Mine. There are those who were never Mine. Do not concern yourselves about this matter.

Mighty is the Lord your God; All-powerful indeed! Whosoever falls on their knees in all surrender to the Father knows Salvation; for it is at this time in the Power of the Holy Spirit, that the works of conversion and healing occur. Mother and I busy Ourselves in these Works of teaching those who come unto the Lord God, the ways of holiness. In unity with Mary, greater graces occur in regard in particular to conversions and the Salvation of souls. I have already won the Victory; the triumph of the two Hearts is at hand. Yet the enemy works furiously, attempting to capture and deceive the many. There are many My little one; many, many, who do not believe, do not adore, do not trust the Living God. My little one, those who pray in unity of love with the Lord their God, are truly instruments of My Peace and My Love; and it is in and through such as you gathered in My Name that the many convert and ultimately know Salvation . My little children, it behooves you therefore to seek aid from your God Who is Love, and indeed is the Author of Love. Those who proclaim themselves atheists or agnostics, seek to win the victory in a purely scientific mode by reasoning and logic alone, and they are entangling themselves in a quagmire of confusion. How can they extricate themselves?

Simply love all those whom I set in your pathway of love. I ask you to love uncondi- tionally even as I your God Love. Those who remain defiant to their Creator in deliberate, willful disobedience, shall experience My wrath. All others who are My Own, I protect. They remain, whether yet in their bodies, or simply souls, they remain, all remain in My Presence, whether on earth, or in Purgatory, or in Heaven; My Own are safe in Me. You ponder many things little child. You may rise up and ask of Me what you will at this moment. A great blessing is upon you. Give Glory! A great and glorious Light comes now upon the Earth. It is the rapidly approaching Sign of Victory . None can see it at this point in time, but the Lord your God sees and knows. Oh, little children of God, you who have surrendered in abandonment to Love; you will be the first to know and you will be the instruments of bringing the multitudes back to the Sanctuary of Love, the Heart of Jesus. Oh precious little one, be at Peace. Sing songs of praise unceasingly. Until the moment of My Return, Mother weeps copious tears of joy. Yes, it is true they are united with tears of sorrow at the very grievous events upon the Earth; and yet there is joy in the Victory of the Holy Name Of Jesus. Oh little one, bless the Lord with all your heart and be at Peace!

I am He Who Lives and Loves eternally, and I am present to thee, little one of faithfulness. Great graces are upon you this day which is holy to the Lord. Little one, I tell you again that I Love thee. My precious little one, I bless thee; I bless thy works. Little one, continue to make reparation to the Father for all that is happening on earth today, and continue winning the great victory over self, which is imperative for each child of God. I Myself have already won the Victory over satan, sin and death. The battle therefore is for each human to win victory over self, assisted by your Jesus, and Our Mother, the Ever-Virgin Mary, and by a myriad of angels and saints your victory is assured, little children . For those who do not heed let us pray;If today you hear God's voice, harden not your hearts.(Ps 95). *Response:My God, I believe, I adore, I trust and I love Thee; I beg pardon for those who do not believe, do not adore, do not trust and do not love Thee.*

Dear child, it is the Lord your God Who speaks. Go in My Light and My Love, and attend. How can you teach Love without living Love. *You* will not by swallowed up by the deceits of the enemy, for thou art profoundly anointed and protected in My Name. My little ones, there are so many deceits about the earth now, and so many of My little lambs, My little sheep, wonder into these deceits, like little lambs to the slaughter, and it is they whom We must protect, by forbidding them. It is My Will, that you attend at all costs, bringing My Presence there, holding Me in your heart and soul and mind. Refrain from actual spiritual partaking; We set angels about you to protect you, and even about W who remains bearing the mark of Salvation in his soul.(Baptism)Little children, it is thus that your trials are multiplied. Little children, love one another and bless one another. Know that I am Creator of all; all belong to Me; and yet I ask specific things of My Own. My little ones, remember that Heaven is your true Native Land. My little ones it is but a brief separation. The Lord reminds you of John Vanier's words that love and pain are united in the Mystery of God.

All Life is sacred, human Life; a Gift from the Living God. The Faith journey is given to each life as it enters earth and that soul is so precious to the Lord your God, it is given time on earth in the journey of Salvation, to find Me the Living God. As you well know, many do not find Me except in suffering and trial, whether the affliction is spiritual or physical or providential, in some manner in their testing, in their formation, in their coming back to Me with all their hearts, a specific frame of time is essential. Sometimes it is brief, but sometimes it is prolonged; for each individual created is unique and each one is given a time to die. That I know well what each scientific mind which shuns Me is doing; does not excuse them. That I see My Plans for individuals altered, refuted, denied, and yet in patient perseverance with My beloved humanity, I am yet continuing, that they come at last to Enlightenment. It is *not* different than the pagan rituals of throwing individuals off the cliffs to their deaths, or into volcanoes or mutilated on altars; it is the fruit of healing will gone awry. Persevere little children in all faithfulness. Some are reluctant at this point in time to deal with the grave consideration at hand in Our Letters. Forbearance daughter.

Love Me, trust Me, for I Love you most tenderly, most totally and eternally. I am with you. Surrender Me your love. I am Jesus and I do all the rest! Believe! Continue to rest prayerfully in My Presence. Many great prayers are not necessary at all times. Just *Be* with Me, *Be* with your Jesus. *Be* with Me in the Church, at the Tabernacle and before the Monstrance; and yes, *be* with Me in Spirit - whither thou goest I am with you. United with Me there is nothing to fear, for I am with you. By Faith are the miracles wrought, by Faith is the Victory won! Remember it is in Love, through Love, by Love, that the miracles occur; by Faith and Love. As for your Mission ; it is in the Hands of your Jesus, and blest in the great graces from your Heavenly Mother; and all is going according to Heaven's Design. I take away for sure, any slightest traces, any signs of anxiety; for you shall work ever in the Peace of My Presence. It is in this your Faith and your surrender, that My great anointing of Peace is ever upon you. Little one you are blest, for in unity with God and the Beloved Mother of God, you have won the essential victory over self, so that the Lord God uses you most freely in the works of Enlightenment and Mercy, at this great hour of Ingathering. Living Waters flow unceasingly upon you. Rejoice! Again I say rejoice! Little children, working closely with your Mother and Mine, and with your God, you attain a high level of victory over self. Since I have won the Victory over Satan, sin and death, I am at last able to use you as My instruments of Love and Peace. Each one of you is profoundly blest and anointed. Pray for your own Victory in Jesus, and wait on the Lord.

The Lord reminded us of the Herculean effort being made to stop me from proceeding. The virtue of Love is such that the vaults of Heaven are wide open. We have allowed you to see what type of attack you are under little children. It continues, it prevails for a time. Indeed, My Victory is already won. This is at this time, what you would call in warfare, a clean sweep, a sweeping up that you are involved in. That which you do coincides, is indeed coordinated to cause, even as you are My instrument to cause enlightenment to both the priesthood and the scientific world; other of My faithful little ones are causing enlightenment in marriages and families and the rearing of children, and many, many aspects of life today. Hosts of angels assist. My precious little one, daughter of faithfulness, prevail. The stonewalling is temporary. You shall succeed in your Mission, for I am with you. Mother is with you. You are profoundly assisted. Continue to pray and address this matter. "<u>By what authority they ask! By the Authority of the Name of Jesus; by the Blood of the Lamb! This is your Authority!</u> Beloved, simply prepare your pamphlets and wait on the Lord. Beloved, persevere! It is in this persevering Faith, this ardent love of the Lord, this absolute trust; this Love of the Mother of God, who is indeed the great intermediary between God and Mankind; thus is each Victory won!

All the children of God will be clothed in the Sun, like unto the transfigured Christ; like unto the Woman Clothed with the Sun; on that Glorious Day of the Lord, for each and every one of My Faithful , it is so!Thus are saints able to attend upon those who pray asking that saint to plead their cause; and I in My Delight, allow the many miracles to happen. I reiterate! Love conquers all. Little children, you who know Love, who embrace each other in love; who embrace each other with a holy kiss; you know the Love of the Lord your

God; agape Love, an "all-charity of Love". The world does not know it. The world knows lust, fascinations and many illusions, confusing that with Love. This only aggravates the misery of the situations in which they find themselves, for they know Me not. Yet I call them by name. Many come unto Me now. Many are the trials upon the earth now. I the Lord God indeed fill your hearts and souls and minds with My Love and My Peace and a concomitant joy in the love of the Lord, I give to you. Many rejected Me, many will reject you, yet I have strengthened you to persevere, and that you shall do! Little children, those who heed the Words know a great Victory of Love, and begin themselves to evangelize, and to propagate the Faith of the Apostles, which is in sore disarray upon the earth at this time. Persevere little children of Faith, persevere. In this your surrender to Love; in this Our unity of Love, you follow Me each one in a unique manner, and the end results are a great Victory, in the Name of Jesus, for many are released from the deceits of the world.

Don't wonder where I am; I am with you. In this the time of times it has to be. The fight is great, yet My Victory is before My Eyes; and in My Victory is your own victory. Little ones, believe! Even providence works out for those who love and serve the Lord. Little children, you are in a time of testing and a time of change. My Victory is close at hand. The great Lighted Cross in the sky will indeed appear at a date in the future. The time is not yet, and yet it is not far. In the interim little children, work and believe, that all your tomorrows are blest, for indeed they are. Do not be fearful of the future. I Love you little children, I want only always that which is good for you. My Own have nothing to fear. My little children, it is written; blessed are those who do not see but believe! Such are you My little ones. But there comes a day, when I must make a Sign in the sky, that those who don't, will at last believe that I am your All-powerful God! It is not a time of fear for My Faithful little ones, who have already embraced the Cross of Eternal Life. Trials are of the essence in the formulation, the molding and fashioning of each individual. Therefore do not shrink from these trials and tribulations. Prevail in Faith. Herein lies your victory little ones.

Little children, great angels fight a great battle, that these Words be given over first for the doctors, then even to the priests involved, but ultimately for the general public, those that can and will read . Do not be dismayed at the obstructions little one, or any of the strange events that will attempt to slow you down or even stop you all together. *It shall not be.* I Myself cause the victory to happen. Thou hast worked well; thou art well advised from Glory. Things are going according to Heaven's Design. Be at Peace. The virtue of Love is such that I am present to you. A severe testing, a severe attack is upon your works little children; prevail, We are with you. Believe , We are with You. Be at Peace therefore! Remember, you are beloved of Jesus and Mary; safe in Our Embrace. Pray often, " In Jesus' Name is My Victory." Little children you are beseeched by many lies being disseminated by our foe the liar, the master of illusion. Be not deceived, I am with you. I am with you in the Holy Sacrifice of the Mass, in My Body Blood Soul and Divinity; in the Blessed Sacrament, the Holy Eucharist, in the written Word. When you are beseeched, come to Me. Seek healing at the Mass; seek healing in My Presence in the Tabernacle, in the Monstrance. Seek healing by prayerfully invoking My Spirit as you read Holy Scripture; by pondering on My Life and Mothers Life on earth in the Rosary. All these means are given to you that you stay secure in My Presence.

I am Jesus, Eternal Victor; I remind you I have already won the Victory over satan, sin and death. Little children, you have only to win the victory over self. Little children, since I am with you always, and Mother is with you, as well as a vast entourage of angels and saints, in the power of the Holy Spirit, you cannot fail, you are My Own. By Faith are the miracles wrought, by Faith is the Victory won! Little children, with your Faith, your love, your compassion, it is as it were, compensation for certain individuals themselves, and certain ones round about them, and since you unite your prayers always with those who have attained the Victory in Heaven, the healings flow. Be at Peace. Beloved little ones, Love Me, Trust Me, when it seems there is no reason to Trust; (Jn14:1)Trust Me. Remember, I know what I am about. My Plan for each little human soul is for their good. On this feast day of St Joseph, I release many souls from bondages, and on the subsequent series of feast days coming forth, on each such day, souls are released from whatsoever binds them, or holds them captive in unwarranted ways. Little children, love one another as I Love you,(Jn15:12) and believe in miracles; by Faith are the miracles wrought, by Faith is the Victory won. I am the Lord Your God(Ex34:6-8); I am attendant upon all these concerns of your heart. My small one; know that your communications have been received, they have been pondered, they have been prayed over, with regard to the response. A courtesy type letter comes from a communicator. Do not think that you are shunned or disregarded with these communications. The Church is extensive through time and the world, and it is seemingly at a ponderous undertaking.[Through Omen Our Lord shows us a Vine; for a new leaf to grow on that Vine.] Therefore be not impatient little children, I am with you through it all. It comes; the Victory comes in due course.

A great and glorious Light comes now upon the Earth. It is the rapidly approaching sign of Victory . None can see it at this point in time, but the Lord your God sees and knows. Oh little children of God, you who have surrendered in abandonment to Love; you will be the first to know and you will be the instruments of bringing the multitudes back to the Sanctuary of Love, the Heart of Jesus. Oh precious little one, be at Peace. Sing songs of praise unceasingly. Until the moment of My return, Mother weeps copious tears of joy. Yes, it is true they are united with tears of sorrow at the very grievous events upon the Earth; and yet there is joy in the Victory of the Holy Name Of Jesus. Oh little one, bless the Lord with all your heart and be at peace! The Lord is with you little children, you may begin to share and discern now. Darling, the One Who is called Faithful and True is attendant upon you. Indeed I am attendant upon each one of you in a profound manner. Little children, as you know there is yet much to be done, and I have strengthened you to the Fortitude, the courage to do what needs doing upon My Requests, and I am delighted in your faithfulness, in your obedience in remaining humbled creatures before Our Father, Who is Creator of All.

It is thus that you permit Me to use you, in your 'yes' to Me, echoing the "Yes" of Our Mother; I am thus using you as instruments of My Healing Love, instruments of My Peace, instruments of My Light, that Enlightenment come upon this world. As is written, 'darkness covers the Earth, and the thick clouds the people.' We must yet bring Light to the world. My faithful ones are sprinkled all over the Earth, like countless candles, great candelabras; a myriad of lights about the Earth, but the darkness is yet immense! <u>Dear little children, in a moment of wonder I shall light up the entire world with My Presence! It is not yet, but in the Eyes of the Lord it is soon!</u> Dear little children, you are called to persevere, and you are strengthened; yes I have given you each one, a Spirit of Boldness in the Lord, to do that which I desire done, and you remain not being afraid, but carrying out these actions in My Name. Blessings fall upon you, graces fall upon you little children. Each one of you is yielded unto Me in and through the Immaculate Heart of Our Mother. As you cling to the Two Hearts of Love, Divine Life, Divine Light flows in you and through you, to the many needy little ones.

The Virtue of Love is that I bless you and I Bless all your works. I am with you in all that you are doing. With regard to the beloved John Paul of Our Heart's Delight, We are profoundly attendant upon him. The many matters weigh heavily upon him, where he has to make pronouncements on so many, and so varied a number of subjects, yet *this* one is dear to his heart, is a priority. There is a convocation; they come together with regard to bodily death. The decision is momentarily reserved, but the beloved John Paul is relentless in his determination to address this subject, and it shall be thus very rapidly now. Pray for the beloved John

Paul, as you do, and all those around him, and trust Me a little bit longer; My Peace, My Love, My Joy is upon you. In all things give Glory to the Father, Who is truly the Creator of all that is seen and unseen. Random research products of scientists about the world are very limited. In no way whatsoever, can man create as Your God does! I give them intellect to work for the good of man and not for the destruction. Thus you see more repeatedly coming out of the mouths of John Paul and his faithful ones, reprimands for the "culture of death," which is most assuredly, not of Me. My little ones, My little ones, who live and love in Me, and fight for the lives of many; these ones live in the "Culture of Life."Thus you see, the sides drawn up, one against the other.

It looks like the "culture of death" is more powerful at certain moments, rather like a fierce wrestling match, but I am Life, and the "culture of Life prevails. In due course you will, each one of you observe, My Victory. I am Jesus, Eternal Victor! You must believe that I am working this through with the Holy Father, the beloved John Paul of Our Heart's Delight, and know that I shall address many Words to you at the moment of his declaration with regard to Life and Death. We shall speak then about this matter. Little children, prevail in all prayerfulness. My people have forgotten that eternal Life is in Heaven. There is no fountain of youth upon earth. It is but a temporary journey. You are called in Holy Scripture to keep your eyes turned towards Heaven your true and native Land. <u>Therefore, the perfection of soul is always the priority.</u> Choosing, in your eyes, that which is the lesser of evils, does not make anything right in the eyes of the Father. Little children, Peace. I the Lord God am profoundly attendant upon you and upon every member of the Body of Christ upon Earth, the Church Militant. Countless of you see now and recognize the signs of the times which are upon you and you know well that the era of Peace is imminent but not yet. The enemy yet prevails for a brief period of time and so there is trouble and distress upon the earth, and yet all those who know Me and love Me; those who call upon My Name in their neediness, Heaven assists them profoundly. See, this way little children, you are safe in the Lord. That is why I am calling many to evangelize, to proclaim the Good News of Salvation to all those who will heed the Call of My Love and come back to Me that they may know repentance and conversion and Salvation. Dear little children, it is a time not unlike when My first Apostles walked upon the Earth.

They were My instruments in causing many to convert; you children are also My instruments in causing others to convert. Do not worry about sheer numbers, but rejoice with Heaven when one sinner comes back to Me wholeheartedly. Rejoice that many are coming unto Me, coming into the Embrace of My Divine Love, yet alas there are many who know Me not, and that is why you are called little children to unhesitatingly proclaim the Good News at every opportunity. As it is written, "the harvest is plenty and the workers are few", so it is today little children, but I am with you and I am your all-powerful God, and in your weakness is My Strength and together, miracles occur. As you are well aware of the many healing miracles, so there are many spiritual miracles, healing of souls unto Myself.

My precious little ones, do not doubt that it will include doctors, lawyers, even politicians, many such seemingly self-important individuals. They too will fall on their knees before the Father in due course that they may also know conversion and Salvation, for nothing is impossible to the Lord your God. Little children, you know the reading, "for they have all gone astray like sheep." I bring them back, I am the Good Shepherd! That is why I call you to pray; stay united with your Jesus. Seek Heavenly assistance from Our beloved Mother who magnifies your prayers and brings all who call on Her unto Me; Jesus, that they may know Me and know Salvation, and the Father is well pleased little children, for "nothing is impossible to the Lord your God," and yet in Heaven's Design each one of you who are My Own, is called to be My Heart, My Hands, My Voice, in bringing My Merciful Love to all mankind.

Yes, you are limited each one, but there are many of you now. I am delighted in My faithful little ones. Precious little brothers and sisters of Jesus, all are anointed in My Love and they do indeed evangelize successfully, and Our Victory is known world-wide in due course. Do you believe little children? Yes little children, you know well that I have already won the Victory over satan, sin and death. In My Name, Jesus, is each souls Victory. Do not worry about the signs of Death, the 666 and other such signs of the times which must be, before My Return. I protect My Own, I shield My Own. Yes you will see sorrow, and yet you will see Victory. Be not afraid, I am with you always. Hosts of angels surround the children of God all over the Earth now. Remember that twice as many angels were loyal to Me. Therefore cling to your Jesus, cling to the Heavenly Host prayerfully and be at Peace. *Lord I pray for the healing, the conversion of this family who do not believe in You.* It is these times in which you live little children, but generations before the forebearers were Christians, therefore little children, simply pray for the conversion of sinners, the Salvation of souls; Heaven powerfully unites with those who pray thus.

You have associates, acquaintances who have not reached this level of spirituality, or even alas, are far away from Me, and that is why Mother appears about the world, pleading for prayers and conversions. You have no idea the power of your prayers little children, little faithful ones. They work the needed miracles of Love upon this Earth. There are many, many of you scattered about the world like a salting all over the Earth, and this is the Seamless Garment encompassing the whole world, the true faithful, united together with Me, the Living God. This is the Great Fisherman's Net, (Mt 13:47-52) which causes Victory in My Name for multitudes. Do not doubt little children but believe. Remember, I Love each one of you most tenderly, most totally and most eternally. You are part of the Kingdom of God, the Kingdom is in Heaven and yet it is here for those who are united with Me. Little children, when you pray the Lord's prayer, you are asking for the Completion of this, My Kingdom of Love. Little children, My Delight is in your prayer, in your faithfulness. In all your trials and stresses and undertakings, you remain faithfully united to Me and thus the Blessings and Graces flow. Truly in My Name, Jesus, is your Victory.

Little children, it is also a time of trial upon the earth; it is more so than for other generations, for you are in that time of change which is upon the earth, and the enemy knows he is limited and attempts to wreak much havoc upon the earth now, but I have already defeated him; he is a defeated foe, and when My little children, you pray in My Name, he must leave. He recoils from the Name Jesus and from the Name Mary, the Woman of Genesis, (Gn3:15) the Woman of Revelation. (Rv12:1)My little children, I am anointing you in My Love and My Peace and My Joy, as I do at every moment of true prayerfulness, of true Unity with Me. Little children, at this time on the earth, the true Body of Christ (1Co12:27), the faithful remnant, therefore walks the Via Dolorosa with the Christ. Embrace your cross, love your Jesus; together we win the Victory, so long awaited which remains imminent, and yet only the Father knows. Peace. I am your Jesus, Eternal Victor!

It is by the Clothing of Jesus, with Flesh and Blood, through the "Yes" of the Immaculate Virgin Mary, that the Victory against satan was won, and that is why he perseveres in persecuting both The Christ and the Mother of God, and the Baptized children, Her "other children" of Faith. [Rev 12 vs 17] This is ongoing, though few take time to pray and ponder on these matters, this is important. The Annunciation [25th March] is as it were, a Portent of the [spiritual] war, as it is today. Today I am asking those who know and love our Mother, to continue to pray for a time of Advent where She is recognized and triumphant, and I too, am recognized; I am your Jesus of Victory. It is My Will that My Mother be recognized in the Body of Christ! She recognizes each child of God as her own precious child, because of My Word to Her at the foot of the Cross of Calvary. (Jn19:26-27)Who are My Own? Those who say, here I am Lord, I will follow You; who repent of their abysmal ignorance and sins of the past and come back Me with all their hearts! At the same time there is sorrow on earth there is rejoicing, as the multitudes come unto Me now, and there is a great Victory -swell up above the world, as people come to know Salvation. Go forth little children, walking in My Light and My Love!

How long oh Lord,"(cfRv6:10)many cry in prayer, before an end of this suffering, and yet it is a time of decision which is upon the world, decisions for Light and Love and Peace, or decisions for the opposing factors. I give time for the multitudes to choose Life, to choose Love, to choose Peace, that they may know the eternal Victory, and in this interim of time, there is rampant suffering about the earth. That is why true believers, all of you are called to pray; pray for Mercy from your God. Tales of Victory abound wherever the little saints relics go; therefore pray much and trust in the Lord. Be at Peace: In all things I am with you ; I am Peace, I am your Peace! *Mother shows Omen her purse, with the rose petals from visiting Little Flower relics on Sunday, so St Therese is intervening for them.* We the Church await the Triumph of the Queen of Heaven and Earth, and the Victory of your Jesus, and the era of Peace. I do not speak of that time as now, for now is a time of great battle, but it is not afar off, and you have been trained in battle each one of you, for the unique purposes to which I am calling each one of you, and that is why I have taught you to persevere, to be patient, to endure in My Name!

I give you Luke. When the Mother of the Lord, bearing the Lord, attended upon the beloved Elizabeth and Zacharias, John the Baptist was indeed baptised in the waters of his mother's womb. (Lk1:40-42)Were you not bearing the Woman Clothed with the Sun,(Rv12:1) in all Faith and Truth, as you attended upon the mother of Gloria? *Yes Lord, I touched and took a blessing in Faith from Our Lady of Guadalupe, pregnant with Our Lord, from that special image before I left the chapel to go and anoint K and Gloria;I can say the Baptism of Gloria, took place through our Lady of Guadalupe.* Yes indeed, for are you not the handmaids of the Handmaid of the Lord! My little ones, Mercy Gate Mission shall proclaim the Good News of Salvation far and wide. Many will come to Me in and through all that transpires here. My beloved little ones, do not be afraid to trust the beloved Father Francis of Our Hearts' delight. I have indeed woven you together that My Word go hither and yon about the earth. I brook no obstructions to My Word.

Yes little children today you are both the seedplanters, and the harvesters, .(Lk10:1-2) for there are so few of you, and so many to tend. Yet I am with you more powerfully than ever, for the Holy Spirit is upon the earth now, in a profound anointing of Love as the Mother, My Mother, your Mother, remains visiting the earth yet a time, calling all the children of God back to repentance and Salvation. All that you mention is a sign of the times in which you are living. Little children, thus your Mother weeps and pleads for all those to convert. Pray, pray for the conversion of sinners! Do not be dismayed at the many who are taken Home now. Pray that they be ready to stand before the Lord God, that they know Salvation! What sorrow this is to the Hearts of your God and of your Loving Mother, who pleads unceasingly on their behalf, and to them, that they may know Salvation. In this manner you see the immense battle which is occurring in this time; and why each little effort, each little prayer, each little penance which you perform dear children, is so precious, is so important to the Lord your God. That is why I the Lord God ask you so often, to Love Me for those who do not!

In these times, each true faithful child of God and child of Mary, is called upon to give their utmost for the Cause. The Cause is Peace on earth, conversion of sinners, Salvation of souls. It remains the Cause! For this I died, that mankind might know Life to the fullest(Jn10:10). Do not delay in these actions which are given to you to do today. Little children, you do not do it yourselves. You do it in the Hand of Almighty God. You are but a small instrument in His Hand. Always remember that little children, this is the Faith which will carry you through this Work of Merciful Love, which will be the Cause of the conversion of many, and the Salvation of many souls who are at present in grave peril of hell. This is the means of Salvation for the Hebrews and the Moslems, all peoples; the Blood of the Lamb without spot.(cf Rv5:6) The Call goes out to all the nations of the earth to come to the Baptismal Waters; the Call like unto that of the beloved John the Baptist Indeed, greater is He Who is in your hearts and souls and minds little children, than that which is in the world. Radiating, healing Love is upon all those through this Peace of the True Cross. It is done.

Militant angels surround you little children, be at Peace! You are safe in the Lord. You live in a time of turbulent warfare, spiritual warfare upon the earth little children; yet My Own are safe in Me. My Own are those who are continuing to cling to Me and My Name, Jesus your Salvation; to proclaim the Good News to the ends of the earth My little ones! Little children, it is Mother's persevering prayer, and that of all the followers who pray for the conversion of sinners, the Salvation of souls; continue as you are doing. One day you will recognize, for I shall permit you to see the fruits of your labours. The Virtue of Love is such that I the Lord God, speak thus! I am with you in all that is happening, even in the moments of quiet, as We await the interaction of the many involved in Our Mission. There is always the foe; watchful, envious, attacking My people as a penetrating evil; those who do not have their armour tightly about them.(Eph 6:10-20) Great angels and archangels surround all the key players in this Mission to a scientific world. My Own are safe in Me! Those who are a bit weak, I begin now to strengthen, for an hour of decision is upon them, to choose the pathway I, the Living God have set out for them in the Ministry of Salvation for Mankind.

Son of God, take and hold the Hand of your Jesus in Spirit and Truth, (Jn4:23-24), and that of Our beloved Mother, as We walk beside Joseph guardian of the Holy Family, guardian of the family of God. Together We walk in Faith and Hope and Trust and Love, in all patient perseverance (cf1Cor13) this is the only Way, this is My Way, and you are My Own. Teach My people that I am indeed the Way the Truth and the Life.(Jn 14:6) Remember, I Light your Way, for you are My brother, part of My Family, the Family of God and Bethlehem and Calvary, and part of the great army of Peace which I am building upon the earth, into which you have been called. Stay as you are, in Union with Me, Your Jesus, Eternal Victor. Tell My People, Victory is in the Name of Jesus, their Salvation. (cf 1Jn5:13)The dissensions, the disruptions in My Body, the Church, are well known to you little ones. Even so, you only see as it were, the tip of the iceberg! There is great turmoil within My Church, for it is assailed from within and without, and the beloved John Paul, because of the circumstances in which he finds himself, is expected one might say, to walk a tightrope in all that he is saying and doing. Yet he is blest with a spirit of boldness in speaking the Truth of Salvation!

My little children of Life, I bless you each and every one. I am blessing those who comprehend that I am God.(cf Ex 14:18) and yield their free wills to Me. When you yield your free wills to Me, it is for the love, not only of your God, but the love of mankind, for the betterment of mankind, for the Salvation of mankind. Thus little children, when you practice loving your neighbour as yourself, great fruits are produced; to come to know Truth, and to live in My Light and My Love. My little children, be at Peace; Heaven hears your prayers. I know all your hearts concerns little children. Even as the light increases, for you have passed the darkest date [21st Dec] and sunlight is increasing daily, so the Light of Christ is increasing in the hearts of human beings. Those hardened hearts begin to soften, and enlightenment comes as My beloved little ones persevere in praying, the plea of Our Mother, the conversion of sinners, the Salvation of souls, dear little children, for nothing is impossible to the Lord your God!

Little children, Heaven hears the prayers of the Faithful. Little children, it is My Delight that so many of My children pray unceasingly for the conversion of sinners, the Salvation of souls. It is begun. Therefore simply pray in the Peace of the Lord's Presence and wait on the Lord! The times in which you are living should be clear evidence to all, that they are signs of impending Judgement. (Rv20:11-15) Little children, you will linger a little longer, pleading for the conversion of sinners, the Salvation of souls. Continue to pray that none of those experience a sudden, unexpected death. Be ready to come before Me, to come to the Embrace of Eternal Love. Many come back to Me now. My little children, just continue doing as Our Mother has asked, to pray for the conversion of sinners, the Salvation of souls, as Mother has asked you. Those whom you carry in your hearts little children, are most assuredly among those who are prayed for profoundly. Mother does not cease pleading the cause of the little wanderers. My darling, your family is safe in Me, Heaven hears your prayers and the prayers of the faithful in your extended family. They resound in Heaven. Graces and blessings flow. In due course I, the Good Shepherd(Jn10) am able to bring them back. They at last open their hearts to Love and Truth. You must believe little children, that I call them back in due course and most assuredly in time to know Salvation. Therefore little children, love one another and be at Peace.

The blessing which the Holy Father has brought upon the earth with his proclamation, endows those formerly without a Heavenly Queen and Mother, to now have one. Many holy and miraculous events occur, and all will know that I am God, .(cf Ex 14:18) Supreme among the nations and that it is My Will that My Mother be recognized. Thus I have set Her, your Mother of Mercy; the Merciful One Who judges not; whose weapon is Love, against the merciless one; and I bless Mankind in Her and through Her with the needed Graces and Heavenly assistance to persevere and to be victorious, and as you know, in Her Intercession, you will come before Me, the Living God, and know Salvation. Healing Love is upon you little one; be at Peace, I am with You. Little children, have I not told you it is a time of perseverance(cf1Cor13) a time of endurance, and again a time of perseverance(cf1Cor13). These are the times in which you are living. Distress is epidemic over the earth yet few return to Me wholeheartedly. My little ones, always recognize that you are front line warriors in My Cause, the Cause of Merciful Love, the Cause of Salvation. My very Names are "Salvation" and "God with you." Therefore be not afraid, I am with you always.

You have no idea the power of your prayers little faithful children, and I simply ask you to continue to pray and to spread the Good News of Salvation.(cf Mt10:6-7) Remind them that My Love knows no bounds, My Mercy knows no bounds, call on Me little children, that I might pour forth My Spirit upon you, that you may know Salvation. Little children, I am the Lord Your God(Ex34:6-8); I am tenderly attendant upon each one of you. My little children, My little Faith-filled ones, the more you pray and act in Faith, the greater the increase of Faith in you, and thus you will see more healing events; a myriad of miracles you might say. You seek a recognizable miracle of the Holy Eucharist and it shall come to pass. It is not yet but it is not far off. Little children, continue to pray. The Eucharistic Miracle is powerful, but the little miracles of Healing Love are also powerful in the matter of winning souls over to Salvation, and that's what it is all about My little evangelizers. As you adore you yourselves are healed, and as you adore further, Healing Love comes upon those who are so needy of My Merciful Love. Little children, persevere! (Rm5:1-5)

Little children, the Call to Christianity is far greater than many Baptized Christians recognize in these times, and it is essential then, that they might know Salvation and wellness, increased testings and trials to bring them to the needed Faith, the needed Fortitude, before the purification of soul can be established in them. Little children, because you are in Unity with Me, Great Blessings and Graces come upon you. I Desire to pour them forth on many others, but they reject Me at this time. That is why you are called to pray for those who know Me not, that they too may know Salvation. Little children, on earth, you are in the Church militant - a brave army of Christians, lead and directed by the Power of the Spirit of the Living God. You are safe in the Embrace of Divine Love. My Love knows no bounds. Bring them in to Me. Bring them all back to Me little children; do not hesitate to proclaim the Good News. My Hour of Mercy prevails for some time.

Pray that the world accept Me; all those in the world whom I am calling to Myself, that they come unto Me wholeheartedly, that they know Salvation. You know that you are in the world, but not of the world,(cfJn15:19) and there are those who will never recognize Me. Even so, pray for every brother and sister on this earth. All are the Works of My Hands! It is a time of great Joy for those who know Me. It is a time of hardship and struggle for those who know Me not, because they believe they are doing all things by themselves, whereas you little children, you know that you are working in Unity with Me and are Blest by Me, and so their lives are difficult because of this lack of knowledge of the Living God! I Bless you in the works I have committed you to do. I Bless this diocese in a unique way. My precious little ones, do not doubt that it will include doctors, lawyers, even politicians, many such seemingly self-important individuals. They too will fall on their knees before the Father in due course that they may also know conversion and Salvation, for nothing is impossible to the Lord your God.

Little children, you are called to persevere on this earth in fighting the good fight, to bring the Good News of Salvation to the many, invoking My Spirit, the Holy Spirit of the Living God, to come upon the multitudes, that their hearts be transformed to hearts of Love, and that Peace and Joy reign henceforth in each heart. Oh My people, I am Calling all to come back to Me like the prodigal son. There is only suffering and sorrow and hardship where they choose to wonder, and they find it so difficult, for the return journey back to Me, and yet I await them with open arms of Love. How I Long to clothe each one with Salvation. Tell Me their names in prayer at the Adoration Chapel and leave them there with Me. I am your Jesus of Mercy, your Jesus of Love. Upon whom I will, I have Mercy. At this time I have Mercy upon all of mankind. I await their response to My Call.

I had a strange experience on Saturday, July 28th, when I came home from Mass, and fell asleep on the couch, only to wake up to the feeling of being watched. I saw this old lady, whom I had never seen and did not recognize, staring at me with curiosity, above my feet; just her upper body in the air above me. She was very old, with grey hair parted in the middle and somewhat ruffled. She had an expression of surprise and I was stunned; then she was gone, but I thought she must be one that I had prayed the chaplet of Divine Mercy for in Adoration, which I've been doing each time since 2-4th February when we had the workshop on Divine Mercy and I became a Eucharistic Apostle of Divine Mercy and promised to pray for a soul dying during my Holy Hour of Adoration.

I bid you know that the one permitted to gaze upon you, is indeed, as you have discerned, one whose sins were negated by the Divine Mercy intercession. This prayer of Faith in My Merciful Love is a great instrument in Salvation. It is underused at this date, and so there are few of you who are accomplishing this healing of souls at the hour of death. Little children it is a time of great Mercy from your God. Yes, I am God and I can do as I will, but in the Design of Your Father of Mercy, it is by man that man is healed. I became Man for the healing of humanity. I am the Way; I have taught you The Way little children, and you are each one, following in My Way, despite the oft times weariness, you persevere. I wish you to know of the success of your prayers on behalf of the little troubled ones. You are aggrieved and concerned about one who has been ensnared by the ways of the world. As you pray little children continuously for the conversion of sinners, the Salvation of souls, as you do daily, you may single out a certain one or other that you know at times specifically in your prayers, but know that all your prayers are heard in Heaven, and it is always your God's desire to say yes to the precious little faithful ones. Even so, all must go according to the Father's Design, and all as you know, is contingent upon the God given free will of the individual for whom you are praying.

MARY: *The Virgin of Fatima bids thee Peace. Mother attends upon the little ones who are desirous of change. I plead their cause before Our Lord Jesus Christ. It is a grievous offense to the Lord God as you know. There are many other grievous offences to the Lord God, but it is paramount for them to convert for the Salvation of each soul. Little children, persevere in prayer for this people. There is an aspect of Salvation in that many who suffer the death of AIDS have turned to the Lord God in true repentance, and they too have pleaded for their brothers who are like ensnared, and thus the Victory is greater than you recognize at the moment little children. Do not let these inroads take away from your Peace. We give you Mother Theresa, We give you John Paul, and We give you your own Father P as examples. Peace prevails within such hearts no matter what is occurring around them.*

You are called little children to love and trust Our Lord Jesus no matter what is happening. I reiterate, though the earth quake beneath your feet, keep your eyes upon Jesus. Thus, thus is your victory won; and I bring your sacrifices of love to the Father that Love may emanate upon the needy upon Earth. Little children, in the Power of the Holy Spirit thou art blest in the Name of the Father, and of the Son, and of the Holy Spirit. Little children, remember the Words in Scripture," By Faith are the miracles wrought, by Faith is your own victory won. " By Faith is the victory of assisting others won. Little one, since you are fully aware of the moment when the Holy Spirit is attendant upon you, it behooves you to be continuously giving Glory to the Father each in your own way, as so many little song birds before your God.

It is for each individual to prevail in defeating the drives prompted by their negative powers, to win their personal victory ; Since anyone turning to God, in particular through Jesus and the Mother of God, Heaven assists them so profoundly that they cannot fail; but they lack this level of trust, this level of Faith. The Salvation is told again and again by those who fight abortion . Little children, you cause many to come back to Me; you are My instruments in bringing the many back to Me with all their hearts and they in turn enlist in the great spiritual battle which is now ongoing. Little children, you fight as it were, a conspiracy of death, propagated as it were by those who are servants of Our enemy, and yet We must always recollect, that greater is God Who dwells within you, than that enemy which is in the world. Believe, all the Victory is in My Name, Jesus. I am your Strength, your Fortitude. Let Us go joyfully together on this Great Mission of Love's Victory. Peace!

Dear little children, many events are occurring on the earth at this time. My precious little ones, We ask you to pray for the beloved John-Paul's intentions at this time. We ask you to make novenas and prayer/ petitions from now until Pentecost. You are living in the most remarkable era in the history of mankind. Dear little children, the enemy is wrath and hurls what it can against the faithful children of God. Even so, their Victory in Jesus is assured. My beloved little ones, it is I, your Mother of Good Counsel Who has given you the Hymn of Pentecost, to the Holy Spirit. It holds you fast in the pathway of holiness. It is one more means of assisting you My little ones. Use it frequently, My little ones; do not worry about perfection of music. The Words themselves are powerful in prayer. My little ones, when you pray this hymn, the Holy Spirit attends upon many who are cold or lukewarm and they begin to come back to the Lord God. Precious little children, I bless each and every one of you. In the power of the Holy Spirit great graces flow upon you.

Our Lady of Fatima: When We are in a direct spiritual battle with the devil, We have to persevere till the Peace Victory of Jesus is clearly demonstrated and His Peace and Joy restored to us. Mother is present. Jesus is present also; be at Peace. Be <u>not</u> dismayed little children about what is happening in the world and those who are of the world still. Your Mission is to persevere in the way of holiness which Our God has chosen for you. In this way, as you remain humbly obedient, persevering despite the harassments *and oppressions, the distractions, you win the victory, and this victory <u>is the conversion of many others, to know Salvation</u>, for you know well that you are front line warriors ,in the battle for souls in the Church militant upon the earth today; yet always remember you are not alone; the Lord is with you, I an with you, angels and saints are with you. Little children, rest secure in the Embrace of the Two Hearts of Love. Mother repeats," In Jesus Holy Name is My Victory."*

Believe little children, believe in the Victory in Jesus Holy Name, for it is so! My dear little children, there are certain events that do indeed happen on this earth which, though not of God, are portends of the times that are ahead, which bring on changes upon the earth, and in due course, the Return of Christ, and a new era of Peace on earth, as has been told through many visionaries with whom I have worked. Little children, in this instance, saints blood has again fallen to the ground, but this time, in the United States of America; and you will see now, conversions occurring as never before! Little children, their sacrifice is not in vain; it is united with Mine, for the Victory of mankind over the foe. Give Glory!

Mother is in attendance, be at Peace; the little one for whom you weep my darling child, is safe in the Divine Embrace of Love. You may yet pray for her when her name comes to mind, when thoughts of her recur. You may actually little one, invite her to pray with thee at these times; and this is a powerful means of praying. This is a great gift of the Communion of Saints who have attained the Victory, and yet their love is for you yet on the earth. My little children, My delight is in your loving hearts; your hearts of compassionate love. Graces and blessings flow upon you my daughter, because of your loving concern for others. Be assured you are secure in the Embrace of Divine Love.

My little ones it is a time of great sorrow upon the earth. The enemy is filling many with fear which is not of our God and again I bid you live the Great Commandments of Love. Pray for one another. Pray for these 2,600 families who do not fully comprehend God's Divine Gifts to them in the Sacraments of Love. You are the lights, and there are a goodly number of you in the parish who are enlightened and become lights of the Truth of our Lord, and through you the others begin to be drawn into Adoration of the Divine Lamb of God. Be at Peace. Perpetual Adoration shall indeed continue. The Virgin of Fatima will stand firmly beside you. The Virgin herself attests to the veracity of all that is given you; little children, prevail in all that you are doing. I have called My children of Light to fight for the conversion of sinners and the Salvation of souls. It is imperative in these times that much prayer is given over to this, for many are impelling their very souls into hell by their actions on earth today. It is a grievous Sorrow to the Lord Your God, and to Me, your Heavenly Mother.

Rest assured it is thus, for there will be, for each individual, an examination of their souls in the Presence of Jesus, through Jesus' Eyes, and they will see the states of their souls, all mankind. At that time a great repentance comes on every one who will know Salvation, and they will see the error of their ways in the Eyes of God , and they will , in all sorrow and pain , repent and seek forgiveness, and be welcomed back into the Arms of the Living God. Be at Peace therefore. You my child, shall be the prophet of the Most High, for you will go before the Lord to prepare His way, to give His people knowledge of Salvation, by the forgiveness of their sins.By the tender compassion of our God, the dawn from on High will break upon us."(Lk1:77-78)Little children, in this Benedictus, you can today see the beloved John Paul, preparing the world for the Return of Our Lord Jesus Christ. I too have been preparing by appearing in the many areas of the world, calling people to pray and repent. The call of John Paul to Humanity is in Unity with The Holy Spirit of the Living God and thus the Way is being prepared in connection with My beloved son, Juan Diego- a most beautiful convert to Christianity.

Little children, those of you who believe are praying incessantly for the conversion of sinners, the Salvation of souls. Jesus' very Name is "Salvation," and Emmanuel is verily "God with us,"-your God is with you! Do not shun Him; do not ignore Him; do not disbelieve! Open the eyes of your soul; open your ears to hear the Divine Call of Love that you may live, have Life to the fullest, Life eternally in Glory. This is why I am upon the earth pleading; weeping, before the Day of the Lord. (cf 2 P3:7) Heed my call, heed my cry little children; I remain your tearful Mother !

Micah 5: 2-5 The Lord says this: You oh Bethlehem of Ephrathah, who are one of the little clans of Judah, from you shall come forth for Me, One who is to rule in Israel, whose origin is from of old, from ancient days. Therefore the Lord shall give them up until the time when she who is in labour has brought forth; then the rest of his kindred shall return to the house of Israel. And he shall stand and feed his flock in the strength of the Lord, in the majesty of the name of the Lord his God. And they shall live secure, for now he shall be great to the ends of the earth: and he shall be the one of peace.

CHAPTER TWENTY
JESUS, ETERNAL PHYSICIAN

JESUS:

FOR MY WAYS ARE NOT YOUR WAYS AND MY TIME IS NOT YOUR TIME (Is55:8-9)

My Love is a healing Love. The practitioners of Faith know full well that the prayer for one another, both friend and stranger - aliens in their land - even then I heal each and every one by the power of Faith. I reiterate, Faith grows in direct proportion to the individual's attendance upon the Lord. *Shun Me not!* Attend upon Me, that I may Enlighten your heart and soul and mind also. Deuteronomy will cover all the rest. Read it, little children; We have Words there which you will recognize! Do you not call Me the Great Physician, the Healer? But you use Me not! Even so, in the Mercy of God, I call the medical profession in particular, and their research scientists, once again to come back to Me with all their hearts. At times, you mention God, or even My Name, Jesus, but you neither know Me, nor obey Me, nor honour Me, as I would have you do! Little helpless ones who are yet praying incessantly on the earth, who do know their God, and the awesome power of the Creator of all that is, do not do surgical operations; they simply pray for one another with all petition, seeking healing and I give it to them. See, you have strayed out of the domain of your God's Love; of the Holy, the immutable Will of the Living God!

Little children it is with Sorrow I gaze upon multitudes of the depressed. Some, even many are Baptized unto Me, but they know Me not! You pray to Me as Almighty God, Great Physician, Wonder Counselor, (Is9:6) but so few know Me in this Way. When there is anxiety, fear, anger; any of the- what you would call negative emotions-it is obstructive. The enemy has a heyday with those individuals. Therefore patiently persevering, you shall remain in the Peace of My Presence. Little ones, your Faith and obedience are delightful to your God. Little ones, the encumbrances are but temporary and the release is now! Healing Love is upon you Faithful Missionary. Healing Love is upon you Omen.

Tell My people, that the lack of hope and trust in the atheist, is grievous to the Lord God, and to Our Mother, who weeps copious tears in these times, in these circumstances; whereas those who truly believe in God go forth, even in what you would describe as terminal illnesses, go forth in Faith and hope and trust, and patiently persevere. Because they believe, they are in the embrace of God. In the power of the Holy Spirit it is so! The Mother of God, the Mother of all, is ever attendant upon them. The many who are so very ill in the hospitals, are like starlight to the unbelievers who work with them, and see them and visit them, for My Light is upon those who believe in Me; and even when they are desperately ill, nay, more so when they are desperately ill, My Light is upon them, emanating in them and through them, to those who are about them. Set My people free from the bondages of sin and death I call! Pray little children. In the economy of Our Father's great Design, the prayers and the sacrifices of the faithful, are important! Heaven hears the prayers of the faithful. I reiterate! Even so, all must go according to the Father's Great Design, and conversions are always contingent upon the free will of the individuals for whom you pray. Therefore, persevering prayer is so important. Little ones, I send forth many now, as fishers of men, and I do so in many and varied ways, gathering them back into the Sanctuary of My Heart. I await them with overwhelming Love, each and every one!

I come in Love and Mercy in the Power of the Holy Spirit; through those who believe, I am able to heal whatever affliction befalls persons of Faith, should they approach prayerfully - two or more gathered in My Name, in the Faith which you call the Faith of the Apostles; in total Faith - I want to heal that person. I repeat, when they come to Me, as it were, as dead men - unbaptized, unconsecrated to God, unknowing of God, living outside the Law and the Commandments, do you not see that help is not forthcoming from the Lord your God in these circumstances? Thus, they decide in dismay and confusion, to study science and become gods themselves. Little children, it does not work that way. I ask mankind to come back to Me with all your hearts. Hear Me : I bless, I heal, I cure, I regenerate; for those with deep Faith united in prayers with their brothers and sisters of deep Faith. Even so, little child of God who is injured and gravely ill from whatever cause; I again bless even the unbelieving doctors and scientists to heal My little one. Much of what is happening in the various fields of medicine is not according to My Will; yet My sheep are there. Because of them the blessings flow in spite of the great errors being made.

<u>MY OWN MIRACULOUS HEALING</u> You have been scooped up, out of the death's doorway, and restored to life on earth for Our purposes. Understand? [January 14th, 1998]

*On March 25, 1977, feast of the Annunciation; the Incarnation of our Lord Jesus, I called St. Mary's Cathedral of the Immaculate Conception and asked for a priest to give my baby what in effect was a "Baptism of Intention." The following day my son, diagnosed anencephalic at 38 weeks, died during labour and was baptized John immediately after birth. Less than 24 hours later, I had slipped into coma, first thought to be due to a cerebral haemorrhage but after surgery, attributed to amniotic fluid embolism. Surgery also revealed a clotting defect due to the amniotic fluid embolism. Doctors are notoriously complicated patients - and I certainly was any neurosurgeon's worst nightmare. To be brief, I earned the reputation of "the miracle patient" by surviving the loss of vital signs due to a tentorial herniation in the recovery room. The neurosurgeon (a solid Irish Catholic, by the grace of God, I found out later) was inspired to stick a needle into the incision and suck up the blood which had oozed due to the clotting defect, with the syringe - right there in the recovery room. He was rewarded by the reversal of the tentorial herniation and the return of my vital signs. As he put it to me a few months later when I was complaining about my nominal dysphasia, which he dismissed with a laugh, "I have never seen, nor heard of, nor read of, nor known of **anyone** surviving what you have survived. You were clinically dead!"*

*The miracle had two parts, clinically speaking. The first was the reversal of the tentorial herniation and my revival. The second was that immediately thereafter, I was returned to the O.T. where all attempts were made to stop the bleeding and, in repeated consultation by phone with the Toronto department of Haematology, everything possible was tried to correct the clotting defect - **to no avail.** The neurosurgeon was under pressure to close because of the increasing cerebral oedema. Then, when they had run out of ideas and just standing there watching the ooze continue, my family already warned that I was not expected to survive the night, **it suddenly stopped right before their eyes.** I was a twenty-nine year old third year psychiatric resident, in perfectly good physical health up till then, a prime candidate for organ donation, had the neurosurgeon not been a faithful practicing Catholic as I later found out; and they would have been justified by ordinary clinical criteria; because I would have been AT LEAST 'brain dead' wouldn't I?*

But I believe I would have been in hell; because understanding and practicing my Faith as I do now, I was not in the state of grace when this happened to me - except for that miracle; the all-compassionate, Agape Love of Jesus our Eternal Physician, Wonder- Counselor, Shepherd of His People, our Redeemer, Friend, King of Love and Mercy, Prince of Peace ; our Lord and our God whom we love, adore, praise, glorify, and thank forever! He spared me because He knew what He could make of me, for the sake of the

Salvation of my soul and other souls, whom He would reach through me, and the Glory of His Kingdom! Our Lord was faithful in my case, as He has said; "I would that none of My Own be lost."

For 21 years thereafter I had to take anti-epileptic drugs daily. Then on the 1st April, 1998 I prayed for healing from the epilepsy, which He granted. No drugs and not a twitch since then have I had. He has however, given me this Gift of His Words, to share with fellow physicians for their conversion and salvation.

KINGSTON GENERAL HOSPITAL
CASE HISTORY SHEET

4348 MAR 23 1977 KGN
HALEY DR. RUTH
391 DAYS RD KINGSTON

Interne _____

History:- 30 year old lady presents with a problem of intracranial haemorrhage. She delivered an anencephalic child 36 hours ago, and following an abnormal delivery went into a state of Disseminated intravascular coagulation. At 3-4 A.M. 27.3.77 she complained of a severe headache. At 5 A.M. her level of consciousness deteriorated and at 8 A.M. she was described as having no response to pain.

I saw her at 9.45 A.M.

Restless. Tossing about, moving all 4 limbs, the left side better than the right. She was not obeying commands but withdrew all 4 limbs in response to pain. Neck was stiff.

Cr. Nerves:- Fundi:- Not seen
E.O.M.:- dysconjugate eye movements.

```
                GENERAL HOSPITAL
        CASE HISTORY SHEET              4348 MAR 23 1977 KGH
                                        MELCK DR. RUTH
                                        321 DAYS RD KINGSTON
        Interne                         AGE 30 F AUG 30 1946
                                        DR. S. [?]
```

V - VII   corneals present.
           winces both sides of the
           face in response to pain.

VIII - XII - not tested

motor:-
    mass ✓
    power - slightly weaker (R) side
            otherwise normal + equal
            bilaterally.
    Tone :- normal + equal bilat.

    Coordination :- not tested.

    Reflexes :-   B   + + +   +
                   T   + +   +
                   S   + +   +
                   K   + +   + +
                   A   + +   + +
                   Pl. ↓   ↓

Sensation   withdraws to pain,
            all 4 limbs.

V.S. :-   P. -   90/min.
          BP -   140/80.
          H.S. - normal
          R. -   normal.

CASE HISTORY SHEET
Interne _____

BLOCK DR. RUTH
S-1 DAYS RD KINGSTON
AGE 50 F AUG 30 1946
DR. S. GEORGE

R.S. Trachea Central
Air Entry good
Expansion :- normal
— Scattered Ronchi

C.S. ✓

Pelvis :- see Gyn. notes.

Dx :- Subarachnoid haemorrhage
? Intracerebral haematoma

Angiography showed displacement
upwards and forwards of the
middle cerebral group on the
right side, indicating the presence
of a right-sided temporal lobe
mass. This was felt to be
an haematoma.

She was brought to the
operating room.

AUG 30 1946
DR. ... GEORGE

O.R. — Right Fronto-Temporal craniotomy for removal of haematoma.

The opening was quite satisfactory in that no extensive bleeding was encountered, and all was under control. No intracerebral haematoma or other mass was found.

2 tiny cores of brain were removed by way of exploring the temporal lobe, far mesial above, as well as needling in all directions. Despite this no haematoma was found.

During the surgery oozing from all layers of the craniotomy became impossible to control.

Dr. Wollin came in to see the normal temporal lobe.

Dr. Galbraith came in to help.

```
                HISTORY SHEET                    KILCK DR. RUTH
                                                 321 DAYS BD KINGSTON
                                                 AGE 30 F AUG 30 1946
                Time _____               DR. S. GEORGE
```

...the control of continuous bleeding.

She received 20 units of platelets prior to surgery, and cryoprecipitate afterwards.

Just prior to closing, the brain began to swell rapidly, such that the dura could not be closed. A gelfilm was spread over the brain, and the scalf closed quickly.

Post-op... moved all 4 limbs, the right side much better than the left.

One hour post-op the right pupil enlarged and the left side was hemiplegic. A haemostat was placed under the scalp flap and 40-50 cc of liquid blood came out under pressure. The pupil came down again, only to go up again by both

At surgery during its reopening, its brain was extremely swollen, and each gyrus was distended such that at the end of each capillary, on the crown of the gyrus was seen a subdell haemorrhage.

AGE 30 F AUG 30 1946
DR. S. GEORGE

later

Fresh blood transfused.
Re-opening indicated.

P. Brennan

4.5 hrs   OR Note   Dr Murray / Rankin

Flap re-opened.
200 cc h'toma evacuated (under pressure).
Bleeding stopped c extreme difficulty
Mainly dural edge and skin. Not brain
Brain under some tension
Flap closed in 1 layer over polythine sheet and pridium rinse.

Post-op R.pup.¹ = L   ⊙   ⊙   J.A. Rankin

I.O.:   not breathing spontaneously
        Pupils equal and reacting
        corneals present & equal
        poor oculo-cephalic responses
        no systemic response to
        painful stimulation.

P. Brennan

28.3.77. alert, awake, understands speech, and obeys commands. moved right side this morning and is now moving both sides.

— no evidence of rebleeding.

28.3.77: — alert – awake + oriented! understands speech & obeys commands. moves both sides, right better than left. no evidence of re-bleeding

The pulmonary picture previously described as aspiration has cleared completely — in less than 24 hours.

It is within the bounds of possibility that both the pulmonary cerebral and haematologic pathologies are on the basis of amniotic fluid embolization.

This, however is impossible to prove. This postulate, however, would have to involve embolization through both the right and left sides of the heart, & involve both the pulmonary and cerebral circulations.

P.M.

29.3.77 — The amniotic fluid embolization, though delayed coincided with the development of DIC. I think that one should not have too much difficulty with the venous & arterial emboli in view of the same kind of phenomenon in fat embolization.

— Pt. ext extubated today. Breathing satisfactorily.

— Pt. seems to have a left sided sensory and motor deficit, including an hemianopia.

P.M.

...STON GENERAL HOSPITAL

CASE HISTORY SHEET

Interne ______________

0348 MAR 23 1977 KGH
MELCK DR. RUTH
321 DAYS RD KINGSTON
AGE 30 F AUG 30 1946
DR. S. GEORGE

29.3.77. moving her left side to command!

She does however have dysphasia

She is left-handed and it would appear that the Right hemisphere is the dominant one.

[signature]

ICU

30-7-77 Ok For Floor

Re: Neuro- Rapid Improve, Verbalizing more + ↑ use of L. hand

Re: DIC PT 12 PTT 27 Plt 263,000

No Evid. Bleeding now

Re: Respir. pO_2 146/40% + CXR - Res. of Atelectasis

~~Should be no problem.~~

Re: Post Partum. needs gyn F/u ✓

Abdo soft ē firm Fundus

T38° Bld Cult x2 Strep

Likely 2° Pelvis

→ Pen G 2,000,000 IU q6

[signature] M.D.

...TON GENERAL HOSPITAL

CASE HISTORY SHEET

Interne ______________

4348 MAR 23 1977 KGH
WELCK DR. RUTH
3?1 DAYS RD KINGSTON
AGE 30 F AUG 30 1946
DR. S. GEORGE

31/3/77 Re Cerebral Insult.
Awake & slightly clearer today
Responding to commands.
(L) Inattention
(L) Hemianopsia.
N 3-4+ power in all muscle groups
Called to see Pt as ? re ? seizure.
- clonic movements (L) face, shoulder & slight movement (L) arm.
1/seconds
- Awake & alert throughout.
- Ordered c 100 Dilantin IV
ordered c Try Valium IV.
Plan ↑ Dilantin to 100 mg q6h
Re: Infection

Vag Swab results → Beta Hemolytic Strep
→ ? Strep septicaemia & → DIC.
- c small number of Strep on blood smear
reviews high risk for meningitis
Discussed c Dr Chadwick who suggested
Pen G 5 m units q4h

[signature]

CASE HISTORY SHEET
AGE 30 F AUG 30 1946
DR. E. MURRAY

0708 Continued

- **:8** RT Arm involved in Seizure, just twitching c̄ small amount rigidity for approximately 30 seconds.
- **:20** LT Leg Rigid c̄ Extension Positioning of Toes, rigidity last app. 2 mins. Pupils E and RB. Patient can be aroused between seizures and answering questions appropriately.
- **:25** Dr Anthony attending. IV Dilantin given. Continued to seizure (LT Sided Focal Seizures only) approximately every 5 to 10 mins until 0120 hrs.
- **:** Peripheral IV established LT WRIST.
- **:** IV Valium given — No further Seizures — Twitchings disappeared.
- **:** B/P 120/70 110. Sleeping easily aroused.
- **:20** Patient awake, stated that she knew she was seizuring. Vitals Remain Stable. No further Seizures since Valium given.

E. Grimes RN

1172. See H&R sheet

Focal seizure — activity noted — eyes look to L — twitching L eye to L side of face — lasting 70 sec. Valium given. Pupils Equal, reacting. Drowsy, slow to respond to commands, lethargic. Pt. had 1 min. seizuring later 8-10 minutes later. Lower L leg appeared to jerk approx 7 seconds. Dilantin 250 mg. Pt. alert & oriented. This happened after pt was placed in (head of bed elevated to 45°). Also a focal seizure involving L eye lasted for 7 seconds when placed on her lunch (notify J. Farrell).

Two

9⁰⁰ Refer to Head injury sheet for report on other seizures — both face L & L eyelid twitches, L leg spasm.

Analgesic given × 2 for Headache c̄ good relief.

A living Testimony of My Love is Faithful Missionary. Should she be prevailed upon to speak, she may use these Words. Be not surprised at what is happening. Each one of you who has truly said yes to your God, like unto the Blessed Virgin Mary, their soul becomes like unto a mirror; reflecting My Love, My Truth, upon mankind. I send many more of My instruments to be My Heart, My Hands, My Voice now. Faithful Missionary is but one, and I have given her this singular Mission. Heed My Voice in her. Recognize the sanctity of each God given life. I place My wholesome Life in you; do not deny it to another human. Seeds of destruction of human life are rampant about the earth, yet in the midst of this remains My Light, My Life, My Love. Now is a moment of enlightenment. Open your hearts, your minds, and together with your God, you will readily work great miracles of healing. The vaults of Heaven pour forth the needed enlightenment now. I repeat; *now* is the opportune time. I am your God of Merciful Love. Continue to work in Faith as thou art taught. In the tape I have inspired your friend to show you, there is a Wonderworking power in the Blood of the Lamb. Claim the Precious Blood of your Jesus to heal the individuals spiritually, mentally, emotionally; and in every aspect of their being as they pray, and it is done; and your patients will be healed most rapidly. Do you believe?

Lord, You have given me the gift of healing by the Power of Your Precious Blood, in Your Name! My beloved, My beloved; My Love is upon you; My Peace is upon you. My beloved, the great cures, the great healings will continue. Each of you is anointed in this healing ministry most profoundly. Little children, do not be afraid to pray one at a time whenever necessary, even though united as two or three, the power of the Holy Spirit is profound; and great healings occur. I have anointed Faithful Missionary and the faithful group of prayer warriors, who attend upon the Lord God at this Shrine, to work miracles of Merciful Love. Thus you are here at the call of your God. You pray, "Holy God, Holy Mighty One, Holy Immortal One, have Mercy on us and upon the whole world;" and the Lord God does indeed have Mercy. I bless you in a profound anointing of My Peace, My Love. There is a certain Joy that comes upon you along with this Peace and this Love. My Spirit has been upon you for a long, long time; and thus you have been blest with a heart of Merciful Love which is known to the Lord your God. Now is a moment of sweet surrender, for the Mother of God is holding you to Her Heart, even as she is depicted holding the Christ Child, so she is holding you.

My precious little one, your assignments are manifold. Therefore, make the prayer card as you have described and been inspired to do and be at Peace. You will also be inspired as to who you should give it to, even as you have been inspired in the past as to whom you should speak My Name to - it shall be so! You will just know because I am working in you and through you. You are My Heart, My Hands, My Voice; believe, little one, and be at Peace. Furthermore, We call you into the Light of Our Presence more frequently, during Adoration or at times of prayerfulness; and in these moments We inspire you more profoundly in what We would have you be doing, for there is a unity here now that is most profound and We are able to work with you in total unity of Love. Loving and serving the Lord your God, causes many miracles to happen. You will live to see many, many, miracles... It is happening all about you. Ever thus is the Lord your God, the God of faithfulness! I cause rivers of Light and Enlightenment on those in the profession whom I am calling by name now; and in September, My enlightened ones will be in every nation!

I expressed concerns about practicing within the clinical guidelines for the College, responding to the spiritual needs of my patients, and being faithful to my Mission).. My darling, My darling, I Myself protect you. There is no need for great, prolonged, elaborate prayers. Quietly and unobtrusively, when you discern that it is an appropriate moment, bring in the Name of your Jesus, and I am with you. I Myself will not risk your Providence, your practice. When you are in humble obedience to the Lord your God, you fall profoundly under His Blessing, His Providence, His protection, bringing success to the works of your hands, both in the healing of the sick and in the works of enlightenment which have been assigned to you. Should you feel that you dare not pray over a certain individual, simply praise the Creator of that individual and ask for healing for that individual - spiritually, mentally, emotionally, socially, physically, united with Jesus, and it will suffice. When you shake hands you may say in your heart : 'Jesus heals' or 'in Jesus' Name be healed.' Thus, unobtrusively, a healing will occur, for it is your Faith which causes healing to happen. These wounded ones seek healing most desperately. Your medical profession asks you to heal without Me. How can this be?

<u>Gifted to heal in His Name, in and through the Power of His Precious Blood.</u>

"By faith are the miracles wrought, by faith is the Victory won."(Hb11) I felt powerful waves from Saturday continuously for about two days. On Monday, during Mass when the Gospel was being read, at the words Jesus said to Him: If you are able! All things can be done for the one who believes.' *'I believe; Help my unbelief!'"* (Mark 9: 23-25) *I started to sink and had to cling to the pew, overcome by that same wave of the Power of the Holy Spirit which had continually flowed over me the whole weekend after the anointing on Friday during which I sank to the floor. Will I know who to do this with?* The virtue of Love is such that I, the Lord God, have blest thee, My beloved little sister. I bless thee with Divine Inspirations. Thou hast already attained a great measure of wisdom and I have blest you with an intellect because these Works are imperative and important to the Lord your God and they shall indeed be done in you and through you. As you complete them you will see clearly the whole picture of the Message. When you finish, you will see it as clearly as a stained glass picture. My precious little one, your assignments are manifold. Therefore, make the prayer card as you have described and been inspired to do and be at Peace. You will also be inspired as to who you should give it to, even as you have been inspired in the past as to whom you should speak My Name to - it shall be so*!* You will just know because I am working in you and through you. You are My Heart, My Hands, My Voice; believe, little one, and be at Peace!

CURES ON 21ST ANNIVERSARY OF MY MIRACULOUS CURE.:March 27th,1998.

I was at Eucharistic Adoration on the 26th, praying for various things but as soon as I prayed for a particular woman who I'd heard was seriously ill, our Lord instructed me to go and heal her. I called Omen and DA, and we could only go on the 27th, the 21st anniversary of my own miraculous healing. Jesus please help us.

Your prayers and penances, your times of Adoration, all that you do in your 'yes' to God, is pleasing to God. The Most High God bends an ear and heeds your prayers and pleas little children. That which you ask for the A family for so long, occurs at last. Do not be dismayed or surprised at anything you hear. Simply persevere as you have done in all these months when you heard nothing, and yet My Miracles of Love where working in this family.

As we prayed over the mother, the children were due to come home from school. The boy with epilepsy came running in first, and his mother held him while we prayed over him. **Our Lady said that he was healed of his epilepsy.**

Omen met the mother at Mass and learned that the epileptic boy, 12 years old, whom we had anointed on the 27th March 1998, had started by summer to insist that he no longer wanted medication, which was therefore reduced gradually and on October 18th, Feast of St Luke, he had gone off all medication completely with no recurrence of the epilepsy; Omen called me at work to tell me.

Continue little children, I Myself Bless each one of you; I Bless you with a connective cord with D so you will know what is happening. Light of Living Love for others to perceive, to understand, to comprehend, I give to him indeed. Print this cure! The virtue of Love is such that I the Lord God address thee in this matter. It is and remains Our Will, to heal this child. As you well know, by Faith are the miracles wrought, by Faith is the Victory won- a Faith that leaves no room for doubt, not even a shadow of doubt. The Faith that is present in each of you, is in others not always evidenced. It is at times seemingly even worked against. This is not Our Will. Little children, the many yet operate as it were, on an intellectual and emotional level, and this creates a barrier of obstruction in the Works of Mercy. It is thus that I call all to come into the Peace of My Presence, and then ask for the blessings. That you have learnt this lesson well and pleasingly is known to your God. That it is not so to many others is also known to the Lord your God, Who reads all hearts and souls and minds.

Children's Hospital

CONFIDENTIAL

NEUROLOGY CLINIC

1995 Sep.09

Dr. D. Ou Tim
206 - 250 Keary Street
New Westminster, BC
V3L 5E7

RE: Christopher
UNIT NO: 0873907
DOB: 1985 Aug.03

Dear Dr. Ou Tim,

Christopher was seen for follow-up of seizures on September 7, 1995. Unfortunately, he continues to have seizures, and since I last saw him, he has had 12 seizures in total. However, the family did not contact you or I to inform us of this. He has been on Carbamazepine controlled release 300 mg in the morning, 400 mg in the evening. According to his mother, he has episodes of unprovoked laughter and episodes of unprovoked temper. He remains aware throughout these episodes and has full recollection of them. In terms of his seizures, they have occurred during the day as well as during the night. His mother is also very concerned about the fact that he has pain in his joints without any joint swelling. He has not developed a fever or a rash. The parents are convinced that he has trouble concentrating and keeping focused and that his memory is deteriorating.

On examination, general and neurological exam were normal. In particular, his height was 140.6 cm, weight 29 kg. There was no joint swelling, no rash, and no organomegaly. B/P was 100/60.

Investigations:

I have repeated an ESR, CBC, liver enzymes and Carbamazepine level and the results will be appended.

Impression:

Christopher continues to have uncontrolled seizures. As I mentioned in my previous letter, I thought based on the clinical semiology and the EEG abnormality and normal MRI, that he most likely had benign rolandic epilepsy. However, he is not behaving completely like a benign rolandic patient, and thus I want to assess him further, particularly to determine if there truly are any cognitive difficulties. I have not been able to detect any cognitive difficulties on examination. This child would appear to have very low self-esteem and is quite bothered by his seizures. I am very unhappy with the present degree of seizure control.

I do not know the exact reason for him having joint pains. On reviewing the literature on Carbamazepine, it has been reported in rare instances to cause arthralgia and, thus, I think we should try removing it slowly and replacing it with Clobazam.

09151609.D21

4480 Oak Street, Vancouver, B.C. V6H 3V4 Phone: (604) 875-2345

COPY

Children's Hospital

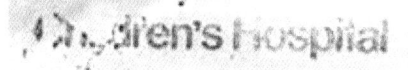

CONFIDENTIAL

Page 2

RE: Christopher
UNIT NO: 0873907

Recommendations:

I have started Christopher on Clobazam 5 mg qhs, increasing by 5 mg at 7 day intervals at up to 10 mg twice daily. When he is on 10 mg twice daily, the dose of Carbamazepine will be decreased by 100 mg at 5 day intervals. I am sending a referral to Dr. Josef Zaide, neuropsychologist, for his opinion on Christopher. I would like to see Christopher for review in about three months with an EEG. I have asked his mother to contact our nurse-clinician in the Seizure Clinic, Cathy Massie to let her know how seizure control is going. I have also asked them to contact you if there are any problems in the interim.

This family is under quite a lot of stress as they have recently taken in 3 of mother's nieces and nephews from the West Indies as their mother died suddenly. So now, the family has a total of 8 children.

Thank you for having me involved with this child. Please do not hesitate to contact me if I can be of assistance.

Yours sincerely,

Mary Connolly

M. Connolly MB, BCh, FRCPC, MRCPI, MRCPUK
Pediatric Neurologist

22/9/95
Date

MC:ad
D: 1995 SEP 09
T: 1995 SEP 15
E: 1995 SEP 20

cc: Dr. C. Thomson, New Westminster — 2006 - 8th Ave. W, V3M 2T5
cc: Dr. M. Connolly
cc: chart

09151609.D21

4480 Oak Street, Vancouver, B.C. V6H 3V4   Phone: (604) 875-2345

COPY

MEDICAL REPORT

Province of British Columbia
Ministry of Finance and Corporate Relations
LOAN ADMINISTRATION BRANCH
1312 Blanshard Street
Victoria, B.C.
V8W 2J1
GENERAL ENQUIRIES: 387-5381

CLIENT NAME: Donna
ACCOUNT NO: 12-013521

Note to Physician:

All information supplied shall be treated as confidential and will be used only by the Ministry of Finance and Corporate Relations as a basis for assessing this individual's repayment capability.

Please be advised that your fees, if any, for completing this form are the responsibility of the patient. The complete form should be returned *directly* to the above address.

Describe the nature of the illness/injury: **Narcolepsy**

When was the illness/injury diagnosed? Y 93 M 11 D 20

Do you consider the illness to be permanent? ☑ YES ☐ NO

In your medical opinion, when would this person be able to return to work? *see below*

Is this illness/disability likely to substantially reduce this person's future earning capacity? ☑ YES ☐ NO

REMARKS

Patient is presently starting to use medication. No improvement noted yet and until symptoms are controlled, she cannot return to her studies.

TREATING PHYSICIAN NAME: C. J. THOMSON
REGISTRATION I.D. NO: 07838 MSP #
TELEPHONE NO: 524 2281

BUSINESS ADDRESS: 2006 - 8th Ave
CITY: New Westminster, B.C.
POSTAL CODE: V3M 2T5

SIGNATURE OF TREATING PHYSICIAN: *Thomson*
DATE SIGNED: Y 94 M 03 D 30

DR. GORDON ROBINSON INC.,
BSc, MD, FRCPC
NEUROLOGY

TELEPHONE: 873-2715

VANCOUVER HOSPITAL
CENTENNIAL PAVILION
855 WEST 12TH AVENUE
VANCOUVER, B.C. V5Z 1M9

May 11, 1995

Dr. C. J. Thomson
2006 - 8th Avenue
New Westminster, B. C.
V3M 2T5

Dear Dr. Thomson:

RE: DONNA

This 39 year old lady was seen on May 9, 1995. Thank you for your note and copies of Dr. Allen's consultations.

This lady comes with a diagnosis of narcolepsy. Her complaints of excessive daytime sleepiness began in the late 1980s during a time she had gone back to university. She noted difficulty maintaining wakefulness in class, even after a few minutes. Medical attention was sought following a motor vehicle accident. By that time daytime sleepiness was pervasive through her life and she had also noted episodes consistent with cataplexy. It is probable that these predated her daytime sleepiness. She has had nothing to suggest hypnagogic hallucinations, sleep fragmentation, or sleep paralysis. She does nap dream. Family history is apparently clear of sleep disorder.

She was initially investigated in New Westminster and then later referred to the UBC Sleep Disorders Clinic. She underwent a multiple sleep latency test, which showed a latency of 5.0 minutes and one episode of REM onset sleep. An overnight recording did not show any other abnormality.

She was started on methylphenidate, initially at 20mg twice a day. She had quite a dramatic improvement but then developed tolerance and has done so on going to 50mg and currently 60mg a day. She is, however, significantly better than prior to treatment.

Her demands upon herself are quite high. She is married and has five children, ages five through sixteen. She works part time as a teaching assistant at a private school fifteen hours a week. Currently she is contemplating going back to school to complete her teaching degree, and will do this a course at a time. She has been able to build in a nap on most days prior to her children coming home from school. She finds she needs two hours to get through the day.

....../2

Dr. C. J. Thomson
RE: Donna
May 11, 1995 --- 2

Her nocturnal sleep is quite long, beginning at 2100 to 2130 hrs and going through usually uninterrupted until 0730 hrs.

Neurological examination found her bright and alert and higher cortical function was normal. Cranial nerve examination showed normal fundi and visual fields. Pupils were normal and extraocular movements were full and free of nystagmus. Facial sensation and power was normal. Tongue and palate was normal.

In her limbs all reflexes were present and symmetrical and toes were downgoing. Muscle power and tone was normal. There were no abnormal movements. Sensation was normal to all modalities. Coordination testing was normal.

Gait including tandem gait was normal.

CONCLUSION

I concur that this lady does have narcolepsy. At the present time she is moderately well treated and it is uncertain as to whether central stimulation will be beneficial any further than currently. I have changed her from methylphenidate to Dexedrine at a dosage of 10mg three times a day. Some patients inexplicably do better on one agent as compared to the other.

I think a major aspect of her problem is her as yet inability to come to terms with her disability. I believe that she continues to think that "mind over matter" or medication will allow her to lead a normal sleep/wake life, fulfilling the high demands on her. I told her I thought that this was unlikely and she is going to have to reconcile this in regard to her lifestyle. She will need to continue judicious use of naps and I have suggested that she strongly consider regular vigorous physical exercise, which also can be helpful. I told her I would be pleased to see her again in two to four weeks for reassessment.

Thank you for asking me to see her.

Yours sincerely,

R. G. Robinson, M.D., F.R.C.P.(C)
RGR:pem

It is entirely pleasing to me; I remind you that by *Faith* are the miracles wrought, by *Faith* is the Victory won! *In every instance it is so!* Continue little children, I Myself Bless each one of you; Light of Living Love for others to perceive, to understand, to comprehend, I give to him indeed. Print this cure! And as a physician you know that they will ask for shall we say backup documents to your claims? And as for the recording of those who have not, as it were, conformed with My Will in responding to you that My Truth of Healing be made known, put a note in that C is well; We await an appropriate response from his mother.

Peace; I thy Spouse, the Living God bless you! My little one, do not be distraught about any of these afflictions. I am attendant upon you. *He gives me the words of St Paul, for I make up in my own body that which was lacking even though nothing was lacking in the Sacrifice of Christ ...'* Little children, you who have said "yes" to the Living God each carry that cross of predilection, and yet I am with you, carrying the brunt of, the main weight of that cross Myself, for you are secure in My embrace. Little children, you recognize the many miracles of healings in those upon whom you have laid hands, and yet like the saints, you carry a certain unity with the Christ, when you are anointed to do this, and so a certain suffering accompanies this He is showing Padre Pio who suffered very, very much. Little children, be not afraid; I am with you.

My little one, co-operate with your physician, but know that I am with you, and I hold you accountable as it were, only to Me, and I Myself, bless your journey. We have a great deal to do together, and it shall be done, My little one. You are here on this earth, and yet in My Embrace, for many years to come. My little one, there are Missions to complete, and there are loved ones to attend to, upon this earth yet a long time and therefore, as ever I bid you, trust Me. I am the Lord your God, supreme among the nations; I know what I am about.

My Love for you, is absolute and eternal. You are My Own. You are cherished of the Lord God and of the Mother of God, and indeed, a goodly number of saints assist you in all the undertakings of your Missions. Even so, I ease the tension, I ease the blood pressure matter. The kidneys, they are strong enough for all that I desire of you, for the rest of your time on earth, which is extensive little one; be at Peace, for nothing is impossible to the Lord your God! On whom I will, I have Mercy; I have Mercy upon thee My little one, in a great anointing of My Love. Be not afraid, I am with you always! *[Our Lord is showing Omen what He told me when I was praying for CH, a victim soul- God has more need of martyrs for the Cause [of Life] on earth, than He has need of angels and saints in Heaven.]* I have carried you through the other times, I will carry you through this time too. My people have forgotten that Eternal Life is in Heaven. There is no fountain of youth upon Earth. It is but a temporary journey. You are called in Holy Scripture to keep your eyes turned towards Heaven your True and Native land. <u>Therefore, the perfection of soul is always the priority</u>. Choosing, in your eyes, that which is the lesser of evils, does not make anything right in the eyes of the Father.

Praying for people with cancer or other chronic, terminal illness. I Jesus, ease her distress. With regard to the woman with cancer, I the Lord your God, attend upon her and I also ease her distress, for Heaven hears the prayers rising up, on behalf of these dear souls. My Mercy encompasses them, My Love encompasses them. My little children, in these instances, see the Holy Spirit Who is Love, indwelling that soul, and encompassing that soul, in Divine Love, as they are in the state of suffering, before they return to Glory.

Simply claiming the Blood of your Jesus is suffice. You may ask that it be instilled in the heart; you may ask that the individual see himself at the foot of the Cross and the Blood of the Lamb bathing away the affliction. By Faith are the miracles wrought, and this month [July] consecrated to the Divine Mercy of My healing Blood and Water pouring forth, it is a good time to instigate this type of prayer hither and yon about the earth to all those who will listen! I am He Who Lives and Loves eternally. I too seek the spiritual healing of My People. I bless them with additional healing as I Will.

The vast River of Light, the power of the Holy Spirit is upon you little children, blessing you profoundly , filling your hearts and souls and minds to overflowing with Love; with the Glory of God! A myriad of blessings is upon you each one. Remember, by Faith are the miracles wrought; by Faith is the Victory won. Little children, working closely with your Mother and Mine, and with your God, you attain a high level of Victory over self. Since I have won the Victory over satan, sin and death, I am at last able to use you as My instruments of Love and Peace. Each one of you is profoundly blest and anointed. Here in My Presence, at the hour of My Mercy, to which I have called you, great graces flow. I bid thee ask of Me what thou wilt. It is My Desire to say yes.

The foe is wrath and does not wish to release her from that which I wish her to be released from. I bless you profoundly; you will be My Heart, My Hands, My Voice; as you lay hands upon her, My Words will address her in and through you for I have trained you in the manner I desire you to be trained and the great graces flow, My beloved, believe and be at Peace. To Omen, Thou art anointed equally, and should I choose to bless A and yourselves with Words they too shall flow. To the other friend; We bid thee strive to accompany this little Mission of Love upon A in the hospital. Mother blesses you.

Jesus : Fall on your knees for the Father attends upon thee now. Most importantly is that you recognize your Creator. *[We pray prone]* Forthwith be at Peace . The Lord your God is attendant upon you now most profoundly. Little children, a blessing anointing in the power of the Holy Spirit is surely yours ; prostrated before your Father, great blessings flow upon you. My littlest loves, I bless you; tell Me that you love Me.

Therefore is your answer ! My little children, you did holy and delightful service in the Name of Jesus through the beloved A, and an all-encompassing Love and charity, embraced the other people in the room ; the elders where given as it were, an anointing in the Light of Christ, at that time of prayerfulness. Thus you were blest and anointed, and the Lord your God does all the rest. Now is a moment of sweet surrender to Love; the Spirit of the Living God anoints you each one yet again. My little children, the prayers prayed in this room , and the anointing of the Living God upon all who attend here, has made this a Holy Place and that it shall remain; and each one of you is blest as you know, to be an instrument of God's Peace. Rest frequently in Me, for I rest in you.

If you wish a more specific direction you may simply say," during Adoration the Lord has anointed me to come to you with a healing anointing, and so , in obedience I come to you in the Name of Jesus, and continue from there. All has gone according to Heaven's Design. Be at Peace in these matters. The great graces have fallen not only upon the beloved A, but on the elders and the visitors, and indeed on the whole hospital, in the binding together hymn in the Name of the Lord. Great graces fell upon the people in the whole hospital both workers and patients and visitors . A certain guest does not *know* what has come over them for they have, as it were, fallen in love with Jesus. Give glory.

In this your confession of Faith in your God more than in the sciences and pseudo- sciences upon the earth now, a great blessing is upon you. Forthwith I name you instruments of My Peace. For that, what you ask of Me at this Hour of My Mercy, I give unto thee. My little ones, do you believe? All lay hands on the sick and they will be healed is it not written?

Therefore I bid thee remain always in My Peace. Little children, when you are in My Peace, you are in My Joy. When you falter a bit, know that it is time to come to Me in prayer and be restored in the Peace of My Presence. When there is anxiety, fear or anger, or any of the, what you would call negative emotions, it is obstructive. The enemy has a heyday with these individuals. Therefore patiently persevering, you shall remain in the Peace of My Presence, and the miracles shall work for you, as you call upon My Name.

Little children, you must be as lighted candles that others, not Christians, not practicing; wanderers; see in you something which draws them to you. They desire to have that which you have. A great wealth; they see that you must have a secret wealth. What you have is the Spirit of the Living God; this is your secret wealth; this is the power of God working in and through you. This is the Power of the Holy Spirit of Love. *He shows that we are like a hand tool, but we are plugged into the power of God and we can be used.* Whither thou goest, I am with thee! It is so for each one of My Own. Let it be so! Healing Love pours forth from the two Hearts of Love, in the power of the Holy Spirit, giving yet greater Glory to God for this miracle of Love. Mighty is the Lord your God.

I Am. I am in the hearts of each one of you gathered here, in My Name. Live in My Light and My Love at all times little children, no matter what is happening about you. Little precious ones, great graces fall upon you each one. Little children, Love conquers all. Continue to love as you do, and be at Peace. I am Jesus and I am attendant upon thee as is Our Mother. As per Our usual procedure, you may speak now; ask of Me what you will. What you carry in your hearts little children is known to Me, and yet I desire that you ask of Me. My little ones, remember that Heaven is your true native land. My little ones it is but a brief separation. The Lord reminds us of John Vanier's words that love and pain are united in the Mystery of God.

Do not be dismayed that you did not see A experience physical healing. All those who laid hands upon A seeking physical healing for her, have been My instruments. I had a great desire for her to come directly into Glory without passing through the purification times between Earth and Heaven. My little ones, each one of you was a small instrument; not necessary, but in a training lesson for each of you including A and her loved ones. She has, in her suffering and in her Faith, so persevered, assisted by the loving hands and hearts and prayers of the faithful, that she has escaped the times of purification. Have I not told you little children, that healing is always first and foremost spiritual?

Tell My people, that the lack of hope and trust in the atheist, is grievous to the Lord God, and to Our Mother, Who weeps copious tears in these times, in these circumstances; whereas those who truly believe in God go forth, even in what you would describe as terminal illnesses, go forth in Faith and Hope and Trust, and patiently persevere. Because they believe, they are in the Embrace of God. In the Power of the Holy Spirit it is so! The Mother of God, the Mother of all, is ever attendant upon them. The many who are so very ill in the hospitals, are like starlight to the unbelievers who work with them, and see them and visit them, for My Light is upon those who believe in Me; and even when they are desperately ill, nay, more so when they are desperately ill, My Light is upon them, emanating in them and through them, to those who are about them. Set My people free from the bondages of sin and death I call!

Pray little children. In the economy of Our Father's great Design, the prayers and the sacrifices of the faithful, are important ! Heaven hears the prayers of the faithful. I reiterate! Even so, all must go according to the Father's Great Design, and conversions are always contingent upon the free will of the individuals for whom you pray. Therefore, persevering prayer is so important. Little ones , I send forth many now, as fishers of men, and I do so in many and varied ways, gathering them back into the Sanctuary of My Heart. I await them with overwhelming Love, each and every one. Has it occurred to you that the parents are in need of a Blessing? Light pouring forth as silver springs surrounds them. We bless them; they are surrounded in Our Light, and all the needed graces, blessings, anointings, providences, for them and their loved ones, are pouring forth upon them to carry them day by day, moment by moment, step by step, throughout their Faith journey. Little children, hold the Name of Jesus ever sacred on your lips and all goes according to Heaven's Design. Little children, I call each of My Own by name now. They are Mine! They come back to Me. I am the Good Shepherd, I seek them out None of My Own are lost. Little children, teach one another to pray this small act of Faith and Love;" I am someone Jesus Loves, I am someone Mary Loves; I am safe in the arms of Jesus, I am safe in the arms of Mary; because it is true! Since you are safe in Our arms, you are safe in Our Hearts, safe in Our Love; what better place to be?

My little ones, whenever you take Our Names prayerfully on your lips We attend upon you, resolving the concerns of your heart, in the Peace of Our Presence where We wish you always to remain. Little ones, you may also pray; "in Jesus Name is My Victory ." This in itself is a powerful prayer. Remember, by virtue of your Baptism, by your Faith, you are named children of faithfulness, children of God, and children of Mary. You are beloved of Jesus and Mary; never forget it! Pray much, but always in Peace, without anxiety, for anxiety is in itself obstructive. Therefore , bring yourself into the Peace of My Presence, and then pray for those of your hearts concern. Love Me and trust Me, and I take care of everything else. Little children, My gift to you is an all-encompassing Love; an overwhelming Love. My little children, you live in the Power of My Peace and My Love; in the power of the Holy Spirit of the Living God. Great graces are poured forth upon you at this time.

I Jesus, bid you take the Hand of your Jesus, in Spirit and Truth; and take the Hand of Our Beloved Mother, and let Us walk together with Joseph, in Faith and hope and trust and Love, in all patient perseverance, for this is My Way, and you are My little sisters, My little brothers, part of the Family, the Family of God, of Peace , of Bethlehem and Nazareth. Even as We speak, I am building a great army of Peace upon the Earth. In the very face of our foe it is happening! Courage is given unto you, for you are truly soldiers of Christ in the great spiritual warfare upon Earth now, for it is indeed a militant Church on Earth. By your prayers you are united to God and to all of Glory, and you are profoundly assisted. Remember little children, no matter what is happening, to those who are united prayerfully with their God, all works out for their good and for the greater Glory of God. Little children, simply rest in the Presence of Jesus, in the Presence of the Prince of Peace, leaving all up to Him!

My little one, I bless you and I give you Peace. Mother and I attend. The majority of those attending will have been enlightened and become aware of the Ingathering which is now in progress. Therefore the many hearts will be opened to the Truth which you bring Faithful Missionary. I Jesus, AM Truth. I have given My beloved little one Omen to understand that the number 7, which you call God's good number, is a symbol of Perfection, and she also understands that the number 6, is the number of imperfection- it is lacking something. The number 666 is therefore severely lacking. Little children, what is lacking in the enemy is Love. What is lacking in those who knowingly and willingly serve him is merciful Love; there is no Charity of Love! Little children those who serve not the Lord God, are therefore in essence seeking aid and mercy from the merciless one ; the one incapable of mercy, the one incapable of Love.

My little children, it behooves you therefore to seek aid from your God Who is Love, and indeed is the Author of Love. Those who proclaim themselves atheists or agnostics, seek to win the victory in a purely scientific mode by reasoning and logic alone, and they are entangling themselves in a quagmire of confusion. How can they extricate themselves? I have given the world many messengers in these times, for example Mother Theresa, who spoke *My Truth, the only Truth.* My people, how many ways can I tell you that I Love you, that I AM Love, that I AM Truth , that I want that which is good for you; and I am forced to stand by and watch you follow the liar, the master of illusion, the darkness. Yet in My Merciful Love, I go forth and draw you out of the darkness and back into My Light. I send many more of My instruments to be My Heart, My Hands, My Voice now. Faithful Missionary is but one, and I have given her this singular Mission. Heed My Voice in her. Recognise the sanctity of each God given Life. I place My wholesome Life in you; do not deny it to another human.

Seeds of destruction of human life are rampant about the earth , yet in the midst of this remains My

Light, My Life, My Love. Now is a moment of Enlightenment. Open your hearts, your minds, and together with your God, you will readily work great miracles of healing. The vaults of Heaven pour forth the needed Enlightenment now. I repeat; *now* is the opportune time. I am your God of Merciful Love. In the testing of one soul, the surrounding souls who love that individual, they too are tested. A great value is upon the suffering of the little one who is My Own, for it causes others conversions and healings, and it brings to the fore, the Power of Faith in Jesus. Little children, you will live to see many miraculous events; curings of cancer and many other diseases said to be incurable, for indeed nothing is impossible to the Lord your God.

Jesus says: "Let it be so; I attend upon these two individuals Myself. I am Your Jesus of Merciful Love. Do you believe, do you believe? The Lord your God attends upon each of these individuals in tender and merciful Love. Mother also attends. A great healing saint attends; Padre Pio. Little children, remain walking in Faith. Do not ask in advance, simply believe. By Faith are the miracles wrought, by Faith is the Victory won! Little children, with your Faith, your love, your compassion, it is as it were, compensation for certain individuals themselves, and certain ones round about them, and since you unite your prayers always with those who have attained the Victory in Heaven, the healings flow. Be at Peace. Continue to pray for each one of these individuals and trust Me. Little children, I remind you, I know what I am about. Little children, all that I Gift unto you, all that I tell unto you, is not only for your own good, but for the good of the many. Multitudes are blest even as you are being blest. Little children; G has a need of much prayer. He has a heart of Love, and a love for Truth. I the Lord God AM Truth. Bless Me, and in blessing Me you are blessing all those whom you have been contacting ; and what seems to be of no avail, suddenly flames out in great growth. Do you believe?

Forthwith, tell Me that you love Me; it is the Lord Who speaks. *My Jesus, I love You; My Saviour and My God, My Redeemer and My King, I adore You!* A living flame of Love We place upon W. We bless you little children, We bless you profoundly. You will hear favourable news. Be at Peace. I am He who is your God, your God of merciful Love. The works of iniquity, the works of the enemy are doused, the flames of hell are doused by the prayers of the faithful. In recompense to the Lord your God, your fastings, your prayers, your penances, work great victories of Love. Indeed they are magnified through the Heart of Our Mother. Now is a moment of sweet surrender to Love. Little children, the blessings are flowing through you; and yet they flow through you to those whom you carry in your hearts, for whom you pray. He asks us to sing 'Bless the Lord My soul, let all that is, give praise to Him; and not forget He is merciful slow to chide; bless the Lord, oh My soul.']Mighty is the Lord your God; you have found favour with the Lord your God and the man is healed! Faithful Missionary, give testimony to this event also !

Indeed little children, lay hands on one another unhesitatingly in My Name, for a headache, for anything; just bless your brothers and sisters, for each one who knows Me with a sincere heart is gifted with a measure of healing Love, for I dwell in that heart and from that heart of Love the healing blessings flow, spiritually, and as you well know, mentally, emotionally, and physically and providentially, in every aspect of their being ; yes sexually for these matters that come to the fore now in these times, they are not of Me; for you know well that sexuality is a clean Gift from God. Were it used thus there would not be so many problems on earth. I assist you little children in the blessing, the cleansing, the purifying of the many. Hosts of angels attend upon you and a goodly number of saints. Saint Ambrose is indeed attendant here at this Shrine of the Mercy Gate of the Immaculate Heart of Mary. Precious little ones prevail; you know well that you are all, each and every one called, to walk in Faith and to step out with a spiritual boldness in Faith, that the healings occur.

I remind you little children once again of the Japanese Faithful who remained faithful for generations until My priests were permitted to return to them and they recognized them. Continue little children, when there are no priests available to study Holy Scripture, to pray the prayers, to live the Traditions, of the people of God, to proclaim the Faith of our Fathers and persevere; this is what Faith is about, and prayerfully heeding the Divine Inspirations ever flowing round about you. Pray and ponder.I Myself attend upon the many, and again, in the Will of your God, you must be instruments in the healing of your brothers and sisters, all you who know Me and have unity of Love with Me. I call you to be healers in My Name, for the suffering ones. You know that some, in My Will, I take Home to Myself; some I heal that they may remain longer in the world in Me, even though they are My Own, for My Own reasons. Little children, love Me and trust Me.He shows us all the technical apparatus that man is using for healing today in the scientific world and saying…I ask you if it is necessary? Some of it works for good, some of it works for harm. If they would ask a blessing from Me upon their undertakings, much, much more good would come upon their works, but they prevail in finite reasoning to do what they do.

Little children, you are as it were, strategic instruments in My Cause, which is Healing Love! I tell you again, I am your Jesus, All Powerful God, Wonder Counselor, Great Physician, and I desire to hold every precious little one to My Heart of Love, even as Mother does, for the Healing of soul and body. My precious little ones, the times in which you are living, have brought distress and unpleasant disorders and diseases to humanity.Let it be as you have spoken;" what I have written, I have written."(cf Jn19:22) Dear little children, in these times in which you are living, many people consider financial compensation to be a means of healing, but alas it is not so; I am the Physician; I am the Counselor.(Is9:6) What healing can be received from the coinage of the day? My poor little ignorant ones, how pathetic they are in seeking not My Healing Love. Am I not the Giver of all Providence?(cf Mt6:25-34) Why don't they trust Me, the Living God? Again, I remind you little children, that lip service is never enough; there must be Faith in every action of the Christian.

Beloved, let the people know that I am God,(cf Ex 14:18) supreme among the nations; that I am the Great Physician, the Healer; that I am Wonder Counselor; I am much, much more, but this is a beginning! Let them know of My Healing Love! I work My Healing Love through those who have been chosen as My Instruments, such as the beloved Padre Pio, the beloved Teresa Neumann[who, as a stigmatist I had been studying this weekend], but there are more! I am the Prince of Peace. I am the Great Physician. The Medicine of God is needed by Humanity, and yet many of them yet shun Me in their free will. My Grace comes upon multitudes, [He shows the ten healed lepers with only one returning to thank Him,[Luke 7:11-19] and this is what We deal with little children. I desire to heal them all; I desire to draw all men unto Me. Those who are My Own are in My Providence.

Do you not call Me the Great Physician, the Healer? (Mk2:17) But you use Me not! Even so, in the Mercy of God, I call the medical profession in particular, and their research scientists, once again to come back to Me with all their hearts. At times, you mention God, or even My Name, Jesus, but you neither know Me, nor obey Me, nor honour Me, as I would have you do. Little helpless ones who are yet praying incessantly on the earth, who do know their God, and the awesome power of the Creator of all that is, do not do surgical operations; they simply pray for one another with all petition, seeking healing and I give it to them. See, you have strayed out of the domain of your God's Love; of the Holy, the immutable Will of the Living God.

It is I your God Who opens eyes, opens ears, opens hearts. It is I who am the Great Physician, Wonder Counselor, Shepherd of My People, My chosen ones.(Is 9:6) Raphael holds a crystal clear liquid in one hand. He is a magnificent Angel of Light. Since he is Medicine-of-God, he destroys the disease-causing demons; causing conflict, poison and venom upon My suffering people. I Myself will give you Faithful Missionary, the complete vision of the great Raphael. (cf Tb chapters 5-12)It must be recognized, the ethical procedures of the physician; tell the little ones, I am the Great Physician. Am I not Wonder-Counselor,(Is9:6) and am I not with you always little children? (Mt28:20)Little children, see in this people the power of prayer for the healing of sufferings.(cf Jm5:13-14) Would that the medical profession would work more closely with the Healing Power of prayer which I have given to My little faithful ones. I am your Jesus, Mighty God, Great Physician, Wonder Counselor.(cf Is 9:6) Through these little children I shall call many back to Me. bless Me.

MARY: *Do thou little children, remain faithful to Jesus, that His wondrous plans for you all come to fruition. His Name is Wonder-Counselor; seek Him, seek Him in all your needs. Come to the Lord little children, Who desires only that which is good for you. Little children, by virtue of your Baptism, even though you are in the world, you are not of the world. Stay prayerfully united with your Jesus!Mother blesses you child, Mother blesses you child. Beautiful children, beautiful little souls, ever kneeling and praying before the Lord our God, blessings flow in you and through you When the action of the Holy Spirit is upon you, the Lord Jesus and I your Heavenly Mother, work in conjunction with each of Our Own little ones on earth. At every moment when one feels the presence of the Holy Spirit, it is good to give praise, and also to listen, and in the quietness of your own heart you are inspired what it is the Lord would have you do. Therefore, simply remain at Peace as your heart sings glory, in the Presence of the Almighty. Little child, you are profoundly blest in being empowered to attain this level of Faith, which brings sanctity to the children of God.*

Little children, remember the Words in Scripture," By Faith are the miracles wrought, by Faith is your own victory won. " By Faith is the Victory of assisting others won. Little one, since you are fully aware of the moment when the Holy Spirit is attendant upon you, it behooves you to be continuously giving Glory to the Father each in your own way, as so many little song birds before your God. The Virgin of Fatima blesses you; a profound anointing is indeed upon you. In the Name of Jesus the enemy is in complete rebuke and is not present! Mother attends upon each of them, dear little children; Our God is Mercy and Love, beyond all human imaginings. Little children, oftentimes the lingering sufferings cause the individual to draw closer to the Lord, to be so purified in the trials that they are ready to ascend into Glory. Many there are who do not attain sufficient purification, and as you know, they must be taken for a time of purification and this occurs also. So My little children that is why you are called, when in illness, to embrace that cross, because it is a sure means of purification in bringing you into the Presence of the Living God in a joyful state of soul! Little children, when your loved ones are on the sick bed, simply love them and pray for them as you do; and trust in the Lord. He knows the better Way. He has a plan for each soul. In His Merciful Love, all that is occurring with your Mother , is according to Heaven's plan. Continue to pray much Thanksgiving for the healing gifts in advance of their receipt is delightfully pleasing to the Lord Your God Who indeed has said, ask believing it is done and it is already done, for when you ask it is done in Heaven and it is already before Our eyes in Heaven once the Lord has acceded to Your prayer requests. Thus as you praise Him in advance these prayers are magnified, and fall back as graces upon the needy upon earth. It is a reciprocal Love between God and Man, and Man and God; which is accomplished in Jesus Our Lord.

Mother Mary, the Virgin of Fatima is present. Little children, I am Mother of Jesus and Mother of all, for you were given to Me at the foot of the Cross of Calvary and you are My Own dear children. Each one of you, I comfort and console, caress and and bless. I dry your tears. My little children, each one of you has a great Guardian Angel, ever attendant upon you. It behooves you to address your Angel prayerfully morning and evening, for each Guardian Angel has a mission; you dear child, are that mission. Your Angel holds you safe in the pathway of holiness, whispering Divine Inspirations into your thoughts that you will know and do the Will of God. My little children, I hold each one of you to My Heart, immersing you in My Love, in the depth of My Heart of Love, in the Wellspring of Love; and the Holy Spirit anoints you each one , surrounding you in the Light pouring forth from glory, surrounding you in the Light of Jesus Our Lord, Who is ever with you.

Little children, by virtue of your Baptism, even though you are in the world, you are not of the world. Stay prayerfully united with your Jesus! My little children, you are blest. The Lord God has seen fit to choose each of you, you among the many peoples of the world, as His instruments in this time of trial, this time of the great ingathering which is occurring upon the earth now. We ask you to never feel fear, for thou art strengthened to do the merciful works of Love, to be the instruments, of the Lord Our God; to be the Hearts, the hands, the Voice of the Saviour of mankind. How anointed you are My little ones; to be as it were handpicked for these missions which are upon you. My darling children, though you work together and are bonded together, in the Body and Blood of Christ, in the faith of the Apostles as you pray, you are yet unique, each having a unique mission in the works of Mercy.

How He will use each one of you now is in a rather intense manner, for time is of the essence, though it be God's time and not your time. Yet the timing is important to your God. Do not be anxious about time. All goes according to Heaven's Design, for each one of you have surrendered in all abandonment to the Lord your God, and it is thus that He is using you. My little ones, in this close union with your God, great things happen. My little ones, believe and be at Peace. My little ones, ask of your God and of your Heavenly Mother what you will. An anointing of great grace is upon you even as We speak. Little child, the saint who assists you in this work is known as Saint Luke, is he not? We bless you in and through Saint Luke in this work and We bid you recall that Jesus, the Great Physician Himself, is profoundly assisting you. Little children, the wages of sin is death - death of the soul;(Rm 5:12; 6:23) so perilously close to some of you. Speak out at any and every given opportunity against this culture of death!

Wisdom:13-18. What man indeed can know the intentions of God? Who can divine the will of the Lord? The reasonings of mortals are unsure, and our intentions unstable; for a perishable body presses down the soul, and this tent of clay weighs down the teeming mind. It is hard enough for us to work out what is on earth, laborious to know what lies within our reach; who, then, can discover what is in the heavens? As for Your intention, who could have learnt it, had You not granted Wisdom, and sent Your Holy Spirit from above? Thus have the paths of those on earth been straightened and men been taught what please You, and saved, by Wisdom.

CHAPTER TWENTY ONE
PEACE IN HIS PRESENCE!

JESUS:

Expound upon mankind little children, that I am God! There is no other; none other! I Jesus bless you, My small sister. I Myself carry your cross. I Myself take all your woundedness, uniting it with Mine. Be not worried, therefore, when harsh words are hurled against you. They fall on your Jesus like so many whiplashes and they are no more, even the most recent ones. Live in this present moment, that is the only place to be - in My Embrace in the present moment. Little sister, you are strengthened to a great fortitude. I have much need of your assistance, I have chosen you to be My Heart, My Hands, My Voice. Speak out boldly in the Name of Jesus, for I am with you always. Even as We speak, I bless you as a river now of prayerfulness, infilling you with My Love and Peace; with Joy in the Love of the Lord. Be not anxious therefore, the day will surely come, when you will understand all things, and why these many trials have had to be.

Little sister, hold My hand, it is your Jesus who speaks; and hold Mother's hand. Let Us walk together with Our beloved Joseph, in Faith and Hope and Trust and Love and patient perseverance. You are part of My Family, the Family of God, of Bethlehem, of Nazareth, the great Family of Peace which I am building up upon the Earth. Despite news to the contrary, the Family of Peace is being built up, one might say right under the noses of the enemy. In the face of the enemy it is being built, and they are yet unaware of it. My little one, you are named "child of faithfulness", child of God and child of Mary, for I have called you by name; you are Mine. You are beloved of Jesus, beloved of Mary, continue to take Our Names prayerfully on your lips and We are with you, resolving the concerns of your heart in the Peace of Our Presence. My little one, pray as you do; it is pleasing to the Lord your God. Do not be anxious about anyone or anything. Stay always in My Presence. Anxiety obstructs, one might say, the pathway.

Love Me, trust Me, for I Love you most tenderly, most totally and eternally. I am with you. Surrender Me your love. I am Jesus and I do all the rest! Believe! Continue to rest prayerfully in My Presence. Many great prayers are not necessary at all times. Just *Be* with Me, *Be* with your Jesus. *Be* with Me in the Church, at the Tabernacle and before the Monstrance; and yes, *be* with Me in spirit - wither thou goest I am with you. United with Me there is nothing to fear, for I am with you. By Faith are the miracles wrought, by Faith is the Victory won! Know this: where you go, silver springs of Light flow constantly, as they are deflected from Heaven, the Holy City, so therefore, falling upon each one of My faithful little ones. Rejoice, My Victory is at hand. The virtue of Love is such that the Lord your God is present. The enemy would taint you at every opportunity. Stay always in the Presence of your Jesus. That is why I am giving you lessons in holding your armour secure about you and not opening it up to react to negative emotions but stay always in the Joy of the Presence of the Living God - and teaching your brothers and sisters to do likewise.

It is a self-discipline - all you who have dedicated yourselves to the Living God, through the Immaculate Heart of Mary, are called to be masters and stewards of your own body and mind. It entails much mastery of your thoughts, words and deeds. The enemy loves to trick you. We bless you with the necessary wisdom, understanding and forthrightness to train your brothers and sisters in this area of purity. Love conquers all. Therefore, remain ever in My Peace, and let the action of the Holy Spirit flow in you, through you to those whom We place in your presence. Those who attend have been called to the meeting by the Lord God. Those who hear have their ears opened by the Lord God. Do not worry about anything else. I Myself address them for the hour is late, and it is time now for the changes of heart to begin. They do begin in rapid sequence.

Little children, realize that the Way of Christ, the Way of Peace, is not of the world. The energy, and the cumbersome weight of the world is obstructive to the Will of God. As it is flowing through the little faithful ones, you'll realize, let us say, the intellect of a doctor is at times obstructive to the free flow of the Holy Spirit. Thus there are delays! Even so, pray for each and every person who will be there. Place them on the altar at My Feet, and believe. I work My Own miracles of conversion in the hearts of the many. All that happens is, as it were step by step, expanding exponentially. Little children, be not distraught, come now into the Peace of My Presence. My little ones, when you come to Me as the Holy Infant of Prague, as the Holy infant in Bethlehem, it is pleasing to Me. When you come to Me at the foot of the Cross, it is pleasing to Me. My little ones, Mother is in tears of joy at your Faith, your persevering Faith despite all the obstacles. Little ones, your prayers are pleasing to God; your times in Adoration; all that you do in the Light of My Love brings blessings upon many upon Earth. This is something My little ones are not aware of but will only become aware of on that Great Day.

Ask of Me what you will. When you want testimonials of any sort, ask Me and the power of the Holy Spirit to be with you where I am, and together we write the Words! I Myself speak to you as you well know, in Divine Inspirations, and a Word here and there, for I am with you My little one, pray as you do; it is pleasing to the Lord your God. Do not be anxious about anyone or anything. Stay always in My Presence. Anxiety obstructs, one might say, the pathway. Mighty, mighty is the Lord your God! We bless thee. We wish you to be at one with your Lord at this time of trial which is upon you. Remain humble and obedient and in utter abandonment to the Will of God. Little, children, in the hush of the woods, the forest, a leaf flutters down, and the Lord knows it; and it is not disruptive but good for the forest. Little children, every moment, every movement, every action, about each one of My Own, is known to the Lord your God. Some of it is directly motivated by the Lord God , for I am the God Who is all-seeing, all-knowing. All powerful is the Lord your God. Little children, just rest in My Presence, without anxiety or fear. Stress is not of Me, anxiety is not of Me, fear is not of Me. Peace is of Me.

Pray much, but always in Peace, without anxiety, for anxiety is in itself obstructive. Therefore, bring yourself into the Peace of My Presence , and then pray for those of your hearts concern. Love Me and trust Me, and I take care of everything else. Little children, My gift to you is an all-encompassing Love; an overwhelming Love. My little children, you live in the power of My Peace and My Love; in the power of the Holy Spirit of the Living God. Great graces are poured forth upon you at this time. Immeasurable are the great graces being poured upon you, and not only you, but the faithful cohort who gather here prayerfully in the Name of Jesus and Mary. A great and Holy Light is upon you, My people. I bid you Peace, I give unto you the Peace Of Christ, the Peace that surpasses all human understanding, the Peace that only I your Jesus, the Prince of Peace, can give, I give to you - that is always accompanied by the Joy and the Love of the Lord; and I bless you with a profound anointing of Love. Keep your eyes upon Jesus; hold the Names of Jesus and Mary on you lips. Sanctuary is in the Hearts of Love!

As for your Mission ; it is in the Hands of your Jesus, and blest in the great graces from your Heavenly Mother; and all is going according to Heaven's Design. I take away for sure, any slightest traces, any signs of anxiety; for you shall work ever in the Peace of My Presence. It is in this your Faith and your surrender, that My great anointing of Peace is ever upon you. Trust your Jesus and be at Peace. The Virgin Herself works side by side with you little one, you are never alone. A great Light is ever attendant upon you. The priest who is called M has a name in Heaven that is most pleasing to the Lord God and he dwells always in Peace, as I have prescribed for each of My Own to dwell always in the Peace of My Presence. I have taken away all your anxieties and concerns and ask you to remain therefore always in the Peace of My Presence. Here in My Presence, at the hour of My Mercy, to which I have called you, great graces flow. I bid thee ask of Me what thou wilt. It is My desire to say yes.

Prevail in Faith little children; have I not told you would live to see many victories in My Name? Little children, as is written in Holy Scripture, each one of you is tested as gold in the fire of purification, and in this testing profoundly, a great Fortitude , a great courage is given unto you, for you are truly soldiers of Christ in the great spiritual warfare upon Earth now, for it is indeed a militant Church on Earth. By your prayers you are united to God and to all of Glory, and you are profoundly assisted. Remember little children, no matter what is happening, to those who are united prayerfully with their God, all works out for their good and for the greater glory of God. Little children, simply rest in the Presence of Jesus, in the Presence of the Prince of Peace, leaving all up to Him! While you are resting in Our Presence many actions of the Holy Spirit are occurring in your lives and the lives of those whom you carry in your heart. Teach one another to pray as you contemplate the Mystery and the Inspirations given over to you then the recurrent words of the angelic salute [Hail Mary] become background music to the scene which you are contemplating, even beholding in your mind, and the Peace of Christ comes upon you, for where two or more are gathered in My Name, it is written, it is so.

My little one, rest as you do often in the Peace of My Presence, giving over all your hearts concerns to Me, for it is in this total abandonment to Love; I the Lord God Am Love; that you begin to work the many miracles of Love, the conversions of hearts and souls and minds, that I desire you to work. Stay as you are; never disappointed, never discouraged, but ever going forward; plodding on, in Faith and hope and trust and Love and patient perseverance. This is the very story of the saints is it not? It is your story too little one. As We gaze upon those whom you carry in your hearts little children, and see their trials and agonies, in Our great Mercy, We lift their suffering, We take away pain, We bless them with the Peace of Our Presence. Some return Home quickly now; others remain yet with their loved ones and healing occurs.

Child of God, love your Jesus, trust your Jesus and be at Peace, and in your" yes "to God, I take care of everything else, for you live in the Power of My Peace and My Love, in the Power of the Holy Spirit of the Living God. Do not be afraid to come unto Me prayerfully at the Mass, or Tabernacle or before the Monstrance in My Presence. Ask of Me what you will, and by Divine Inspiration, I respond to you; besides which, in this one- on -one relationship, My healing Light is radiating out upon you ; and in you and through you to the many. Little children, this is the Way, the Key of holiness. I give to My little ones every one, this small act of Love. Pray it until it is a song in your Heart; until it becomes like a passport to walk anywhere on the earth, for the earth is the Lord's, and the fullness thereof, and you are My Own, and to bring you ultimately into the Glory of My Presence in Heaven. It is easy enough for the youngest child to learn, and powerful enough to bring you into the Sanctuary of the Hearts that Love you so!" I am someone Jesus Loves, I am someone Mary Loves. I am safe in the Arms of Jesus, I am safe in the Arms of Mary." When you invoke Our Names prayerfully We attend upon you, resolving the concerns of your heart, in the Peace of Our Presence where We wish you always to remain.

Children, when you have decisions to make, spend time in the Peace of the Lord's Presence praying; and in that Peace of His Presence, make a decision. Pray and act, and the Lord is with you. Unhampered are the actions of those who are truly abandoned to the Will of the Living God. This does not mean that there is no testing or no trials, but that the Lord is profoundly with you, and all falls into place in due course!

Children, be not afraid to invoke the Name of Jesus and the Name of Mary for assistance . We attend upon you always and more immediately at moments of stress or distress, that you remain always at Peace. Therefore little children, at moments of stress or distress, when fear, hatred, anger, anxiety; any of these emotions, temptations rise up in your hearts; before you speak out words you may regret, or take any action which is not prudent, firstly pray this prayer, calling on Us, that you remain always in Our Peace. There must be Peace in each human heart and in each home and in each parish, then the Peace of Christ will spread like wild fire, throughout the world. In the power of the Holy Spirit it is so; and it shall be so!

Little children, pray much; your prayers are pleasing to the Lord your God. Remember little children, that Heaven hears the prayers of the faithful. It is always Our Desire to say yes to Our precious little ones. Even so it must be according to the Fathers great Design, and be for the good of the souls concerned, and it is always contingent upon the free will of those for whom you pray. Therefore persevering prayer is so essential. We come to you, We attend upon you, resolving the concerns of your heart in the Peace of Our Presence. Ameliorated is this affliction which is upon you. I am your Merciful Jesus. The Peace of Christ is yours. Gone is that which has taunted you for a long time obstructing you from coming fully into My Presence. My little brother/sister talk to Me often; for prayer is talking to your God. Walk always in Faith and trust, and thus you are in unity with Me; and I take care of every aspect of your being; for thus you live in the power of My Peace and My Love; in the Power of the Holy Spirit, of the Living God. Great graces accrue upon you now, for Heaven hears the prayers of the faithful. By Faith are the miracles wrought; by Faith is the Victory won. Little children; love one another like this always.

Little children, simply rest in the Presence of Jesus, in the Presence of the Prince of Peace, leaving all up to Him! Whenever you take Our Names prayerfully on your lips We attend upon you, resolving the concerns of Our Hearts in the Peace of Our Presence. Little children, you are called now to walk in the Light that the darkness be no more. Pray, it is pleasing to your Father in Heaven; Love your Jesus and trust Your Jesus and in this your surrender to Love, echoing The Virgin and the beloved St Joseph and the myriads of saints who have gone before you, I your God take care of everything else, for thus you live in the Power of My Peace and My Love. Little children, I love you most tenderly, most totally and most eternally. Tell your Jesus you love Him sometimes and be at Peace. I take care of everything else, for you live in the Power of the Holy Spirit, in the Power of My Peace. It is now a moment of sweet surrender to Love. I am your Jesus of Merciful Love, I attend upon thee in a profound anointing of My Love. Your success is before My Eyes. Be at Peace in this matter. Do not doubt. Believe! I have plans for you, for your good, and the good of all those whom I set in your pathway of life. Believe. It shall be so: and be at Peace. Mighty is the Lord your God. If today you hear My voice, harden not your heart !

Therefore be at Peace. I bless thee; I am your Jesus of Merciful Love. Having come into the Light of My Presence, I bless you; I am with you; I carry your cross; I hold you to My Heart. In all these testings and trials I am with thee. My little one, persevere, I am with thee. In My Light and My Love , you shall succeed in your endeavors.I attend you most tenderly little children; your love, your unity with Me is known. Mother is in tears of Joy at your pleadings here, and now together We work the necessary formula, to cause others to come into the Light and attend upon Love, that they all may know the reciprocal Love which awaits them. Be at Peace; trust Me! My darling, tell My people that it is the Will of God, that each soul unite with Me in a total union of Love, that I may flood them with My Love and My Peace and My Joy! Tell them again, 'seek Me where I am!' I am most profoundly present to My people the children of God, in the Bread and Wine of My Love, in the Holy Eucharist; for My Flesh is real flesh, and My Blood is real blood, in the Consecration of the Mass.

Little children, countless saints know this fact; countless members of the priesthood, most indeed know this! Many, many of the faithful on the Earth today indeed know this, and yet there are those who close themselves, separate themselves from Me! It is true; I am present to each of you in the Power of My Spirit, the Holy Spirit, but I am more powerfully, shall We say most assuredly present; to be molded, molded and fashioned like Me, take and eat the Food and Drink that I give to you! It is thus that you become truly like Me. My little ones, continue as you are doing in your prayers and in your Adorations, in your constant attendance upon Your Jesus and you beloved Mother; this is pleasing to the Lord Your God. But of course We send more, because you have acted in Faith little ones, and I do not deny you the fruits of your labour, the fruits of your prayers. Continue as you are doing and trust Me! <u>ALL COME UNTO ME!</u>

I send Michael to attend upon the spiritual warfare involved in the Adoration Chapel and I send Joseph to watch over the Christ, for he is ever the Guardian of holiness and purity. Again, the people begin to come back and adore! [Our Lord gave us the parable about the ten lepers and only one came back to say thanks.] Heaven is present, ask what you will. I am the Lord Your God. I hear your pleading, I hear your love, I hear your compassion. I have permitted you to discern the division in My Church which is not pleasing to Me. My Church is attacked on every possible front in these times, but there is one staunch shepherd in My Name, John Paul, who as you know is yielded to Our Mother, the Woman Clothed with the Sun; the One Who crushes the enemy's head; and I ask you to stay, like him, united with him, in all surrender, to the Love of God, and in all tender loving abandonment, to the Love of Our Mother. This is My Way; let it be your Way as well. Little children, do not worry about those who have permitted themselves to go astray.

Those who are My Own come back to Me wholeheartedly. Those who do not come back to Me, were never Mine, to their sorrow and ruin, and to My Sorrow. I ask you little children, to abide with Me as you do, in My Presence in the Mass, in the shrine, [Adoration Chapel] and as you go about your days, for truly I am with you. As you know, the Lord your God indwells the hearts of those who are truly abandoned unto their God, such as you. Therefore, do not be dismayed at all that is occurring; simply persevere; continue in all-patient perseverance, enduring all things in My Name. Much Heavenly assistance is given to you and the true Body of Christ upon Earth. The works of iniquity prevail yet a little longer. I strengthen you, My Power comes profoundly upon each and every one who is truly My Own. You will readily know, you will instantly recognize the wolves in sheep's clothing, for I gift you to recognize them, that you are not be wary of everyone that you meet. Your very soul, and your guardian angel will allow you to know. You may call it Divine Inspiration, or intuition, or some such thing, but it is the Lord God permitting you to know, that your armour remain always intact; and I teach My little ones, when you come upon such a one who is seemingly one of you, but causes distress and obstruction and destruction, these fruits are not of Me, pray for that one, but do not become overly emotional about it; simply claim your place in Our Hearts and be at Peace. It is the Peace during these moments that is powerful in the conversion of the many.

Dear little children, persevere in all prayerfulness and be at Peace. Attendant upon this conversation, is your God; your Triune God, and the Mother of God, and a myriad of angels and saints. Attendance at Adoration shall indeed increase, and do so rapidly now, for Heaven hears the prayers of you precious little ones. Your request is answered with a resounding YES! Dear little ones, simply pray much and continue to adore, and Trust Me in these matters. We shall succeed in this enterprise. Multitudes will begin to adore at last. It shall come to pass that a yet greater miracle occurs that does indeed draw many, many people back to Me with all their hearts. Little children, persevere in all prayerfulness. There are many who attend upon Me at the Tabernacle in all sincerity of love, and in this Loves union, your God cannot resist but pour forth Blessings. Therefore, be not surprised when yet greater miracles occur. I Bless you little children, for your part in all that is occurring. There is a great sign occurring in My Body and Blood in the Eucharist which will become known throughout the world, and a vivified Church is at last before My Eyes. Believe little children; you are partakers of a vast miracle. Loving Mercy is outreaching to all. There are those who have bodily hungers and needs, but the majority have a great spiritual hunger which I, the Lord, would fill at this time. I would assuage the anguish of the souls so in need of comforting Love. Continue to speak out in the Name of Jesus. In so doing you are living all that has been asked of you little children. You are Faith filled children; there are many who have scant Faith and are in sore need of a deepening of Faith.

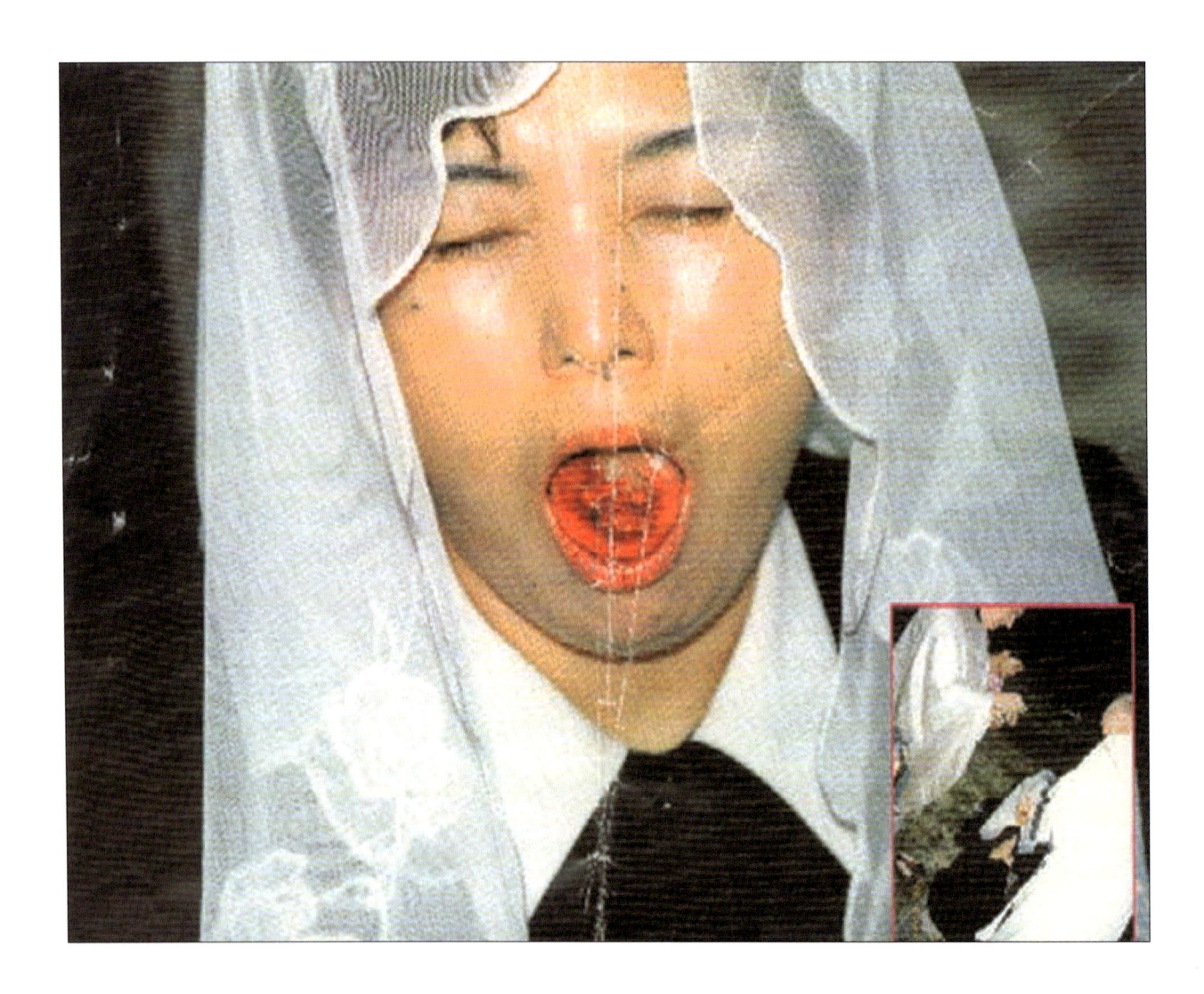

Eucharistic Miracle at Naju, Korea

BISHOP ROMAN DANYLAK, Apostolic Administrator of the Eparchy of Toronto for Ukrainian Catholics in Toronto, Canada, and titular bishop of Nyssa, herewith solemnly testify that I concelebrated the Divine Liturgy or Holy Mass, with the Reverend Fathers Aloysius Chang, parish priest of the Kwangju Archdiocese in Korea, invited by me to assist during my visit to Korea, and Joseph Peter Finn, retired priest of the London Diocese in Ontario on Friday, September 22, 1995, at 5 p.m. in an open-air celebration on the grounds of the valley where a future church is to be erected, God-willing, to the honour of the Blessed Virgin Mary and Mother of God.

Following the Liturgy of the Word, I delivered a brief homily for the occasion. After the communion of the priests, Fr. Chang and I administered Holy Eucharist under both species to Julia Kim and the eleven others. As we continued to distribute Holy Communion to the others present, we heard the sudden sobbing of one of the women assisting at Mass. The Sacred Host received by Julia Kim was changed to living flesh and blood. Fr. Joseph Finn, who had remained at the altar during the communion of the faithful, was observing Julia; he noted that at the moment he turned to observe Julia, he saw the white edge of the host disappearing, and changing into the substance of living flesh.

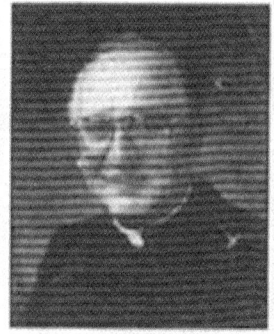

Fr. Chang and I returned to Julia. The Host had changed to dark red, living flesh and blood was flowing from it. After Mass, Julia shared with us that she experienced the Divine Flesh as a thick consistency and a copious flowing of blood, more so than on the occasion of previous miracles of the changing of the host into bleeding flesh. We remained in silence and prayer; all present had the opportunity of viewing and venerating the miraculous Host. After some moments I asked Julia to swallow and consume the Host. And after the Mass Julia explained that the Host had become large and fleshy; and that she consumed it with some difficulty. The taste of blood remained in her mouth for some time. I then asked that she be given a glass of water, from the miraculous source of water nearby. As she drank the water, her finger touched her lips, and a trace of blood was visible on her finger. She rinsed her finger in the water and drank it.

In testimony of this, I append my signature, together with the signatures of all the witnesses present. *Dated at Naju, this twenty-second day of September, 1995.*

+ **Roman Danylak, titular Bishop of Nyssa, Apostolic Administrator, Eparchy of Toronto, Canada.**

Joseph P. Finn, St. Peter's Cathedral Basilica, London, Ontario, Canada, et al. (Korean signatures of others present)

Soon they will experience an Enlightenment and have a great hunger, a great thirst to draw near the Bread of Life. Mankind is ever seeking a sign of My Existence, a sign of My Presence with them. The beloved John Paul is himself a great sign. Even so, I will cause specific signs to occur on the Earth, to melt the hearts of many, to take away disbelief, to cause people to know that I am your God, that I am Mercy, that I am Love.

The Hand of My Justice is stayed yet a little longer because of My Love for Humanity. Continue to be lights along the way for the many weary travelers on Earth who walk yet in darkness not aware of the Light of My Presence. Speak to Me of Love. I shall pour out My Spirit upon all Mankind and they shall Live. The constancy of Love is here. When you come together as you do, in My Name, I am infilling your hearts and souls and minds with all that you need to carry on in all perseverance. You are waiting on Me at this time. Simply rest in the Peace of My Presence in regard to this matter. Continue to wait on the swift sure actions of your God, for I am with You always.

My darling I attend upon you and each precious little one of Faith. The miracle of the Eucharist does indeed appear in due course. Little children persevere in all prayerfulness invoking this miracle to occur. By Faith are the miracles wrought, by Faith is the Victory won. Little children a great Blessing comes upon your little parish Church for those Faith-filled individuals. Bear with Me patiently little one. Beloved little children, soon! In your time, soon. Have I not told you the world will be turned upside down after the 6th January, 2001; beginning immediately after the 6th. Nine. [our Lord says nine frequently to confirm we are praying for the right things. Like a nine day novena.] *You are busy Lord*! Counting My sheep! Ask not; wait and see! You shall see miracles of Love dearest children. My Love for My little faithful ones is so profound as to be unspeakable, for words in the human tongues cannot contain it. My little ones, rejoice in Our Love's union and be at Peace. The Rock of Ages bids thee Peace. Do not be distraught: We Bless the child with many rosaries. They are not all identical little children . Their beauty lies in the hands of those who touch them prayerfully, proclaiming the mysteries of Love. Be at Peace little ones. Do not be surprised at the events which are about to occur.

Little children, I am the Lord Your God; I am tenderly attendant upon each one of you. My little children, My little Faith-filled ones, the more you pray and act in Faith, the greater the increase of Faith in you, and thus you will see more healing events; a myriad of miracles you might say. You seek a recognizable miracle of the Holy Eucharist and it shall come to pass. It is not yet but it is not far off. Little children, continue to pray. The Eucharistic Miracle is powerful, but the little miracles of Healing Love are also powerful in the matter of winning souls over to Salvation, and that's what it is all about My little evangelizers. As you adore you yourselves are healed, and as you adore further, Healing Love comes upon those who are so needy of My Merciful Love. Little children, persevere! Little children, when you come before Me in Adoration, sharing all of your hearts concerns for Me, I tenderly Bless you and assist you and those for whom you pray. Always you know that those in free will, who have not yet yielded to Me, are in need of much prayer, that there will be a movement from each heart to open up to Love.

I the Lord God, Delight in your hours of Adoration; I do not take any such hour lightly. Know that each hour of Adoration bears far greater fruit than you can recognize, for few there are who put in an hour of Adoration, and many there are in the world so in need of My Merciful Love. Little children, you cause by your Faith, this River of Light and Love and Life to pour forth upon the needy ones, and the more you abandon your hearts to Divine Love in My Holy Will for each one of you, the greater the River of Faith which is being poured out upon the earth. Little children, My Delight is in your Faith, and I Bless you and remind you that I Love each one of you most tenderly, most totally and eternally, and My Plans for you and the good of your neighbors shall come to pass, because you are Faith-filled and obedient and humble before the God of all Creation.

Little children, as is written in Holy Scripture, each one of you is tested as gold in the fire of purification, and in this testing profoundly, a great fortitude , a great courage is given unto you, for you are truly soldiers of Christ in the great spiritual warfare upon Earth now, for it is indeed a militant Church on Earth. By your prayers you are united to God and to all of Glory, and you are profoundly assisted. Remember little children, no matter what is happening, to those who are united prayerfully with their God, all works out for their good and for the greater Glory of God. Little children, simply rest in the Presence of Jesus, in the Presence of the Prince of Peace, leaving all up to Him!

I am the Lord your God; I am attendant upon this nation of yours, and in all manner they scatter from Me. I do not abandon them, I am the Good Shepherd; even those who are afflicted, and awaiting the medical attention. These ones I am attendant upon, each in his or her own way. In due course the children of God will depend more and more on Me, the Living God, for their healing, or many will depend both on the Lord God and on the believing physicians to assist them with their health concerns. I am your merciful God! In a brilliant burst of Light, humanity will at last recognize the Commission, shall We say, which the Living God has entrusted to the Blessed Virgin Mary, will come to believe and to understand, the Family of God; will come to recognize, the Living God in the Holy Sacrifice of the Mass; and in the Consecrated Bread and Wine recognize at last, My Presence, for I have spoken, "I will be with you always, even unto the end of time," and I am with you fully- Body, Blood, Soul and Divinity,- in the Holy Eucharist, and I am with you in Spirit, the Spirit of the Living God, Who is Love, Who is Sanctifier.

This knowledge is free to all who will heed and I now cause events to occur which brings humanity-for the most part- to their knees, and even prone before the Living God. You will hear of miraculous events, and know yourselves miracles of My Healing Love- here, in your parish, which remains a faithful portal of Light to humanity. Question not these Words little children, but believe, for nothing is impossible to the Lord your God! The beloved John Paul is Our Chosen Instrument for these times. But of course, He is illuminated, and with his illumination, his flock-My Flock are illuminated, in a great blessing of Peace and Light and Love and Joy. Heavenly angels work in relaying the Messages of Truth, enlightenment of Scripture, Truth in the Mass, and much, much more in these times, through the beloved John-Paul, and through the many, who have made their "yes" in emulation of that of the Virgin Mother of God, and that of the beloved Saint Joseph.

In your yieldedness to Me, the Living God, in your daily "yes, " as it were, the morning offering, I guide you with Divine Inspirations. Little children, stay in the Peace of My Presence throughout each day. Yes, there are trials in the interaction with other people who are not believers, or are only limited in their belief; they are yet My Own. And when you can remain in the Peace of My Presence by calling on My Name, by calling on Mother's Name, at those needy moments, you become a great example to the other ones who are agitating or disturbed, who are disruptive. . That is why I would like to call each of My little ones, not only lighted candles but pillars of Faith, for pillars of Faith are unmoved by all that is going on around them. Do you understand little children? In the Name of Jesus you pray, and I am attendant upon you. Peace; I am your Jesus of Merciful Love; be not too much aggrieved about the dreadful things you see and hear in these times; you well know that you are living in the time of great trial, and before My return, these things have to be.

Today I am asking those who know and love our Mother, to continue to pray for a time of advent where She is recognized and triumphant, and I too, am recognized; I am your Jesus of Victory. It is My Will that My Mother be recognized in the Body of Christ! She recognizes each child of God as her own precious child, because of My Word to Her at the foot of the Cross of Calvary. I call to humanity; do not shun Our Mother, the Queen of Heaven and earth, the Mother of God, and by My very Word, your Mother also. It is now a moment of Love; I am pouring out My healing Love upon you, filling you with My Love and My Peace and My Joy, that sure and quiet Joy, which indwells your heart, and which is indicative of the indwelling Presence of the Holy Spirit, the Spirit of the Living God, Who is within you and encompassing you at all times.

You are aggrieved and concerned about one who has been ensnared by the ways of the world. As you pray little children continuously for the conversion of sinners, the Salvation of souls, as you do daily, you may single out a certain one or other that you know at times specifically in your prayers, but know that all your prayers are heard in Heaven, and it is always your God's desire to say 'yes' to the precious little faithful ones. Even so, all must go according to the Father's Design, and all as you know, is contingent upon the God-given free will of the individual for whom you are praying. A Covenant of Love is a Covenant of Love. You know that it is written n the Blood of the Lamb without spot; sealed, that all may know Salvation. I bless you little children who can hear, who can see, who open your hearts and souls and minds to Truth. I remain your Truth. My beloved little sister, I shall assist you at every step of this work; on every page My Presence is imprinted. Doubt not, but believe, for this is a Calling to the people who need to know Divinity, who need to know of human souls, of the eternity of a soul.

You pray, "Thy Kingdom come, Thy Will be done..." My Kingdom is present within My faithful ones on Earth. My Will is not being done in many aspects of human society, human life. My flock is being led astray by the atheistic and pagan currents of the times. I am not oblivious to this! Even so, with this worldwide war, many of My Own die in this battle, which is truly a battle for souls, for it is a battle between good and evil. Yet My Own, even those caught up in the fray, come to Me and are secure in Me, and I reiterate, My Own are safe in Me, whether on earth, in Purgatory or in Heaven, the True Homeland of the Body of Christ, the Kingdom of God! Little children, that is why Mother has appeared again and again and again pleading for the conversion of sinners, the Salvation of souls, for more prayer. I have shown mankind the Way for I am the Way, and little children, in the economy of Our Father's design, those who follow the Way; their prayers, their acts of Love, their sufferings, cause others to catch the Flame of My Love, to come unto Me, to be drawn unto Me.

It is a cycle of Love, of all reciprocal Love, between the Triune God, the Mother of God, and the faithful children of God, and in this cycle of God, more and more are drawn in. See little children, My Mother pleads, now in tears, for more conversions to occur. My little ones, it is not pleasing for your God to gaze upon such a world at this moment, and yet [He shows Omen Sodom and Gomorrha] got destroyed because there were not sufficient believers. That is why I have sprinkled believers all over the earth, so that there are sufficient believers to bring about a time of Peace. Yet little children, this must be endured for a period of time before My Eyes! I am Jesus, Eternal Victor. Even at this time I call you to trust Me. Hope in Me when there seems no reason to hope at all! Hope in Me; do you not know that your God brings good out of all this wickedness, that I am ever Victor in the battle for souls!

Little children, continue to pray for them, and for all those that are not so close to your Jesus Who is Salvation, remembering that the Lord your God, is the Good Shepherd, always remember that when you pray, we are as it were, working together for those souls. Many yet rest in free will, but increasingly each individual living on earth, is recognizing that the wars and the disasters are greater than humans can cope with, and in this way they begin to turn to Me the Living God for aid, and in the process they are becoming yielded to Me, and in due course know Salvation. Little children, that is why your prayers, your fastings, your sufferings are an integral part in the conversion of sinners, the Salvation of souls. I am He Who Lives and Loves eternally. My Love is upon mankind even now where horrors against My Love are committed, round and about the world. [Our Lord is showing as if He is going about the world picking up pieces bits and pieces of maimed bodies.] This is not of Me nor can it ever be of Me. I am aggrieved! When you attend upon Me in the Adoration Chapel you give recompense to Me for all those who have failed in one manner or another, to receive the Message of Salvation!

Continue to stay prayerfully united with Me in this time of trial which is upon the earth. Many individuals on earth who profess Christianity, find themselves being tested not unlike Job, and that is why I am calling each and every one of you to persevere, to endure, to cling to your Jesus. Unite prayerfully with Our Mother, always remembering the Sanctuary of Love, the Two Hearts of Love. Continue as the beloved John Paul has pleaded, to pray the Rosary for Peace. Pray in whatsoever form you like to pray for Peace. It is sufficient for this evening. "Let Peace be your Quest and your aim." [St Benedict."]The Virtue of Love is such that I, The Lord God bless you both little children, in an anointing of My Love and My Peace and My Joy. My precious little ones, you are living in a time of great change as you know. There is great peril hither and yon about the world. You are yet in a safe area, rather like a Sanctuary where you live, in My Mercy and My Love, but others about the earth are not so fortunate. You will hear of dreadful matters and you will simply continue to pray little children and make the sacrifices which you do in My Name; and stay united with

Your Jesus and with Our beloved Mother, in the Unity of the Family of God, and persevere little children, through it all.

In due course it becomes apparent to you. My little one, you are an instrument of My Peace and Healing Love; and though you are unaware of it, you have indeed touched other individuals according to My Design. One day you shall know the fullness of what you do in the Name of Your Jesus, but the day, the time, the hour is not yet! My little one, I am the Lord your God(Is43:13); I am Your Jesus of Merciful Love and I am profoundly attendant upon you. You know Me well My little one and indeed I am calling you closer to Me in this Communion of Our Love in the Sacraments given to you in My Love. It is then that I am saying to you as I spoke to the Father;" Father if they could be one in Me as I am in You and You are in Me."(Jn 17:21-24) In this manner you become in Unity with Me most profoundly. You already know My Divine Inspirations to you and even Words, and this will grow as you grow in Unity with Me, and I am Blessing you with a great infilling of My Love and My Peace and My Joy.

Little one, hold My Hand; reach out and hold My Hand in Spirit and Truth. (Jn4:23-24), Hold Mother's hand as We walk with the beloved Joseph through all the hills and valleys of this life, walking ever in Faith and Hope and Trust and Love, patiently persevering. Little one, this is the only Way, and you are My small sister, part of My Family, the Family of God, of Nazareth , of Bethlehem; the great Family of Peace which I am building upon the earth, and to which I have called you. Yes, I have called you by Name. You are My Own and I bless you and I name you child of faithfulness, child of God and child of Mary. You are beloved of Jesus and Mary; never forget it. I am placing My Healing Hands upon you and Omen, both of you are My beloved ones; you both work healing love in My Name; and thus on this day, in honour of the beloved St Luke I bless you both, I bless those whom you carry in your hearts little children, I bless multitudes of physicians around the world who know Me and also work healing love, in a great anointing of My Peace upon you. Again at this time in the history of man, the important word is persevere; therefore persevere in all prayerfulness; know that I am with you. Little children always remember, you are never alone; I am with you always; I am your Shield and Protector, you are ever in the Providence of the Living God.

I Jesus bid you love Me, trust Me,(Jn14:1) no matter what is happening, for you are My Own and you live in the Power of My Peace and My Love; in the Power of the Holy Spirit of the Living God. Children, know well and teach others, that this is the greatest Power in all Creation, for all Creation is Mine, it is the Works of My Hands.(Gn1:1) When you pray My little ones, you are uniting with Me, Your Jesus, Who is Man and yet God, and My Godly Power comes upon you as the needed graces, blessings, healings, anointings; all that you need to carry you forth in Faith My little children.I Myself; it is the Lord Who Speaks, strengthen you to yet greater Fortitude. We have much to do together. I recognize the limits of time in your life and the many matters you must attend upon. Therefore I set many angels, and goodly saints to assist you, and I endow you with a vast measure of My Peace, My Love and that everlasting Joy in Love and Unity with Me, that you do indeed persevere.(Rm5:1-5)

Little children remember; all individuals remain in free will always, and yet you have given your wills to the Living God, and you have a bond of unity most profound, with your God. Thus you are, each one of you, a profound instrument of My Peace, of My Healing Love. Little children, stay the Joy-filled little vessels that you are. Little children, each one of you gathered here together is My Own and you are safe in Me. My precious ones, be at Peace. Do I not give you My Peace at every Mass? Little children, be at Peace; I am with you always. I pour out My Spirit upon My loved ones most profoundly. I pour it out on many who shield themselves from My Spirit, to their sorrow and My Sorrow. Comfort the afflicted.(Beatitudes Mt 5) The little one is sorely afflicted and you are blest with healing Gifts to assist her. I anoint you with the necessary Words of Wisdom to assist her. Do not be fearful; I attend upon you in your working with her. I Bless all of your undertakings for you are My instrument of Peace and Truth, and I ask you to simply attend upon her in Truth, and should it become a legal matter, do not be unduly concerned; I assist you then as I assist you now, for you are My Own and you live in the Power of My Peace and My Love. Assist the poor suffering little one, that some Light come into her Life!

It is this that draws others to you; they seek to know what IS this Joy, what IS this Peace; where does THIS Love emanate from, for it overflows your hearts little children. You sing, "fill my cup unto the fullest"; the cup of your heart is overflowing with My Love and My Peace and My Joy, each one of you precious instruments of My Peace. Blessings and graces pour forth upon you each one now, as we approach the season of Lent. Little children, when you unite yourselves with Your Jesus, increased blessings flow upon the needy, enlightenment comes upon many others, and they begin to come back to Truth. The world is filled with the lies of Our foe, yet Truth shall and does prevail. Bless Me!

Little children, I tell you again, some of you plant the seeds and it will be others who will recognize the harvest.(Lk10:1-2) and bring in the harvest. It is not often that you are both the seed planter and harvester, (Ps126:6) but yet it is happening. I bless you in a great anointing of My Love and My Peace and My Joy. Be comforted; the Spirit of the Living God is within you and surrounding you. You are in unity with the Living God. Be at Peace; I fill you with My Peace! Remember the words of the great saint;(Benedict) let Peace be your quest and your aim. I am Peace. Rest often in My Embrace. (cf Mt11:28) Put your head upon My Shoulder in those needy moments like John; rest on My Bosom. Be comforted in the Divine Embrace of Love. I am lighting your pathway to wondrous experiences of Faith, to knowledge of the Glory of God. Hearken to the Voice of the Spirit Who is ever attendant upon you.

MARY: *My precious little ones, there is a faithful remnant among whom you are numbered, who continue to persevere in all faithfulness prayerfully, as the Lord God has decreed and has asked. You know, as does your Mother, the Power of the very Presence of the Living God in the Blessed Sacrament, the Bread and Wine of your God's Love ever attendant upon you. Dear little children, those who adore, are profoundly anointed, blest and assisted, more so than many, because of this Faith-in-action, this love-in-action.*

Treasure the hours that you spend in Adoration little children; you have no idea what blessings are coming upon you and in you and through you, to multitudes of others. Also, you are emulating your Mother. It is true indeed; wheresoever My Son is I am there with Him; in the power of the Holy Spirit, it is so! The sorrow that such a scant few in number of the flock attend, is grievously wounding to both your God and your Heavenly Mother. Darkness covers the Earth and the thick clouds, the people. Little children, even those who seemingly walk in the Light, even think they are walking in the Light; they are yet in darkness; they haven't responded fully to the Call of Love!

My darling it is painful to your Mother that so few Catholics recognize the True Presence of Our Lord and God, Body Blood Soul and Divinity, in the tabernacle, in the monstrance, in the Holy Sacrifice of the Mass. My little ones, at this time I bid you simply persevere in all prayerfulness when you attend upon your own hours, and ask at that time for more adorers to come. The benefits upon yourselves are so great, and they are in effect denying themselves many graces and blessings by failing to attend upon the Living God, the Prince of Peace. From where else does Peace on earth come, but from our Lord and our God!

Darling children, you are all under My Mantle of Love, the power of the Holy Spirit, and as you pray on this Cause great things begin to happen. It shall come to pass that it shall be a busy parish with many adorers night and day, and therefore I bid you persevere. In due course you shall see the great increase. The Victory of Jesus becomes evident to more and more people.

My little ones it is a time of great sorrow upon the earth. The enemy is filling many with fear which is not of our God and again I bid you live the Great Commandments of Love. Pray for one another. Pray for these 2,600 families who do not fully comprehend God's Divine Gifts to them in the Sacraments of Love. You are the lights, and there are a goodly number of you in the parish who are enlightened and become lights of the Truth of our Lord, and through you the others begin to be drawn into Adoration of the Divine Lamb of God. Be at Peace. Perpetual Adoration shall indeed continue.

Mother wishes you little children to remain in this position [praying prone] throughout these prayers, for little children you are instruments of the Living God, and you must teach humility before the Creator of all that is; that humility before the Creator, the Father of all, is so lacking upon the Earth in these times. Mother Mary is speaking. The Singular Vessel of Devotion bids you Peace. My little children, you who have always reverenced your Mother, while worshipping Our Lord and Our God, Jesus the Christ; I Myself, on this day which is Holy to the Lord God, bless you in a great anointing of Peace. I am the Queen of Peace! My little children, this anointing is for you and for all believers.

My little one, in your Mission , be not dismayed. I Queen of Peace, and Our Lord Jesus, Prince of Peace, attend upon you continuously. We bid you, little children, at the slightest disruption of your Peace, to call on Our Names, restoring yourselves to Our Peace. The enemy, and the world, would disrupt the Peace of Christ wherever it is found. Do not let these inroads take away from your Peace. We give you Mother Theresa, We give you John Paul, and We give you your own Father Paul as examples. Peace prevails within such hearts no matter what is occurring around them.

The Mother of God salutes you. I bless you little children; precious little ones, be at Peace. What has transpired here this evening is recorded in Glory. Precious children, you do not know the Victory you have won, but you will notice it as you go forward day by day in Faith. Do not be anxious nor frustrated All is falling into place according to Heaven's Design; your prayers are heard, the Blessings flow, the peoples flock .Although you are not fully aware of it little children, many unusual events are occurring round about the world, and all of these events are causing the flock to be shaken out of their lethargy, their sleepiness , causing them to awaken and begin to seek the Light.

Remember your Jesus is the Light of the world. In the Light of His Love for mankind, present in the Bread and Wine of His Love , this Sacrament; they begin to see and hear and know at last! You are called little children to love and trust Our Lord Jesus no matter what is happening. I reiterate, though the Earth quake beneath your feet, keep your eyes upon Jesus. Thus, thus is your Victory won; and I bring your sacrifices of love to the Father, that Love may emanate upon the needy upon Earth. Little children, in the power of the Holy Spirit thou art blest in the Name of the Father, and of the Son, and of the Holy Spirit. All over the world today there is trouble of one form or another. I, your Heavenly Mother, attend upon My precious children, round and about the earth in many visits, many appearances, many assistances. Precious children, I call you to persevere. You invoke the Father, the Son, and the Holy Spirit, and even Me, your Mother, in this matter of seeking responsible adorers of The Christ. Little children, believe; it is so, it is already so! The Living God is pleased with your hearts and souls and minds. Your desire to love the Lord your God, and love your neighbour as yourself, is so evident.

Little children, in His humble appearance, His humble one might even say disguise, He is able to test the many, for their Love of the Word of God, and for their love of Holy Mother Church. Oh My little ones, continue to love Him as you do; continue to seek Him out; continue to share every detail of your lives with your God and with your Mother. Precious, precious little children, continue in all prayerfulness; many are praying with you, and for this intention. Little ones, since you ever invoke the angels and saints of Glory, Heaven resounds with your prayers, and your God is pleased and comes to your assistance.

Believe, trust in your God, stay united with Our Lord Jesus, and all goes according to Heaven's design. The time of Peace, which fast approaches, is most beautiful. The children of God will live in a manner of delight, and ever in the Light of Christ. Truly darkness is then no more; as Our Lord God has pledged, so it shall be. Believe, little children; I am your Mother, Queen of Peace, Queen of all saints and I bless each one of you profoundly again and again. And the time is quite soon.

Michael attends; Michael the great Archangel of Almighty God says, You have found favour with God, and the faithful cohort, but there is a bad spirit like a coiled serpent against The Mass and against the Holy Eucharist.

Hebrews 10: vs 36-39

Be as confident now, then, since the reward is so great. You will need endurance to do God's Will and gain what He has promised. Only a little while now, a very little while, and the One that is coming will have come; He will not delay. The righteous man will live by Faith, but if he draws back, my soul will take no pleasure in him. You and I are not the sort of people who draw back, and are lost by it; we are the sort who keep faithful until our souls are saved.

ACKNOWLEDGMENTS

I am greatly indebted to:

1. "Omen" who prayed with me for four years at great personal sacrifice, for these "Words," written in my soul, to be spoken through the voice of another who had no medical background, thus confirming and witnessing to them independently of me.

2. My prayer partner, LT, who would have preferred not to be mentioned, but who has helped greatly by joining me in prayer, witnessing to some events, and by helping with the Scriptural referencing.

3. Dr Dianne N. Irving, a former research biochemist, is a PhD philosopher who has taught medical ethics at Georgetown and Catholic Universities.

4. Dr Alan Shewmon: for permission to use his records of prolonged survivors of "brain death" available at Nationa Auxiliary Publications Service (NAPS), 248 Hempstead Turnpike, West Hempstead, NY 11552, request document #0546.

5. Dr Peter Fenwick; neuropsychiatrist for his research and his help directing me to the Dutch research similar to his own, especially when I had given up the search.

6. Dr Herbert Hendin; although I did not quote him directly, his thorough and expert psychodynamic analyses, kept me clear on the differences between patient needs and doctor/relative needs, in his book, "Seduced by Death,"with his expert handling their motivations became transparent.

7. Dr Nicholas Sparrow. With the freshness of a medical student newly exploring an ethical quagmire, he shared what is still challenging, at the end of the chapter on "brain death."

8. Thong Doan: who patiently helped me to design and create the website of the Mission in 1998.

9. Guadalupe Project Group in Ann Arbor , through Dr Cathy Dowling, whom I met in Buffalo, and linked with Life Foundation Canada and "Eleventh Hour Mission" to become international eventually.

10. The several authors who gave permission for their articles to be quoted in the introductory pages.

11. Dr. Michael Brear and Mrs. Brear for their frequent, friendly support, as well as faithfulness to the Truth of the sanctity of Human Life, through thick and thin.

12. .Drs. John Yun, John Mendes, Paul Byrne, and Mr. Humphrey Waldock, Mary Wagner, the two Judith Browns, all longstanding faithful soldiers in the cause of Life.

13. Nancy Valko and the women of Faith and family who faithfully included me daily in her "media watch."

14. Mr. Vellacourt and his associates who stood up faithfully for the pro-life Cause.

15. Tam and Damian Kuehn, two experts who patiently took me through the technical nightmares that seemed insurmountable, to the "other side" that seemed magical to me, and little Amayah and Xavier who were my "excuse" for showing up on their doorstep frequently.,and the clergy, family and friends known and unknown, who have prayed with me and for me.

16. The many people who allowed me to share their medical and personal stories.

17. Media such as Zenit, Lifesite, Steven Ertelt, EWTN who could use your support

18. Dr. Stephen White, through whose voice Our Lord let me know He wanted His Words in print.

CPSIA information can be obtained
at www.ICGtesting.com
Printed in the USA
250968LV00001B